MEDICINAL AND AROMATIC PLANTS:

Essentials Oils and Pharmaceutical Use

About the Book

This book may be able to provide a lucid discourse on the subject to the person seeking a brief information on the topics. Medicinal plants are nature's hidden and to a large extent unexplored treasure. Although they have been used as a source of safe and effective medicine since time immemorial, this potential resource has hardly been commercially tapped. India is endowed with about 8000 species of medicinal plants. According to a recent estimate of the Planning Commission, Government of India, the potential for plant-based crude drugs is about Rs. 400 billion. Globally, the demand for medicinal plants and their derivatives is growing at a rate of 7-15%.

About the Author

Dr. Jaspreet Gogia. PhD, is an Assistant Professor of Botany in ACEAS, Gujrat, India and she has teaching Experience of more than 11 years. She is a biotechnologist with a several years of wet lab research experience, worked at International Center for Genetic Engineering and Biotechnology, New Delhi. She has also worked for Advance Enzyme Technologies as a scientist. Jaspreet has published papers in Journals and submitted a numbers of annotated Geminiviral Genome Sequences in the Genbank, She did her Higher studies from (IRNAS-CSIC) Sevilla. She is also Chief Editor of Bioinformatics Review and a Co-founder/Executive Chief Editor of a Science. She is in role of the Arabidopsis Na+/H+ antiporter SOS1 in the regulation of Na+ and K+ homeostasis since 2012.

MEDICINAL AND AROMATIC PLANTS:
Essentials Oils and Pharmaceutical Use

Dr. Jaspreet Gogia

AMIGA PRESS INC.

DELHI (INDIA)

AMIGA PRESS INC.
H.O.: 28-A, Indra Park,
Chander Nagar, Delhi-110051 (India)
Tel.: 011-22504028, +91-98736-57000
E-mail: amigapress@gmail.com
amigaeditorial@gmail.com
amigapub@gmail.com
info@amigapress.co.in
Website : www.amigapress.co.in

This edition is published by Amiga Press Inc.

ISBN: 978-93-84533-49-6

First Published 2019

Printed and bound in India by Replika Press Pvt. Ltd.

Preface

Medicinal plants as a group comprise approximately 8000 species and account for around 50per cent of all the higher flowering plant species of India. Millions of rural households use medicinal plants in a self-help mode. Over one and a half million practitioners of the Indian System of Medicine in the oral and codified streams use medicinal plants in preventive, promotive and curative applications. There are estimated to be over 7800 manufacturing units in India. In recent years, the growing demand for herbal product has led to a quantum jump in volume of plant materials traded within and across the countries. An estimate of the EXIM Bank puts the international market of medicinal plants related trade at US$ 60 billion per year growing at the rate of 7per cent only. Though India has a rich biodiversity, the growing demand is putting a heavy strain on the existing resources. While the demand for medicinal plants is growing, some of them are increasingly being threatened in their natural habitat. For meeting the future needs cultivation of medicinal plant has to be encouraged. According to an all India ethnobiological survey carried out by the Ministry of Environment and Forests, Government of India, there are over 8000 species of plants being used by the people of India.

Today we find a renewed interest in traditional medicine. During the past decade there have been an ever increasing demand especially from developed countries for more and more drugs from plant sources. This revival of interest in plant derived drugs is mainly due to the current widespread belief that `green medicine' is safe and more dependable than the costly synthetic drug many of which have adverse side effects. This resurgence of interest in the plant based drugs have necessitated an increased demand of medicinal plants leading to over- exploitation, unsustainable harvesting and finally to the virtual decimation of several valuable plant species in the wild.

Moreover, the habitat degradation due to increased human activities (human settlements, agriculture and other developmental programmes), illegal trade in rare and endangered medicinal plants, and loss of regeneration potential of the degraded forests have further accelerated the current rate of extinction of plants particularly the medicinal plants.

Ayurveda, the Science of life, has its foundation in a sound philosophy (Sankhaya) of origin of life on earth. Ayurvedic system defines the state of health as equilibrium of tridoshashas (Vat, Pitta, Kapha) combined with a satisfied and happy state of mind. The simple technique of healthful life, according to this system, is to follow a middle course of Ahar (balanced &optimum food intake), Vihar (exposure to nature i.e. sun, cold etc.) and Achar (living a disciplined life following yama and niyama). This wonderful treatment evolved progressed and spread to other parts of the world in pre-Christian era. It has some distinctions which still provide glory and excellence. These are use of poisons in the treatment, use of rasa (mercurial preparations) and rasayana (Rasayanam tad geyam jara vyadhi nashnam) use of bhashma (metallic ashes) and excellent surgery. Unfortunately time took turn the patronage provided by the Kings to this system disappeared and other systems (unani &Allopathic) dominated the scene.

Ayurveda have already mentioned herbal remediation for a number of human ailments. Among Indian traditional medicinal plants several potential anti-diabetic plants and herbs are being used as part of our diet since prehistoric time. India has a long list of native medicinal plants with confirmed blood sugar lowering property. Some of these have proved remarkable for cure of diabetes and its complications. Medicinal Plants is the outcome of a national seminar held to address challenging opportunities in the field.

This book may be able to provide a lucid discourse on the subject to the person seeking a brief information on the topics.

—Editor

Contents

Introduction

Ayurveda, the Science of life, has its foundation in a sound philosophy (Sankhaya) of origin of life on earth. Ayurvedic system defines the state of health as equilibrium of tridoshashas (Vat, Pitta, Kapha) combined with a satisfied and happy state of mind. The simple technique of healthful life, according to this system, is to follow a middle course of Ahar (balanced & optimum food intake), Vihar (exposure to nature i.e. sun, cold etc.) and Achar (living a disciplined life following yama and niyama). This wonderful treatment evolved progressed and spread to other parts of the world in pre-Christian era. It has some distinctions which still provide glory and excellence. These are use of poisons in the treatment, use of rasa (mercurial preparations) and rasayana (Rasayanam tad geyam jara vyadhi nashnam) use of bhashma (metallic ashes) and excellent surgery. Unfortunately time took turn the patronage provided by the Kings to this system disappeared and other systems (unani &Allopathic) dominated the scene.

The introduced systems of treatment could not spread to rural India where millions of people always saw ray of hope in this system However the system of Ayurveda suffered a great setback because educational institutions declined in quality and quantity. The system could not receive any reward/ award for its promotion or further research. All this resulted in making the system most of the time as family heritage or few clever and incompetent persons in the field adding many wrong information in the literature. A glaring example is the information on herbal medicines where multiple synonyms were added without making an effort to provide proper identification or description. People started keeping the information on use as secret may be due to fear of losing this as sole source of income or prestige. There had been a great invention in the ancient India by the Aswani Kumars which was tested on Rishi Chayavan. This was searching for Jeevaniya (Vitality enhancing), vyasthapan (revival of youthful condition), body nourishing, antioxidant and invigorating group of 8 plants popularly known as Astavarga plants and prepared the famous "CHAYAVANPRASH " for the cure of ailing frail old body of Chayavan Rishi who, in turn, regained youthful vitality and vigour. From that time onwards till 15th or 16th century A. D. there was no printing and much of the information orally maintained and written records were difficult to preserve over centuries. The original methods of goshthies (seminars) involving discussions disappeared overtime. There was loss of much valuable information. That is why today we find much confusion over the correct identity of medicinal plants.

The information on Astavarga plants of Chayavanprash has undergone the same course. There is no mention of Astavarga plants in the Atharva Veda. Paniniya Astadhayi and Vedic literature (Sharma, 1981). In Dhanwantri Nighantu, there is mention of Astavarga and these plants are Rdhi, Vrdhi, Jeevak, Rishbhak, Kakoli, Kshirkakoli, Meda and Mahameda. The great Ayurvedic sages Charak and Sushrut made a mention of 5 of Astaverga plants for use in Chayavanprash.

These were Rdhi, Jeevak, Rishbhak, Meda and Kakoli (Charak samhita of Agnivesa, Chikitsa Sthanam). In another Charak Samhita by Vidyadhar Shukla and Ravidutta Tripathi there is mention of three groups of plants –

(i) Jeevaniya which includes Jeevak, Rishbhak, Meda and Mahameda,
(ii) Brhnayiya – Kakoli and Kshirkakoli
(iii) Vayasthapna –Rdhi.

It is difficult to mention all works in their Chronological order. For reference purpose, various works are cited here below. In "Abhinav Nighantu " compiled and translated by Pandit Duttaram Chaube on page 44 all the Astavarga plants have been listed referring Rishi Charak and others. Shaligram Nighantu also mentions all the Astaverga plants with some vague description of these plants. Acharya Vishwnath Dwivedi had made commentary on "Raj Nighantu " which mentions only Meda, Mahameda, Rdhi and Vrdhi with out any identifying characters. The important early literature is of Shri Vagbhatta Virachitam "Astanghridya " with commentary of Shri Lal Chand Vaidya and includes Jeevak, Rishbhak, Meda, Kakoli and Kshirkakoli among the forty one ingredients of Chayavanprash Avaleh. The Shaligram Nighantu describes Astavarga plants in a vague manner based on old works. Thakur Balwant Singh in his "Glossary of Vegetable Drugs in Brhattrayi " gave confusing botanical identity of four plants of Astavarga. Kirtikar and Basu did not include any of the Astavarga plants in their treatise on Indian Medicinal plants. Similarly Dr. Ram Sushil Singh prepared "Vanaushadhi Nidarshika " with—out any mention of Astavarga. Kaidev Nighantu edited and translated by P. V. Sharma and Guru Prasad Sharma gave botanical nomenclature of four plants only. In work of Shri Chakarpani dutta (11th century) includes Rdhi, Jeevak, Rishbhak, Meda and Kakoli in Chayavanprash but mentions 6 plants in Jeevaniya gana.

In Sharangadhar Samhita Rdhi, Jeevak, Rishbhak, Kakoli, Kshirkakoli, Meda and Mahameda had been used along-with 38 other ingredients. In Bhava Prakash Nighantu with commentary of Vishwanath Dwivedi, the Astavarga has been included in Jeevaniya gana. Obviously therefore Astavarga plants have much confusion with regard to their identity.

MEDICINAL PLANTS

- Conservation of natural resources and the capability to utilize them in sustained manner are essential for the well being and continued survival of man.
- Under the duress of over exploration and habitat degradation a number of wild plants are essentially facing a constant threat of extinction.
- Out of the 60, 000 plant species that are listed as threatened of extinction, over 20, 000 (or more) are from India alone.
- The botanical survey of India has prepared a provisional list of threatened plants which includes a large number wild (or) wild relatives of food, horticultural, medicinal and aromatic plants.
- India is endowed with a unique wealth of biota which inlcude a large number of medicinal and aromatic plants.
- Many of these plants are rare and endemic and found only in wild sources.
- The population explosion coupled with the improved standard of living led to ruthless exploitation, resulting in the imminent danger of extinction of these plants.
- Most of these wild medicinal and aromatic plants are highly habitual specific, found only in forests and occupying highly specialized ecological niche with restricted distribution.
- There are neither biological informations nor adequate knowledge of casual factors that led to their rarity in the habital.
- There is however, now an urgent need to evolve a sound strategy for the management and conservation of these plants on a long term basis.
- To evolve suitable strategies for conservation (or) the domestication/ cultivation of medicinal plants, it is very essential to study the complete biological and ecological back ground of these species.
- Under domestication outside their normal ecological range (or) under the distributed eco-system conditions may of the wild medicinal and aromatic plants tend to behave differently.
- In some cases it becomes difficult to grow them (or) it may not even survive.
- In certain other cases if survives and grows but may not be producing the desired traits.
- A through understanding on their reproductive and growth biology as well as identification of the biological and ecological constraints leading to their reduced fitness, restricted distribution (or) even extinction etc., is therefore, necessary.

- An understanding of the biological and ecological back ground of the species in their normal habitat is also essential to understand their conservation biology as well as to predict their behaviour under artificial cultivation.

Strategies for conservation of medicinal plants:

- The conservation of the wild medicinal plants or any other such threatened species can be tackled by scientific techniques as well as social actions.
- There are basically two scientific techniques of conservation of genetic diversity of these plants.
- They are the in situ and ex situ method of conservation. In Situ conservation:
- It is only in nature that plant diversity at the genetic, species and eco-system level can be conserved on long-term basis.
- Unless plant populations are conserved in the wild, that is in natural habitats, in viable breeding populations, they run the risk of extinction.
- It is necessary to conserve in distinct, representative biogeographic zones inter and intraspecific genetic variation.

Current status:

- In Karnataka, Kerala and Tamil nadu and more recently in Maharashtra the forest department in collaboration with FRUHT (Foundation for Rural Revitalization of Local Health Tradition) have established a network of 33 "Medicinal Plants Conservation Areas" (MPCAs) across the entire altitudinal range of south India.
- Each of these reserves is around 200 ha in size. Regulation and wild collection:
- Regulating the harvest of medicinal plants from the wild for commercial purposes.
- Particularly those species whose harvest inevitably involves destructive collection.
- Local communities can develop a stake in sustainable harvesting of medicinal plants from the forest and village, district and state level co- operative are set up to manage collection, storage and marketing.

Current status:

- LAMP societies as they function at present neither benefit the primary tribal collectors nor provides adequate powers (or) accountability of the LAMPs with regard to protection and management of forests.
- The marketing function of LAMPs is also weak, so that collectors do not get remunerative prices through LAMP sales.

EX situ conservation

A. Ethno-medicinal plant gardens:

- Creation of a network of regional and sub-regional ethno-medicinal plant gardens which should contain accessions of all the medicinal plants known to the various ethnic communities in different regions of India.
- This chain of gardens will act as regional repositories of our cultural and ethno-medicinal history and embody the living traditions of our socity's knowledge of medicinal plants.

Current status:

- There are estimated to be around 50 such gardens in the country ranging from acre to 40 acres some of them were set up by an All India Health Network.
- More recently a network of 15 such gardens have been set up in 3 states of South India with the initiative of FRLHT. One of the gardens is located in TBGRI, (Tropical botanical garden research institute) Palode at Thiruvananthapuram.

B. Gene banks:

- While it is known that the largest proportion of local bio-diversity in all our eco-system is used for medicinal purposes, very little is known about their conservation status in the wild.
- What is likely is that a large number of medicinal plant species are under various degrees of threat.
- Theprecautionaryprincipleswouldsuggestthatanimmediateandcountry-wide exercise be taken up to deposit seeds of wild medicinal plants with a first priority to known Red listed species and endemic species.

Current status:

- The department of bio-technology, Government of India has recently taken the initiative to establish 3 gene banks in the country.
- One is with ICAR at the NBPGR (National Bureau of plant genetic Resources) Campus, the second is with CIMAPs, (Cental Institute of Medicinal and Aromatic plants) Lucknow and the third with TBFRI in Thiruvananthapuram.

C. Nursery network:

- The most urgent and primary task in order to ensure immediate availability of plants and planting materials to various user groups is to promote a nation wide network of medicinal plant nurseries, which will multiply all the regional specific plants that are used in the current practice of traditional medicine.
- These nurseries should become the primary sources of supply of plants and seed material that can be subsequently multiplied by the various users.

Current status:

- Planting material for 40 odd species of medicinal and aromatic plants is reportedly available in the ICAR and CSIR (CIMAP) network.
- In South India FRLHT has recently set up a network of 55 supply nurseries.

D. Cultivation:

- Figures projecting demand and trade in medicinal plant species globally indicate a step upward trend in the near future.
- One estimate puts the figure of world trade in medicinal plants and related products at US $ 5 trillion by A. D. 2050 (world bank report, 1996).
- The demand so far has been met mainly from wild sources.
- This can't go on for much longer; policy intervention is urgently needed to encourage and facilitate investments into commercial cultivation of medicinal plants.
- Cultivation of medicinal plants however, is inversely linked to prevalence of easy and cheap collection from the wild, lack of regulation in trade, cornering of the profits from wild collection by a vast network of traders and middlemen and absence of industry's interest in providing buy-back guarantees to growers.

Current status:

- In the Govt. sector agro-technology of 40 odd species has been developed by ICAR-Agricultural University System and CSIR (CIMAOs & RRL, Jammu and Jorhat).
- In recent years industries like Dabur, Zandu, Indian Herbs, Arya Vaidya Shala, and Arya Vaidya Pharmacy and others have made some symbolic efforts to initiate cultivation.
- Since 1984 NABARD (National Bank of Agricultural and Rural Development) has formulated schemes for financing cultivation and processing of medicinal plants.

E. Community based enterprises:

- The income generated by the traditional medicine industry benefits small section of the socity.
- A strong case exists for promotion of community level enterprises for value addition to medicinal plants through simple, on site techniques like drying, cleaning, crushing, powdering, grading, packaging etc.
- This will also increase the stake of rural communities in conservation and change the skewed nature of income distribution of the industry.

Current status:

- Three community based enterprises are known in south India, one in Gandhigram Trust, (Dindigul), Preemade development Society (Peermade) Kerala and the third by VGKK in B. R. Hills, Mysore.

IMPORTANCE OF MEDICINAL PLANTS

Important Medicinal Plants and their active constituents

Plant	Active principle	Pharmacological activity
1 Rauvolfia serpentina	Reserpine	Hypotensive
2 Catharanthus roseus	Ajmalicine	Vasodilator
	Vinblastine	Anticancer
	Vincristine	Anticancer
3 Cassia angustifolia, Cassia acutifolia	Sennosides	Laxative
4 Plantago ovata	Psyllium mucilage	laxative
5 Glycyrrhiza glabra	Glycyrrhizic acid	Antiinflammatory
6 Berberis sp.	Berberin	Antidiarrhoeal
7 Digitalis lanata	Digitoxin Lanatoside	Cardiotonic
8 Taxus baccata	Taxol	Anticancer
9 Podophyllum emodi Etoposide	Podophyllotoxin	
Tenoposide	Anticancer	
10 Datura species,		
Hyocymus musticus,		
Duboisia myoporoides	Hyoscine	
Syoscyamina		
Atropine	Parasympatholytic	
11 Artemisai annua	Artemisinin	Antimalarial
12 Mappia foetida	Camptothecine	Anticancer

Medicinal Plants used as Crude Extracts/Tinctures in Medicines

Botanical Name	Common Name
1 Belladonna	Atropa belladonna
2 Ipecac	Cephaelis ipecacuanha
3 Opium	Papaver somniferum
4 Henbane	Hyoscyamus niger
5 Stramonium	Datura stramonium
6 Liquorice	Glycyrrhiza glabra
7 Rhubarb	Rheum officinale
8 Podophyllum	Podophyllium emodi
9 Capscicum olcoresin	Capsicum annum

10 Digitalis	Digitalis lanata, Digitalis purpurea
11 Aloe	Aloe vera

Important Plant Products having great potential in Medicine

Plant Product	Source	Pharmacological activity
1 Valepotriates	Valeriana wallichii	Sedative, tranquilizer
2 Silymarin	Silybum marianum	Antihepatoxic
3 Podophyllotoxin (Etoposide/tenoposide)	Podophyllum emodi, P. pellatum ,	Anticancer
4 Taxol	Taxus baccata	Anticancer
5 Guggul saponins Cormmiphora wiightii	Hypolipidaemic	
6 Artemisinin	Artemisai annua	Antimalarial

Some important medicinal plants suggested for cultivation :

Botanical name of the plant	Common
Aegle marmalos	Bilva (Hindi); Maredu (Telugu)
Glycyrrhiza glabra	Mulethi (Hindi); Athimadhuramu (Telugu)
Gmelina arborea	Gambhiri (Hindi); Gummadi (Telugu)
Mesua ferrea	Nagkesara (Hindi); Keearamu (Telugu)
Piper longum	Pipli (Hindi); Pippali (Telugu)
Picrorhiza kurroa	Kutki (Hindi); Katukarogani (Telugu)
Phyllanthus niruri	Jar-amla (Hindi); Nelausiri (Telugu)
Saraca indica	Ashoka (Hindi); Asokachettu (Telugu)
Swertia chirayata	Chirayata (Hindi); Nilavemyu (Telugu)
Andrographis paniculata	Kalmegha (Hindi); Nelavemu (Telugu)
Terminalia arjuna	Arjuna (Hindi); Tellamaddi (Telugu)
Valeriana wallichii	Tagar (Hindi)
Tinospora cordifolia	Gulancha (Hindi); Thippatheega (Telugu)
Asparagus racemosus	Shatavar (Hindi); Pillitheegalu (Telugu)
Plumbago zeylanica	Chita (Hindi); Chitramulamu (Telugu)
Conuniphora wightii	Guggul (Hindi, Telugu)
Boerhaavia diffusa	Punarnava, Sant (Hindi, Telugu)
Withania somnifera	Ashwagandha (Hindi, Telugu)
Bacopa monnieri	Brahmi (Hindi, Telugu)

Systems of Medicine

- There are mainly 3 systems of medicine practised in the world today. They are :

Modern System or Allopathy

- This system was developed in the Western countries. In this system drugs (tablets, capsules, injections, tonics etc.) are manufactured using synthetic chemicals and/or chemicals derived from natural products like plants, animals, minerals etc. This system also uses modern equipment for diagnosis, analysis, surgery etc.
- Medicines or drugs of this system is often criticised for its treatment of the symptoms rather than the cause of the disease, harmful side effects of certain drugs and for being out of reach of common/poor people due to the high cost of drugs and treatment.
- This system is used in all the countries of the world today.

Alternative Medicine or Traditional System

- Different countries of the world developed independently their own traditional systems of medicine using locally available materials like minerals and products of plants and animals.
- The World Health Organisation is giving considerable importance to these alternate medicine (as they act as alternative to allopathy) systems to provide Primary Health Care to millions of people in the developing countries.
- China developed the Chinese system of medicine, which is practised in China, Singapore, Taiwan, Japan and other countries.
- In Indonesia, Jamu and in South Africa, Zulu systems of herbal medicine are practised. The Unani or Tibb system was developed in the Middle Eastern Arab countries and is practised in India and in many countries.
- In India, Ayurveda (developed in North India), Siddha (developed in Tamil Nadu) and Nagarjuna (developed in Andhra Pradesh) systems of medicine were developed. Ayurveda is practised in Sri Lanka, Pakistan and Bangladesh also. Herbo-mineral is another traditional system used in India and other neighbouring countries.
- Drugs (balms, oils, pills, tonics, paste etc) are manufactured and marketed in these systems. The major advantage of these systems is that they are within the reach of the people, particularly rural poor.
- These systems are claimed to be pollution free, eco-freindly and have minimal or no harmful side effects. Ayurveda claims to cure the cause of the disease rather than the symptoms and is wholistic in its approach.
- In this system a disease is conceived as an imbalance in the systems of the body and the treatment aims at restoring the balance in the various systems of the body.

Folk Medicine

- The medicinal systems followed by various tribals/aborigins of different countries is popularly known as folk or tribal medicine.
- In the system, the "medicine man" or the "doctor " of the tribe who has the knowledge of treating diseases, keeps this knowledge as a closely guarded secret and passes it to the next generation by word of mouth.
- No written texts on these systems are available and different tribes follow different time tested methods. The treatment is often associated with lengthy and mystic rituals, in addition to prescription of drugs (decoctions, pastes, powders, oils, ashed materials etc.).
- Mostly locally available natural materials are used for the preparation of drugs, which are not commercially made and marketed. Generally speaking, folk medicine can also be regarded as a traditional system of medicine.
- The basic aim of all the above systems of medicine is to alleviate the sufferings of human beings and their domesticated animals.
- The knowledge of the traditional systems is undergoing close scientific scrutiny and is being increasingly incorporated into the modern system.

Other Systems

- Yoga, Acupressure, Acupuncture, Reiki, Magneto therepy, Pyramid therapy, Flower therapy, Homeopathy, Nature Cure or Naturopathy etc. are some of the other systems of medicine practised in different parts of the world today.

Utilization of Medicinal Plants

- The utility of medicinal plants has four major segments:
  - o Medicinal plants utilised in indigenous or traditional systems of medicines (ISM) -Ayurveda, Siddha, Unani and Homeopathy systems of medicines.
  - o OTC (over the country, non-prescription) items/products involving plant parts, extracts galenicals etc.
  - o Essential oils
  - o Phyto-pharmaceuticals or plants used in modern systems of medicine.

Medicinal plants used in Traditional Systems of Medicine

- Traditional medicine is widespread through the world and it comprises of those practices based on beliefs that were in existence, often for hundreds of years, before the development and spread of modern scientific medicines and which are still in use today.
- As its name implies, it is the part of tradition of each country which employs practices that have been handed down from generation to

generation. Its acceptance by a population is largely conditioned by cultural factors and much of traditional medicine, therefore, may not be easily transferable from one culture to another.

- An important feature of traditional therapy is the preference of practitioner for compound prescriptions over single substance/drug as it is being held that some constituents are effective only in the presence of others.
- This renders assessment of efficacy and eventually identification of active principles as required in international standards much difficult than for simple preparation.
- In India, earlier the medicines used in indigenous systems of medicines were generally prepared by the practicing physicians by themselves, but now this practice has been largely replaced by the establishment of organised indigenous drug industries.
- It is estimated that at present there are more than 1, 00, 000 licensed registered practitioners of Ayurveda, Siddha, Unani medicine or Homeopathy.
- As far as the Ayurveda system of medicine is concerned, it does not rule out any substances being used as potential source of medicine.
- Presently about 10 00 single drugs and 8000 compound drug formulations of recognised merit are in vogue.
- In fact reliable data on availability in different regions of country as well as supply and demand of medicinal plants used in production of indigenous medicines are not available.
- However, annual herbal drug market has been estimated around 2200 crores and is expected to reach up to 4000 crores by the year 2000.

Plants-parts, extracts and galenicals

- The direct utilisation of plant material is not only a feature of ISM in the developing world but also in developed countries like USA, UK, Germany etc., the various herbal formulations are sold on health food shops.
- Preparation of decoctions, tinctures, galenicals and total extracts of plants also form a part of many pharmacopoeias of the world.
- The current trend of medicinal plants based drug industry is to procedure standard extracts of plants as raw material.

Essential Oils from plants

- The essential oil industry was traditionally a cottage industry in India. Since 1947, a number of industrial companies have been established for large scale production of essential oils, oleoresins and perfumes.
- The essential oil from plants includes Ajowan oil, Eucalyptus oil,

Geranium oil, Lavender oil, Palmarosa oil, Patchouli oil, Rose oil, Sandalwood oil, Turpentine oil and Vetiver oil.

Phyto-pharmaceuticals

- During the past decades, bulk production of plant based drugs has become an important segment of Indian pharmaceutical industry.
- Some of the phyto-pharmaceuticals which are produced in India at present include
  1. morphone,
  2. codeine,
  3. papaverine (Papaver somniferum),
  4. quinine,
  5. quinidine,
  6. cinchonine and cinchonidine (Cinchona sp., C. calisaya, C. ledgeriana, C. officinais and C. succirubra);
  7. hyoscine,
  8. hyoscyamine (Hyocyamus niger and H. muticus),
  9. colchicine (Gloriosa superbad, Colchicum luteum and Iphigenia stellata),
  10. cephaeline and emetin (Cephalis ipacacuanha),
  11. sennosides A & B (Cassia angustifolia and C. acutifolia),
  12. reserpine,
  13. rescinnamine,
  14. ajmalicine and ajmaline (Rauvolfia serpentina);
  15. vinblastine and vincristine,
  16. ajmalicine (raubacine) (Catharanthus roseus);
  17. guggul lipid (Commiphora wightii);
  18. taxol (Taxus baccata);
  19. artemisinin (Artemisai annua) etc.
- For alll these segments of drug, perfumery, flavouring and cosmetic industries, mostly the higher plants are one of the raw materials and comes from the natural resources i.e. forests through forest contractors employing local or tribal people or from the drug farms maintained by the growers of aromatic and medicinal plants.

REVIEW OF LITERATURE ON IDENTITY OF ASTAVARGA PLANTS

As has been pointed out earlier, the identity of Astavarga plants suffer lot of confusion and doubts in the Ayurvedic literature till the introduction of taxonomic nomenclature. It will be of worth to cite few examples in this regard. Before proceeding to this it is also proper to know the ancient methodology of identification of medicinal plants and their implications. The Nighantus describe a plant with multi-synonyms each of which describe its one or more characters and these names ascribed to a plant were mostly related to other creations of nature. This was befitting to the time as during that period people were very close to nature. During the Vedic period the knowledge of medicinal plants was not much confusing because Gurukul education was in forests and much of it was practical and oral communication. However there was a period may be called as Samhita Kal during which large number of Samhitas were composed and orally passed on or were written. These were Atreya Samhita, Brahma Samhita, Dhanwantri Samhita, Agnivesh Samhita, Bhel Samhita, Jatukaran Samhita, Parashar Samhita, Ashwani Kumar Samhita, Atri Samhita, Ksarpani Samhita, Viswmitra Samhita, Hareet Samhita & Aupeghenava Samhita etc. Many of these in original form are not available now. Synonyms and homonyms (name used for more than one medicinal plant) were used in the post samhita period. For acquiring knowledge of medicinal plants following steps were followed:

Identification of plants-should be done with the help of tribal people, cow herdsmen, hermits etc. living in forests and other experts.

The above information should be compared and confirmed in the light of standard text books i.e. Nighantus.

These plants should there after be subjected to study their properties (Rasa, Veerya, Vipaka and Prabhava). This method of identification of medicinal plants require good competence of a physician at physical, mental, intellectual and spiritual levels. This is further supported by Sushrut by saying that "the Physician gets confused without the knowledge of names (which vary in different regions, according to habitat, shape, colour, properties, use etc.) and is unable to identify medicinal plants even on seeing them." By the time the Dhanwantri Nighantu was composed, a number of medicinal plants had become controversial because of the large number of synonyms and homonyms. In the absence of original Nighantus of Samhita Kal, the later written or composed Nighantus form the base of knowledge contained in them. Unfortunately slowly over centuries Dravyaguna teachers mostly did not have practical knowledge of medicinal plants, as a result most of the practical knowledge were restricted either to Ayurved practitioners or herbal traders only. Due to lack of competent back up here also the knowledge have further eroded and the system of using substitutes and related species have increased. The confusion and doubts went on over past many centuries of rule by Yavanas and Britishers. This is evident from the following examples particularly with reference to Astavarga plants.

Dhanwantri Nighantu provides following information on Astavarga plants which were included in Guruchayaadi varga.

Jeevak: Jeevak had been described by giving nine different synonyms. These are Shringak, Ksveda, Dirghayu, Kurchashirsa, Hraswang, Madhur, Swadu, Pranada, Chiranjivi. Then the medicinal qualities of Jeevak has been given such as it is sweet (madhur), sheeta (cooling), curing rakta pitta, vata, burning (dah), fever and tuberculosis (ksaya) and aggravates Kapha, increases seminal fluid.

Rishbhak : Various synonyms attributed to Rishbhak are Durdhar, Dheer, Matrik, Vrishabha, Vrisha, Vishani, Kakud, Indraksa, Bandhur and Gopati. It is sweet (Madhur), vitiates pitta, rakta, vata and controls Ksaya (Phthisis), Fever and is Kaphvardhak shukrajanan (aphrodisiac).

Meda, Mahameda: Synonyms of meda are Manichhidra, Shalya Parni and dharaa and it is sweet, cooling, destroys consumption, burning, fever pacifies pitta dosha and increases vitatlity. Mahameda has the similar medicinal properties and its synonyms are Devamani and Vasuchhidra, and is tasty, cooling, increases kapha and shukra (seminal fluid) and destroys burning sensation due to pitta, consumption and fever owing to vatta vitiction.

Kakoli: Various synonyms of Kakoli are Madhura, Shukla, Ksheera, Dhwan ksoklika, vaysastha, swadumansi, Vayasoli and Karanika and is sweet (Madhur) refrigerant, destroys vata, pitta, fever, burning and consumptions and has aphrodisiac properties.

Kshirkakoli: Kshirshukla, Payaswani, Vayastha, Kshir Madhura, veera and Kshirvishanika are synonyms of Ksirkokoli and its medicinal properties include good taste, tonic and destroys phthisis, pacifies vata pitta, disorders of blood, heart diseases and respiratory problems.

Rdhi, Vrdhi: Both have been dealt together and synonyms of both are also same such as Sukh, Sidhi, Rathanga, Mangal, Vasu, Rishisrista, Yuga, Laksami and Sarvajanapriya. They have sweet taste and are refrigerant, doshas.

They are useful in phthisis and fevers. It is evident from the above description that during the period of Dhanwantri there was more emphasis on imparting practical knowledge, as plant description is not given it is implied in synonyms and their medicinal properties only. The Ayurvedic students during that period must be observing them in their natural habitats.

The same shalokas have been repeated in various Ayurvedic Nighantu texts over the period of time. In certain cases some additions have been made as pointed out below:-

Shaligram Nighantu Bhushana: He wrote that Astavarga plants are even rare to kings, therefore their substitutes (having similar drug properties) should be used and he suggested that Shatavar should replace Meda- Mahameda; Vidarikand should replace Jeevak —Rishbhak; Aswagandha should substitute Kakoli-Kshirkakoli, and Rdhi —Vrdhi may be substituted by Varahikand. He has mentioned that Rdhi —Vrdhi occur in Koshal Mountain and these both are vines which bear white hairy growth and have some holes on them. Rdhi bear fruits resembling cotton boll and arranged in leftward placement on stem.

This arrangement is right moving in case of Vrdhi.

Kakoli–Kshirkakoli: It is mentioned that Kakoli and Kshirkakoli are found in the same habitat where Mahameda could be found. He has added a confusion by saying that rhizome of Kshir Kakoli are like satavar (Asparagus roots) and they exudate a kind of scented milk and the only difference between these two is that Kakoli is blackish in colour. Further it was mentioned that Jeevak and Rishbhak both of these are found in Himalayan mountain peaks, their tubers are like garlic bulbs without any juice and have small leaves.

Meda & Mahameda: Among these meda is attributed to possess under ground part (used in medicine) which is white and a scratch by nail causes exudation of grey white coloured juice. Mahameda occur in Maurang countries its rhizome looks like white ginger and its stem is viny. The author (Shri Shaligram) says that availability of Astavarga is even rare to kings therefore these should be substituted by similar property drugs. He has further commented that except Sanskrit names their names in other Indian languages are never heard even if some body had mentioned, they are unfamiliar to local people. Bhavmishra and Abhinava Nighantu have repeated the same and there is much similarity in both authors for description of Astavarga plants and about their availability for drug use. Bhavmishra in his Bhav Prakash Nighantu has further Mentioned that none of the Astavarga drugs are true or right kind in the market in spite of large number of firms/traders claiming Astavarga drug material in the market. Among these Dehradun market has earned the reputation of Astavarga drug material sale or trade. However none of these sold drug materials satisfy the proper drug quality properties.

In "Brithatryi " there is no mention of Astavarga plants. In fact Astavarga is included in Jeevaniya gana (Jeevak, Rishbhak, Kakoli, Kshirkakoli, Meda and Mahameda), Brihaniya (Kakoli, Kshirkakoli) and both these are also treated under vayaasthapan-age process regulators.

Susrut has included all the Astavarga plants in Kakoliyaadivarga (Sharma 1993). In "Bhav Prakash of Sri Bhav Mishra" with vidyotani Hindi commentary by Shri Brahma Shankar Mishra and Shri Ruplal ji Vaidya (1984) same story has been reproduced.

SHASTROKTA & TAXONOMIC (ESTABLISHED) IDENTITY OF ASTAVARGA PLANT SPECIES

P. V. Sharma and Guru Prasad Sharma (1998) in his translation of Dhanwantri—Nighantu has identified the Astavarga plant species as follows—

Jeevak-Microstylis wallichii Lindl. F. Orchidaceae
Rishbhak-Microstylis muscifera Ridley F. Orchidaceae
Meda and MahaMeda-Polygonatum verticillatum All. Family Liliaceae
Kakoli-Roscoea procera Wall. Family Zingiberaceae
Kshirkakoli-Roscoea sp. F. Zingiberaceae
Rdhi, Vrdhi-Habenaria spp. Family Orchidaceae

Acharya Priyavrata Sharma 1998). In "Dravyaguna —Vijnana Vol I (P. 408) has identified —

Jeevak-Microstylis wallichii Lindl. F. Orchidaceae
Meda-Polygonatum Verticillatum All. F. Liliaceae

Family name is wrong for Microstylis wallichii which belongs to family Orchidaceae. Dr. S. D. Kamat (2002) in his book on "Studies on Medicinal Plants and Drugs in Dhanwantri — Nighantu" identified Jeevak ((Microstylis wallichii Lindl, Rishbhak (Microstylis muscifera Ridley), Meda (Polygonatum verticillatum All.), Mahameda (Polygonatum cirrifolium Royle), Kakoli (Roscoea procera wall.) Kshirkakoli wrongly identified as Roscoea alpina Royle which is Kakoli only. Rdhi has been identified with reference to Dr. Chunekar as Habenaria intermedia. D. Don.

Thakur Balwant Singh and K. C. Chunekar (1972) in their "Glossary of Vegetable Drugs in Brhattrayi " identified some of Astavarga plant species as Kakoli (Roscoea procera), Jeevak (Microstylis wallichii Lindl), Rdhi (Habenaria Sp.), Vrdhi (Habenaria Sp.), Mahameda wrongly identified as Polygonatum verticilliatum Allioni. Acharya P. V. Sharma (1976) in "Introduction to Dravyaguna " has mentioned botanical names of the plants under Mahakasyayas and ganas of charak and Susrut where he had given the identification as follows:

Jeevak-Microstylis wallichii Lindl.
Rishbhak-Microstylis, muscifera Ridley
Meda-Polygonatum Verticillatum All.
Mahameda-Polygonatum sp.
Kakoli-Roscoea procera
Kshirkakoli-Roscoea sp.

In this description Khikrkakoli has been wrongly ascribed to genus Roscoea and species of genus Polygonatum is not mentioned thus Mahameda remains unidentified species of Polygonatum.

In " Vaanaspatika Anusandha n Darshika 196 6-68 " Dr.. Krishna Chandra Chunekar (1969) has given the following details of Astavarga plant species;

(1) Rdhi-Vrdhi-Habenaria intermedia D. Don
(2) Kshirkakoli-Lilium polyphyllum D. Don
(3) Jeevak-Rishbhak-Jeevak —Microstylis wallichii Ridley
(4) Meda-Polygonatum verticillatum All.
(5) Mahameda-Polygonatum cirrifolium Royle
(6) Kakoli-Roscoea alpina Royle and Roscoea procera Wall.

In "Kaiyadeva Nighantu edited and translated by P. V. Sharma and Guru Prasad Sharma (1979)," they have given the identity to Astavarga plants as below:-

(i) Kakoli-Kshirkakoli-Roscoea procera Wall. (Family: Zingiberaceae)
(ii) Meda-Mahameda-Polygonatum verticillatum All. (Family: Liliaceae)
(iii) Jeevak-Rishbhak-Microstylis wallichii Lindl. Microstylis muscifera Ridley
(iv) Rdhi —Vrdhi-Habenaria spp.

Acharya Raghvir Prasad Trivedi (1985) in his book "Sandigdha Vanaushadhi Darshika " mentioned from the Anandakandam following resemblences of Astavarga plants;

1. Jeevak resembles the tongue.
2. Rshabhak resembes a finger.
3. Meda resembles a nail.
4. Mahameda resembles the skin.
5. Kakoli resembles an eye.
6. Ksheerkakoli resembles an ear.
7. Rddhi resembles the nose.
8. Vrddhi resembles the leg.

In a separate description of each plant, he mentions the following details-

Rshabhak or Rshabha-It is Carpopogon pruriens found in Gauradesh and Kashmir. Bhavamishra prescribes Vidareekanda as a substitiute of it. Balbant Singh & K. C. Chunekar mentions that it is Microstylis Wallichi Lindl. He says it was well known in Sushruta's times.

Kakoli-Ashwagandha and Kali Musali (Curculigo orchioides Gaertn.) are mentioned as substitutes. A disagreement about the use of Roscoea procera Wall has been mentioned but no basis has been given. Kshirkakoli-Different authors have been quoted increasing confusion about its identity. Safed Musali (Chlorophytum arundinaceum) has been mentioned as its substitute. Roscoca procera Wall. has been suggested to be used for both Kakoliees. He has also cited a sanskrit verse indicating thereby that it is a latex bearing creeper and its tuberous roots are used. Jeevak-Bhavamishra had mentioned its two *Substitutes*-Vidarikanda and Shatawari. Another author Surendra Mohan has suggested Bahamana Safed (Centaurea behen) as substitute. Even while quoting Microstylis wallichi Lindl. as Jeevak doubts persist.

Meda-Polygonatum verticillatum has been mentioned its name and two substitutes such as Shatavari, Salabmishri (Orchis latifolia Lam. =Dactylorhiza hatagirea) have been suggested in a confused end quote.

Mahameda-Its botanical name has been mentioned as Polygonatum cirricifolium Roylc quoting Mayaram Uniyal. Thc substitutes are given as Shakaakul (Trachydium lehmanni Benth.) and Shatavari and also Polygonatum verticillatum All.

Rddhi-Different authors have given different substitutes such as Varahikanda, Shravanee, Vaidyak-shabdasindhu, Chiraikanda or Malakanda (Eulophia nuda Lindl.). He mentions the use of Habenaria.

Vrddhi-In this case also use of substitutes has been mentioned. These are Varahikanda (Tacca aspera Roxb.) Beejbanda (Seeds of Sida Cordifolia). He mentions use of Habenaria.

In "Medicinal Flora of Garhwal Himalayas " written by Dr.. M. R. Uniyal (1989) has described the Astaverga as follows —

Taxonomic Nomenclature Hindi Name Family

1. Habenaria inter media D. Don Rdhi Orchidaceae
2. Malaxis acuminata D. Don (=Microstylis wallichii Lindl) Rshbhak Orchidaceae
3. Microstylis muscifera Lindl Jeevak Orchidaceae

4. Roscoea alpina Royle Kakoli Zingiberaceae (Scitamineae Sensu Benth & Hook)
5. Roscoea procera Wall. Kakoli Zingiberaceae (Scitamineae Sensu Benth & Hook)
6. Lilium polyphyllum D. Don Kshirkakoli Zingiberaceae (Scitamineae Sensu Benth &Hook)
7. Polygonatum cirrifolium Royle Mahameda Zingiberaceae (Scitamineae Sensu Benth &Hook)
8. Polygonatum verticillatum All. Meda Zingiberaceae (Scitamineae Sensu Benth &Hook)

Dr Uniyal has identified M. accuminata as Rsbhak and Microstylis muscifera as Jeevak where as these should be reverse.

In recent years another important and good treatise on Indian medicinal plants is that from Vaidyaratnam P. S. Varier 's Arya Vaidyasala Kottakal (Kerla) published in 1994 and 1995. It covers 500 medicinal plants. The diagrams or paintings of Astavarga plants does not represent true to the type specimen and moreover there is some confusion in the nomenclature also, as shown below:-

S. Scientific name Hindi/Sanskrit

Family Prominent Character (s)

1. Habenaria intermedia D. Don Rdhi Orchidaceae intermedia, D. Don Large white flowers (2-6) in a raceme distant
2. Habenaria acuminata Lindl. (=Habenaria edgeworthii H. f. ex. Collett) Vrdhi Orchidaceae Spur upturned, petals &lip yellow
3. Malaxis acuminata D. Don (=Microstylis wallichii Lindl.) Jeevaka Orchidaceae Sides of the apical part of the lip with straight edges.
4. Malaxis muscifera (Lindl.) O. Ktze. (=Microstylis muscifera Lindl.) Rshbhak Orchidaceae Leaves two, lip-3, lobedby a notch near the centre.
5. Polygonatum verticillatum All. Meda Liliaceae Leaves in whorles of 4-8 tips usually actue.
6. Polygonatum cirrifolium Royle Mahameda Liliaceae Leaves in Whorls of 3-6 tendril-like tips of the leaves.
7. Roscoea alpina Royle Roscoea procera Wall. Kakoli Zingiberaceae (Scitamineae) Anthers notched at the top
8. Lilium polyphyllum Don Kshirkakoli Liliaceae Flowers scented greenish white the inside purple dotted.

The literature review clearly brings out one fact that authors of various Nighantus or Various Commentators have relied most of the time on the information provided by the herbal traders. In "A Dictionary of the flowering Plants in India "Santapau and Henry with assistance of Bela Roy and Partha Basu (1973) has given following details about the genera belonging to Astavarga Plants.

1. Habenaria Willd, (Orchidaceae) has about 600 species in the world of which 100 species occur in India. These are terresterial leafy herbs bearing flowers in spikes of racemes. Two species (Vrdhi) H. accuminata Lindl. (=Habenaria edgeworthii H. f. ex collett) and (Rdhi) H. intermedia D. Don. are found in temperate Himalaya.
2. Malaxis Soland ex Sw. (Orchindaceac) genus contain about 300 species distributed all over the world out of which 17 species occur in India. These are mainly terrestrial, rarely epiphytic or lithophytic herbs. The colour of the plant bears a striking relation to the kind of light under which it grown. Malaxis acuminata D. Don (=Microslylis wallichii Lindl.) know as Jeevak and Malaxis muscifera (Lindl.) O. Ktze. (=Microstylis muscifera Lindl.) named as Rsbhak occurring temperate Himalaya and are included under the genus Malaxis.
3. Lilium Linn. (Liliaceae) : About 80 species occur under this genus the worldover of which 10 species are found in India. These are perennial, erect, leafy steamed herbs which bear flowers in axillary or terminal racemes. A temperate Himalayan species Lilium polyphyllum belongs to Astavarga group of plants and is known as ksirkakoli.
4. Roscoea Smith (Zingiberaceae) include about 15 species found in different parts of the world. Only 4 species occur in India. These are perennial herbs with thick fleshky roots. The species under this genus are R. alpina Royle, R. purpurea Smith., R. procera Wall. R. Capitata Smith and these are know as Kakoli.
5. Ploygonatum Mill. (Liliaceae) About 50 species occur in the world of which 15 species are found in India. These herbs have creeping root stocks and leafy stems above which bear drooping white, green or purplish flowers. Two species, P. cirrifolium (Wallich.) All known as Mahameda and P. verticillatum (L.) All known as Meda, are included in the Astavarga of Chayavanprash.

HIMALAYAN HABITATS OF ASTAVARGA PLANTS AND THEIR GRADUAL DECLINE

The doubtful identify of Astavarga plants has been mainly because of their specific habitat conditions which are always found in small patches. It requires much travelling in the Himalayas particularly the North —Western Himalaya to collect even a small number of plants of at least four species as has been pointed out.

Roscoea: Two species R. alpina and R. procera are used in Astavarga, but there are four species and the other two are R. purpurea which has dark purple stems and flowers also have deeper shade; R. capitata which has dense head of flowers borne on a leafless long stalk and plants are also taller than other species. These occur mostly in forest edges shrubberies, open slopes on altitudes ranging from 1500 to 3000 m except R. alpina which is alpine species and is found between 2500m to 4000m above MSL. The species occurrence is quite common at present.

Polygonatum: Four species are commonly found. These are P. hookeri Baker, P. multiflorum (L.) All., P. verticillatum (L.) All. and P. Cirrifolium (Wallich.) Royle and out of these P. cirrifolium and P. Verticillatum are used in Astavarga. These grow in shrubberies open grassy slopes, and as under growth in forests on altitudes varying between 1500m to 3700m in temperate Himalaya.

Malaxis: Three species are found distributed in N-W Himalaya. These are M. acuminata, M. musicfera, M. cylindrostachya. These grow as undergrowth in forests over the altitudes varying from 600m to 4000m. They prefer shrubberies and grassy slopes, moist and humus rich soil and shady rocks. Another M. mackinnoni Duthie also occurrs in Uttaranchal State.

Lilium: At least 5 to 6 species occur in Himalayas. Medicinally most important among these are Lilium polyphyllum Don and Lilium wallichianu m Schult. & Schult. f. These are generally found in open slopes, grassy lands in forests. These are rare and occur between 1800m to 3800m altitudes. The other closely related plant is Fritillaria royle and Fritillaria cirrhosa D. Don. Their bulbs are also used as tonic and are employed as substitute.

Habenaria: Occur in temperate Himalaya on grassy slopes between 1800m to 2900m altitudes. Habenaria have 4 species, but medicinally most important are H. intermedia D. Don and H. acuminata Lindl. The other species are H. griffithi H. f., H. goodyeroides D. Don. There is scope of mixing bulbs of Eulophia compestris Wall., and Eulophia herbacea Lindl. which are also considered as aphrodisiac and tonic.

Gradual Decline in Natural Habitats: The Rapid destruction of forests, various developmental actives such as roads, buildings, orchards etc. and climatic changes (due to human intervention) inducing ecological changes in the habitat conditions are all responsible for severe loss in plant populations and as a consequence, these species, which have specific habitat requirements, are becoming rare. This is at least true for Lilium polyphyllum D. Don which was common in Shimla forests about 100 years ago when Flora Simlensis was written by Col. Henry Collett (1902). Other Astavarga plants such as Habenaria intermedia, H. acuminata, Malaxis muscifera have undergone the same fate and it is difficult to find spots rich in their populations. The early grazing and forest fires are the other hazardous causes. The other potent cause is grass for the domestic animals, the area under which have shrunk greatly, clear the grass lands bushes etc. by burning and also go for early grass cutting. This removal of above ground parts do not allow seed set or seed maturity causing severe decline in plant populations.

MEDICINAL PROPERTIES OF ASTAVARGA PLANTS

Various Ayurvedic Nighantu books composed or commented by different Vaidyas over several centuries describe the medicinal properties of all the Astavarga plants either as a group or alone are reproduced hereunder. Till date none has tried their chemical evaluation in the modern laboratories. Certainly, as is evident, they need further investigation on scientific lines to add value to their excellent text described qualities. The Astavarga plants have been described under three Ayurvedic terms that is Jeevniya, Brhneeya, Vayaasthapan. It is therefore essential to explain them before proceeding to give their medicinal properties.

Jeevaniya are those plant drugs which strengthen the bodily Vitality (Prana Shakti) through their action on three humours (three doshas —vata, Pitta, Kapha) bringing them into equilibrium state — described in Ayurveda as a state of perfect health.. Plants described as Jeevaniya, in various Nighantus are Jeevak, Rishbhak, Meda, Mahameda, Kakoli, Kshirkakoli, Mugdaparni, Mashaparni, Jeevanti and Yastimadhu. These medicines also enchance anabolic activities over the catabolism in the body.

Brhneeya **:**The drugs which promote the formation of mansa dhatu that is flesh formation. Such drug plants are ksirini, Dugdhika, Aswagandha, Kakoli, Kshirkakoli, Sweta Bala, Peet Bala, Van Kapas, Vidari, Vidhara.

Vaya Sthapan (Gerontologic): These plant drugs clears the body of three doshas and particularly the Vata dosha and thus does not allow progressive growth changes to occur or if they occur it is at a very slow rate. This means that the immunity system becomes strong and metabolic processes are growth promoting. The plant drugs in this category are Meda, Mahameda, Rdhi, Vrdhi, Amalaka, Guruchi, Punarnava, Shatavari, Jeevanti, Haritaki, Sweta Aprajita, Mandukaparni and Shalparni.

Jeevaka: Is sweet (madhur), refrigerant, pacifies pitta, Rakta and vata doshas. It is useful in burning sensation, fever and consumption, increases kapha dosha and sukra (seminal fluid) (Gana Nighantu). Nighantu Ratnakar states that it is madhur, sheetal, shukrajanak, kaphakarak, Rakta pitta nashak, Balkarak (tonic) and is useful in treating vata, pitta, fever (jvar), Krsta (emanciation), phthisis, burning sansation and blood disorders.

Rshbhak is sweet in taste and pacifies pitta, vata and rakta doshas. It is useful in consumption, burning sensation in the body, fever and increases kapha dosha and Shukradhatu (Nighantu Ratnakar).

Both Jeevak and Rishbhak are nutritious, tonic, refrigerant, viryavardhaka, madhur and are useful in pitta dosha, burning, blood disorder, vata dosha and consumption (Bhava Prakash).

Meda **:**In Nighantu Churamani it is stated that meda is sweet, sheetvirya, it pacifies pitta dosha, increases kapha and shukra. It is useful in phthisis, burning sensation in the body and fever. Nighantu Rantnakar describes its properties as sweet in taste, sheetal, guru, dhatuvardhaka, increases milk in ladies, Snigdha, kaphakarak and is useful in vata, pitta, rakta vikar, consumption, fever, burning sensation in body and cough.

Mahameda is madhur in taste, sheetal, increases kapha and shukra. It pacifies pitta dosha, and is useful in burning sensation of the body, blood disorders, consumption and fever due to vata dosha (Dhanwantri Nighantu, Raj Nighantu). Both Meda and Mahameda increases meda dhatu in the body.

Rdhi is paustik, tridoshnashak, Shukrajanak, madhur, guru, vitality enhancing prana (Pranaprada). Aishwarya janak and is useful in epilepsy, rakta —pitta doshas —(Bhava Prakash). In Nighantu Ratnakar it is written that it is sweet in taste, unctous, medha janak, sheetal, kaphakarak, sukravardhaka, pranadayaka, Balkarak, Rakta shodhak, Ruchikarka, guru and is useful in leprosy, worm infestation, epilepsy, raktapitta thirst, consumption, pitta, vata, rakta dosha and fever.

Vrdhi is cooling nutritious, causing conception, Shukra vardhaka, pacifies rakta pitta doshas, ulcers in stomach, cough and consumption ("Shaligram Nighantu ").

Kakoli : The roots are sweet in taste, slightly bitter, refrigerant, galactagogue, fatty and is useful in phthisis, pitta, pains due to vata aggravation, blood problems, burning sensation in the body and fever. It increases kapha and shukra dhatu. (Dhanwantri Nighantu). It is vata —pittahar, Sheetal, Brhna and cures emaciation due to consumption (Madan Pal Nighantu). In Nighantu Ratnakar, it is mentioned that it is Sheetal, Vrsya, madhura, tikta, kaphakari, guru, destroys phthisis, pitta, thirst and is beneficial in rakta dosha, raktapitta, emaciation, visam jwar, and aggravated vata-pitta.

Kshirkakoli: The bulbs are sweet slightly bitter, refrigerant, expectorant, antipyretic, aphrodisiac, galactagogue and tonic. It is useful in cough, general debility, fever, vitiated condition of pitta, seminal weakness, burning sensation, increases vitality (Madan Vinod Nighantu, Sodhal Nighantu, Raj Nighantu, Kaidev Nighantu, Dhanwantri Nighantu).

Astavarga is cooling, tasty, nutritious tonic, aphrodisiac, nourishes body and increases kapha. It is beneficial in seminal weakness, increases fat in the body, heals bone fracture and cures vata, pitta, and rakta doshas, abnormal thirst, burning sensation in the body, consumption, fever and diabetic condition.

It is one of the excellent combination of herbal drugs which restores health immediately, strengthens immunity system and rectifies defects in anabolism or body growth processes and works as antioxidant in the body. That is why Aswani Kumars invented it for curing the frail, emaciated sick body of Chayavan Rishi who regained youthful condition it is claimed. There is need to grow these species on large scale to take up clinical trials and chemical investigations. The tissue culture programme may be advantageous to save these species and achieve fast multiplication.

Botanical Description with Characters of Drug Part of Astavarga Plants

Vrdhi – (Habenaria acuminata Lindl. syn. Habenaria edgeworthii Hook. f. ex Collett) :

Stem – 30 to 60 cm.. high. leafy, stout

Leaves – Ovate, oblong-lanceolate, 4-10 cm long acute, acuminate thick, upper leaves gradually smaller, nerves 5-7, base sheathing.

Flowering Spike – 7cm to 25cm long,, bearing many flowers.

Flowers – Yellow – green 1 to 1. 5cm across with lanceolate acute bracts, the lower shorter, the upper longer, than the ovary sepals green, pubescent, the margins slightly fringed; petals yellow thick, erect; lip yellow, longer than the sepals concave narrowing to a long strap shaped limb; Spur about twice the length of ovary, yellowish –green curving upwards with tip curved down.

Flowering & Fruiting time – July –August.

Characteristics of usable drug part – Tubers are in pair the older becomes Shrivelled as the growing period proceeds. The shape of the tuber is oval to ovate and slightly tapering at the opposite end giving it a shape resembling to cotton boll. Skin dull white, flesh white and sweetish-bitter in taste.

Distribution

Himachal – Summer Hills,, Shimla; Mountains near Manali, Rahla Forest, Kothi, Manali, Sarahan, Nirmand-Annu, Rwanda, Kamarunag peak, Saptasar above Rawalsar (Mandi), Chansel, Churdhar, Jangtoo, Chamba, Narkanda.

Uttaranchal-Mussoorie-Jaberkhet, Mussoorie, Kyarphulli, Company Bagh, Deoban, Tehri-Nagtibba West of Dhanolti; Uttarkashi-Jamuna Valley, Kharshali, Har-Ki-Dun; Chamoli-Valley of flowers, Gobindghat, Khirsu; Pithoragarh- Tejam Jankhola Vally, Kali Valley, Sarju Valley, Nainital-Nainital, Bhowali, Ramgarh, Fatehgarh, Above Malli Tal; Almora-Binsar, Almora, Lorakhet, Ranikhet to Chaubatia.

Ayurvedic drug properties: It is emollient, aphrodisiac, rejuvenating and tonic and is beneficial in aggravated vata and pitta, burning sensation in the body, hyperdipsia, fever, cough, epilepsy, insanity, emanciation and general debility (Bhav Prakash, kai, Nirs, so, Ni, Ni, Ra)

Substitutes-Varahi Kand ((Tacca aspera Roxb.) salam panja (Dactylorhiza hatagirea) Mahabala (Sida acuta, seeds of Sida cordifolia).

Status- It is a rare species because grows in assocaiton with grasses and is being cut in early stages before seeds are mature.

Rdhi– (Habenaria intermedia D. Don)

Stem- Erect, 25-60cm high, terete, robust, leafy.

Leaves- Scattered usually 5-nerved, ovate-lanceolate acuminate, cordate at the base.

Raceme- 2-6 flowered.

Flowers- 5cm across white or greenish-white few, distant. Bracts leaf like lanceolate, acuminate, equal or more than ovary. Sepals persistent, 20-25mm long, green, spreading tips reflexed, upper one white inside. Petals white, 5-

nerved. Lip 3-lobed, longer than sepals, green spur 5-6cm stout, longer than ovary more or less curved. Side lobes deeply fringed. Flowering time-July-August Characteristics Usable Drug Part-Tubers are round at the opposite end but tapering towards stem joint. Skin is dirty white, flesh white and is slightly bitter in taste.

Distribution- Himanchal Pradesh, Koti (Shimla) Summer Hill Indian Institute of Advance study, Kamana Hill), Rwanda and Kamarunag (Karsog), Rewalsar hills (Mandi), Shimla (Fagu), Dalhousie (Chamba), Kinnaur.

Jammu &Kashmir- Azmabad, Poonch, Pirpanjal Range.

Uttaranchal- Dehradun-Mussoorie (Jaberkhet), Camel back road, company bagh, Bhatta Fall, Kampty fall; Tehri (Nagtibba) Suakholi, Chamoli-on way to Kedarnath, Jangal chatti, way to valley of flowers, Gaurikund (Rambera); Utarrkashi-Tons Valley, Bhagirathi valley and way to Dodital.

Ayurvedic Medicinal Properties

Rdhi is Sheetvirya, pacifies vata, pitta, rakta doshas. It is useful in consumption and fevers. It increases kapha dosha and shukra dhatu. It is intellect promoting, aphrodisiac, rejuvenating, tonic and cures emaciation, epilepsy, cough, skin diseases, haematemesis and general debility.

Substitutes: Varahi Kand (Tacca aspera Roxb.) Utangan seeds (Blepharis edulis Pers.) Bala (Sida cordifolia), Chiriya Musali (Asparagus filicinus Buch. -Ham.)

Jeevak —(Malaxis acuminata D. Don)

Syn. Microstylis wallichii Lindl.

Stem- 5 to 25 cm, ribbed bearing pseudo bulbs

Leaves– Usually 3 may be more,, 5-10cm ovate-lanceolate, acute with prominent veins and light green.

Flowers– Shortly stalked about 10mm in diameter, yellowish-green with purple centre. Sepals oblong, 2 lateral rather shorter than the dorsal, margins recurved. Petals linear longer than sepals, margin recurved. Lip shied-like, slightly convex, tip notched or bilobulate, auricles straight and slightly over lapping.

Flowering Time- July-August.

Characteristics of Usable Drug Part

Pseudo bulbs are in pair and new formation looks like a garlic clove (hence called rasona kand vat). Colour is green white and these remain alive over long period. Flesh is bitterish in taste.

Distribution: Himalaya, Khasihills (Meghalaya) Andaman Islands, Travencore, Mdhya Pradesh. In Himalaya 1850 m to 2300 m Himachal Pradesh to Arunachal Pradesh, Assam, Nagaland, Manipur, Mizoram, Tripura.

Himachal Pradesh:- Shimla-Glen, Boileaugunj, Elysium Hill in forests, way to Rani forest, way from Khajiar to Chmba, Chail, Hattoo, Narkanda.

Uttaranchal: Dehradun-Camel back road, Below Mussoorie bypass road, above barlowgunj, chakrata, Jaunsar, Tehri (Magra); Pauri-Pode khal, Chamoli-Nagnath; Ukhimath, Gopeshwar, Pithoragarh-Sarju Valley, Berenag, Thal Kedar; Nainital, Bhowali, Ramagarh, Almora-Ranikhet, Between Ranikhet-Chaubatia.

Ayurvedic Medicinal Properties: It is sheet virya and calms down vata, rakta and pitta doshas and is beneficial in burning sensation of the body, fever, and consumption. It increases kapha and Shukra dhatu. It is aphrodisiac and tonic. It cures haematemesis, aggravated vata and pitta doshas, seminal weakness, dipsia, emaciation, tuberculosis and general body weakness. It increases body flesh and is jeevniya.

Substitutes: Vidari kand, Bahaman Safed (Centaurea behen Linn.), Guruchi (Tinospora cordifolia)

Rshbhak- (Malaxis muscifera (Lindl.)

Kuntze- Synonym Microstylis muscifera Lindl.

Stem – 3 to 25cm high with ovoid pseudo bulbs

Leaves- One or two (unequal) 3-10 x 2-4cm sessile, ovate to ovate-lanceolate obtuse, narrowed at base to sheathing petiole.

Inflorescence- 10 to 25 cm. long.

Flowers: 3-4 mm long, pale-yellow-green, Bracts lanceolate shorter than ovary sepals broadly lanceolate. Petals linear Shorter than sepals. Lip ovate abruptly pointed, margins thickened.

Flowering Time- July –August.

Characteristics of the usable drug Part- Tubers round, shining white bearing stem giving shape of bullock horn having a similar curvature. The taste is slightly bitter with mucilaginous substance.

Distribution- Himalaya between 1800-3500m eastward to Sikkim.

Himachal Pradesh- Shimla (Mashobra, Fagu, Hattoo forests) Rahala forest, Dhanchoo, Sangla, chamba.

Jammu & Kashmir- Gulmarg, Datni, Leh.

Uttaranchal- Pithoragarh-Tejum Haya, Bakariudiyar, Ralam Valley, Palangarh, Ralam, Almora-Dwali, Dehradun-Chakrata, Deoban Tehri-Masartal, Bokhills, Dhanolti, way to Nagtibba; Chamoli-Vasukital, Bajmora, Jumma Area, Dunagiri, Valley of flowers, Rambara, Hemkund; Uttarkashi-Jamuna Valley above village kharsil.

Ayurvedic Medicinal Properties- Tubers are efficacious cure for pitta, rakta, vata doshas. It is useful in phthisis, burning sensation in the body, fever and increases Kapha and shukra. It is styptic, aphrodisiac and tonic. It is an effective cure in vitiated pitta and vata, seminal weakness, dysentery, emaciation and general debility.

Substitutes: Vida ri Kanda (Pueraria tuberosa DC.) Ba haman Lal (Centaurium roxburghii (G. Don) Druce), Vansalochan.

Status: Malaxis muscifera is also a rare species and at present its reasons are not clear.

Kakoli: (Roscoea alpina Royle, Roscoea procera Wall.)

Stem- 6-20cm and 30-60cm, robust.

Leaves- 2-6 lanceolate, 15x3 cm.

Flowers- Several lilak, purple or white, corolla tube much longer than the calyx, borne in a short stem with or without leaves, upper lobe (petal) rounded, hooded and narrower reflexed lateral petals. Lower staminode 5x3cm obscurly 3-lobed spreading, notched at the tip.

Flowering Time- July –August or June for R. alpina.

Characteristics of the usable drug part- Fingers replacing roots are thickened 3-4 and have sickle shape, white and flesh inside is also white, tastes sweet resembling shatavar.

Distribution- Western Himalaya 1000 to 2700m commonly found in these altitudes in Himachal Pradesh, Jammu and Uttaranchal (Joshi Math, Mussoorie) and in other all districts.

Ayurvedic Medicinal Properties- Root fingers are sweet sheetvirya, pacifies vata pitta, fever due to vitiated vata-pitta. It is beneficial in consumption, burning sensation in body, increases Kapha dosa and shukra. It is also an effective cure for pains due to pitta, vata, rakta dosha, thirst due to pitta, rakta pitta etc.

Substitutes- Aswagandha (Withania somnifera) Curculigo orchioides (Kali musali)

Kshirkakoli: (Lilium polyphyllum D. Don)

Stem- 30 to 100cm high, erect.

Leaves- Sessile, alternate or nearly opposite or whorled, narrow lanceolate or linear 7cm-13cmx 5mm-12mm. Bracts leaf like whorled.

Flowers- Solitary, racemed or whorled stalked (3cm-10cm), Perianth 6cm-8cm long, green-white with purple dots inside. Stigma 3-lobed, capsule 2cm to 3cm.

Flowering Time- 15June-15 July

Characteristics of Usable Drug Part- The bulb is a loose mass of fleshy scales white in colour and is sweetish bitter in taste.

Distribution- Himachal-Hattoo peak, Narkanda forests, Chail (Solan district), Sungari-Bahli on Rampur Road.

Jammu & Kashmir- Gulmarg, Liddar Valley.

Uttaranchal- Gangotri, Rainthal, Amardhar, Kedarnath, Madmaheshwar. It is a rare species and its populations are very small that is 10-15 plants.

Ayurvedic Medicinal Properties- It promotes appetite and pacifies vata, pitta, rakta dosas. It is efficacious in bleeding disorders, cardiac diseases, dyspnoea, cough, consumption and diseases of urine system and is vrsya (tonic). Bulbs are refrigerant, galactagogue, expectorant and aphrodisiac. They are useful in bronchitis, burning sensation, hyperdipsia, rheumatalgia and general weakness in the body.

Substitutes- Aswagandha (Withania somnifera Dunal), swet musali (Chlorophytum arundinaceum), Fritillaria roylei Hook. f., Fritillaria oxypetala

Royle.

Comments on Lilum Polyphyllum Don-Sir Col. Henry Collett (1902) wrote Flora Simlensis and in frontispiece he gave a diagram of this plant species and also mentioned under the description of species in family Orchidaceae that it is common in Shimla woods. But a search of this plant species in forests in and around was futile because even a single plant specimen was not found. This is because of disturbance in natural habitat and changing ecological conditions. Similar experience was felt in some other habitats in Uttaranchal especially in Ponwali Kanta, Rainthal area. The species has become rare and need immediate action for its conservation.

Meda— (Polygonatum verticillatum Allioni)

Stem- 30cm to 1. 20m, erect, angled, grooved and sometimes mottled. Leaves-in whorls of 4-8 sessile, linear, 10-20cm long and 5-13mm broad or lanceolate 8cm x 18mm, tips usually acute, sometimes obtuse or slightly enrolled to the midrib.

Raceme-whorled 2-3 flowered.

Parianth-5mm white often greenish

Berry-6-7mm in diameter green and red or orange on ripening.

Flowering & Fruiting Time-July-September

Characteristics of the Usable Drug Part- Plants bear rhizomes as under ground part which resemble ginger but comparatively much less thick except in very old (7-8 years) plants. The rhizomes are white or dull white in colour but flesh inside is white and is sweet in taste when dried.

Distribution- The species is widely distributed in temperate Himalaya between 1600m and 3500m.

Himachal Pradesh – Shimla,, Narkanda, Hattoo, Churdhar, Janjelli, Sikari Tibba, Kamarunagh.

Jammu & Kashmir- Trikuta Hills, Udhampur, Doda area.

Uttaranchal- Ponwalikanta, Tali, Amardhar, Ganganani dhar, Rainthal, Kedarnath, Gangotri, Madmaheshwar.

Ayurvedic Medicinal Properties- Meda rhizomes are sweet in taste sheetvirya, pacify pitta dosh and increase kapha and shukra dhatu. They are beneficial in phthisis, burning sensation in the body, and fever (Dhan. Ni.). They are emollient, aphrodisiac, tonic, galactagogue, and beneficial in aggravation of pitta, cough, ulcers, skin diseases, general debility and vulnerary.

Substitutes- Asparagus racemosus Dunal (Shatavari), Salam misri (Eulophia campestris Wall).

Mahameda —(Polygonatum cirrifolium Royle)

Stem- 30 to 130cm tall, terete, round or grooved, climbing by means of tendril like tips of the leaves and grow generally in association with bushes. leaves-are always in whorls of 3-6, sessile, linear, 5cm to 8cm long and 3-5mm broad, lower surface glaucus, the margins usually inrolled to the midrib.

Racemes- Whorled 2-4 flowered.

Parianth- 5mm white often greenish or slightly purple.

Berry- 6-7mm in diameter, green and on ripening Orange-Red.

Flowering & Fruiting Time = July-September

Characteristics of the usable Drug Part- The rhizomes generally look like ginger but less thick, white or dull white in colour and are sweet in taste on drying.

Distribution- Temperate Himalaya 1500m to 2700m

Himachal Pradesh- Shimla, Matiana, Narkanda.

Uttaranchal- Mussoorie, Chakrata, Gaurikund, Rambara, Harshal, Ganganani, Devban, Rainthal, Mandakini Ghati, Bhilangana Ghati, Ponwali, Kalimath.

Ayurvedic Medicinal Properties- According to Dhanwantri Nighantu, Mahameda is sweet in taste, sheet virya, increases Kapha and shukra dhatu and is beneficial in consumption burning sensation, and fever. Various Nighantus describe its properties as emollient aphrodisiac, galactagoue, tonic and useful invitiation of vata-pitta, strangury seminal weakness, anorexia and general body weakness.

Substitutes- Shatavari (Asparagus racemosus Willd.) Nagbala (S. Veronicaefolia Linn.) Shakaakul mishri (Polygonatum multiflorum (Linn.) All.), Paederia foetida Linn. (Prasarani).

Status- It is also a rare species because of early cutting before Seeds are mature and burning of grassy plots for removal of bushes.

Henbane: Qualities and Benefits

Family name: Solanaceae. black colored henbane Latin name: Hyoscyamus Niger Linn

Sanskrit: Prasik Yamani, Madakarani, Turushka

Hindi: Khurasani Ajwain

Gujarati: Khurasani Ajmo

Marathi: Khuasani Oba

Bengali: Khurasani Yamani

Telangi: Khurasani Vamu

Dravidi: Kurishani Vanam

Arabian: Teralbanj, Bajul

French: Tukhme Bunj, Bunj

Punjabi: Khurasani Ajwain

The plants of Henbane are found in the Garhwal regions of northern India and grow up to a height of 800 to 10, 000 feet. They are cultivated in Saharanpur, Kolkata, Agra, Ajmer, Pune and government parks and fields.

Chemical Composition

The seeds have 25 to 30 per cent oil; the leaves and flowers have hiosimine and alkaline called hiosan along with atopin and scopin in little quantities. The biannual atropine plants grow in mud.

External Form

The plants are longer than the plants of thymol seeds, annual or biannual. The roots have fibres and round in shape, straight and strong. The leaves are broad and long, with sharp edges, green in colour. The branches also have fibres. The flowers grow in bunches in yellowish colors with violet stripes. The fruits are small, there are two segments at a distance of half inch and each section has black coloured henbane with flat shape.

Qualities

1. It is dry, bitter and pungent, hot. It has alcoholic affect and causes anxiety. It cures kapha, respiratory problems, heart pain and sexual problems.
2. It is curative hence beneficial in case of piles, pain in the stomach early ejaculation, dreams, menses. painful discharge of menses and irregular menstrual cycle. It calms down the sexual desire as well.
3. Henbane has alcoholic tendency and causes urination. If taken in small doses it reduces the pace of heart beat at night and strengthens but excess quantity is harmful for the heart.
4. The weariness effect is seen on the brain, genital organs and intestines. Opium and thorn apple are similar medicines but opium causes constipation, whereas henbane is free from this quality. Thorn apple leads to drowsiness and illusions but this herb does not have any such effect hence henbane is considered to be a betzer medicine. It is the best medicine for sleepiness and getting rid off weariness.
5. It has an effect on the nervous system. It calms down the mind, gives good sleep.

Medicinal Use

Toothache: Grind henbane with leaves and keep it on the cavity to get rid off toothache.

Joint pain: Boil it in sesame oil. Massage the painful area to cure joint pain. sciatica pain and backache etc.

Ear pain: Boil henbane in sesame oil and our feu drops in the ear to cure ear pain.

Liver pain: Lep with this oil cures chronic liver er pain and chest pain.

Bleeding gums: Rinsing the mouth With the kwath (decoction) of henbane leaves stops bleeding from the gums.

Urinary Problems: The extract of henbane seeds is beneficial in case of stones, pain or burning sensation. It causes urination and thereby reduces the pain.

Anxiety: Add 30 drops of henbane juice in 25ml of water and should be administered to patients at an interval of one hour. This is very effective in case of hysteria, lunacy and other vata related doshas.

Worms: The male having worms in the stomach should eat jaggery on empty stomach and then take henbane churna with stale water. The worms present in the intestines will come out through stools.

Uterus pain: Make a long stick with the henbane powder and insert it in the vagina.

Stomachache: Make a pill with jaggery and henbane and take to control stomachache. Alternatively add black salt in henbane churna and take it.

Add one gram dry ginger powder in two to four drops of henbane oil and eat it and drink hot aniseed extract over it, this controls stomachache immediately or add little amount of jaggery in its kwath and take it.

Cough, hiccups and vomiting

1. Keep henbane and sugar candy in a betel leaf and suck the juice to cure dry cough caused due to vata.
2. Keep the henbane seeds in mouth and suck the juice to stop hiccups caused after meals.
3. Grind the top portion of henbane and clove and lick with honey to cure vomiting.

Dysentery: Take equal quantities of henbane, ginger, tea and mochrasa, make a fine powder. Take 2 to 3 grams with water less curd, it stops dysentery.

Stones: Take 5 gm of henbane churna with 20 gm of radish juice to dissolve stones.

Worms: Grind the henbane or give its fumigation in the rectum of children to get rid off small white worms.

Leprosy: Take henbane churna with jaggery for seven days and maintain strict diet.

Piles: Make a poultice of henbane and give fomentation on the piles and with salt it calms down the urinary pain.

Fever due to indigestion: Swallow four henbane seeds with cold water without chewing it. It can also be taken with honey.

Wounds: Grind it with little jaggery and tie a poultice with rapeseed oil to heal the wounds quickly.

❐

Properties of Astavarga Plants

Various Ayurvedic Nighantu books composed or commented by different Vaidyas over several centuries describe the medicinal properties of all the Astavarga plants either as a group or alone are reproduced hereunder. Till date none has tried their chemical evaluation in the modern laboratories. Certainly, as is evident, they need further investigation on scientific lines to add value to their excellent text described qualities. The Astavarga plants have been described under three Ayurvedic terms that is Jeevniya, Brhneeya, Vayaasthapan. It is therefore essential to explain them before proceeding to give their medicinal properties.

Jeevaniya are those plant drugs which strengthen the bodily Vitality (Prana Shakti) through their action on three humours (three doshas —vata, Pitta, Kapha) bringing them into equilibrium state — described in Ayurveda as a state of perfect health.. Plants described as Jeevaniya, in various Nighantus are Jeevak, Rishbhak, Meda, Mahameda, Kakoli, Kshirkakoli, Mugdaparni, Mashaparni, Jeevanti and Yastimadhu. These medicines also enchance anabolic activities over the catabolism in the body.

Brhneeya :The drugs which promote the formation of mansa dhatu that is flesh formation. Such drug plants are ksirini, Dugdhika, Aswagandha, Kakoli, Kshirkakoli, Sweta Bala, Peet Bala, Van Kapas, Vidari, Vidhara.

Vaya Sthapan (Gerontologic) :These plant drugs clears the body of three doshas and particularly the Vata dosha and thus does not allow progressive growth changes to occur or if they occur it is at a very slow rate. This means that the immunity system becomes strong and metabolic processes are growth promoting. The plant drugs in this category are Meda, Mahameda, Rdhi, Vrdhi, Amalaka, Guruchi, Punarnava, Shatavari, Jeevanti, Haritaki, Sweta Aprajita, Mandukaparni and Shalparni.

Jeevaka :is sweet (madhur), refrigerant, pacifies pitta, Rakta and vata doshas. It is useful in burning sensation, fever and consumption, increases kapha dosha and sukra (seminal fluid) (Gana Nighantu). Nighantu Ratnakar states that it is madhur, sheetal, shukrajanak, kaphakarak, Rakta pitta nashak, Balkarak (tonic) and is useful in treating vata, pitta, fever (jvar), Krsta (emanciation), phthisis, burning sansation and blood disorders.

Rshbhak is sweet in taste and pacifies pitta, vata and rakta doshas. It is useful in consumption, burning sensation in the body, fever and increases kapha dosha and Shukradhatu (Nighantu Ratnakar).

Both Jeevak and Rishbhak are nutritious, tonic, refrigerant, viryavardhaka, madhur and are useful in pitta dosha, burning, blood disorder, vata dosha and consumption (Bhava Prakash).

Meda :In Nighantu Churamani it is stated that meda is sweet, sheetvirya, it pacifies pitta dosha, increases kapha and shukra. It is useful in phthisis, burning sensation in the body and fever. Nighantu Rantnakar describes its properties as sweet in taste, sheetal, guru, dhatuvardhaka, increases milk in ladies, Snigdha, kaphakarak and is useful in vata, pitta, rakta vikar, consumption, fever, burning sensation in body and cough.

Mahameda is madhur in taste, sheetal, increases kapha and shukra. It pacifies pitta dosha, and is useful in burning sensation of the body, blood disorders, consumption and fever due to vata dosha (Dhanwantri Nighantu, Raj Nighantu). Both Meda and Mahameda increases meda dhatu in the body.

Rdhi is paustik, tridoshnashak, Shukrajanak, madhur, guru, vitality enhancing prana (Pranaprada). Aishwarya janak and is useful in epilepsy, rakta —pitta doshas —(Bhava Prakash). In Nighantu Ratnakar it is written that it is sweet in taste, unctous, medha janak, sheetal, kaphakarak, sukravardhaka, pranadayaka, Balkarak, Rakta shodhak, Ruchikarka, guru and is useful in leprosy, worm infestation, epilepsy, raktapitta thirst, consumption, pitta, vata, rakta dosha and fever.

Vrdhi is cooling nutritious, causing conception, Shukra vardhaka, pacifies rakta pitta doshas, ulcers in stomach, cough and consumption ("Shaligram Nighantu ").

Kakoli :The roots are sweet in taste, slightly bitter, refrigerant, galactagogue, fatty and is useful in phthisis, pitta, pains due to vata aggravation, blood problems, burning sensation in the body and fever. It increases kapha and shukra dhatu. (Dhanwantri Nighantu). It is vata —pittahar, Sheetal, Brhna and cures emaciation due to consumption (Madan Pal Nighantu). In Nighantu Ratnakar, it is mentioned that it is Sheetal, Vrsya, madhura, tikta, kaphakari, guru, destroys phthisis, pitta, thirst and is beneficial in rakta dosha, raktapitta, emaciation, visam jwar, and aggravated vata-pitta.

Kshirkakoli :The bulbs are sweet slightly bitter, refrigerant, expectorant, antipyretic, aphrodisiac, galactagogue and tonic. It is useful in cough, general debility, fever, vitiated condition of pitta, seminal weakness, burning sensation, increases vitality (Madan Vinod Nighantu, Sodhal Nighantu, Raj Nighantu, Kaidev Nighantu, Dhanwantri Nighantu).

Astavarga is cooling, tasty, nutritious tonic, aphrodisiac, nourishes body and increases kapha. It is beneficial in seminal weakness, increases fat in the body, heals bone fracture and cures vata, pitta, and rakta doshas, abnormal thirst, burning sensation in the body, consumption, fever and diabetic condition. It is one of the excellent combination of herbal drugs which restores health immediately, strengthens immunity system and rectifies defects in anabolism or body growth processes and works as antioxidant in the body. That is why Aswani Kumars invented it for curing the frail, emaciated sick body of Chayavan Rishi who regained youthful condition it is claimed. There is need to grow these species on large scale to take up clinical trials and chemical investigations. The tissue culture programme may be advantageous to save these species and achieve fast multiplication.

Botanical Description with Characters of Drug Part of Astavarga Plants

Vrdhi – (Habenaria acuminata Lindl. syn. Habenaria edgeworthii Hook. f. ex Collett) : Stem – 30 to 60 cm.. high. leafy, stout

Leaves – Ovate, oblong-lanceolate, 4-10 cm long acute, acuminate thick, upper leaves gradually smaller, nerves 5-7, base sheathing.

Flowering Spike – 7cm to 25cm long,, bearing many flowers.

Flowers – Yellow – green 1 to 1. 5cm across with lanceolate acute bracts, the lower shorter, the upper longer, than the ovary sepals green, pubescent, the margins slightly fringed; petals yellow thick, erect; lip yellow, longer than the sepals concave narrowing to a long strap shaped limb; Spur about twice the length of ovary, yellowish –green curving upwards with tip curved down.

Flowering & Fruiting time – July –August.

Characteristics of usable drug part – Tubers are in pair the older becomes Shrivelled as the growing period proceeds. The shape of the tuber is oval to ovate and slightly tapering at the opposite end giving it a shape resembling to cotton boll. Skin dull white, flesh white and sweetish-bitter in taste.

Distribution

Himachal – Summer Hills,, Shimla; Mountains near Manali, Rahla Forest, Kothi, Manali, Sarahan, Nirmand-Annu, Rwanda, Kamarunag peak, Saptasar above Rawalsar (Mandi), Chansel, Churdhar, Jangtoo, Chamba, Narkanda.

Uttaranchal-Mussoorie-Jaberkhet, Mussoorie, Kyarphulli, Company Bagh, Deoban, Tehri-Nagtibba West of Dhanolti; Uttarkashi-Jamuna Valley, Kharshali, Har-Ki-Dun; Chamoli-Valley of flowers, Gobindghat, Khirsu; Pithoragarh-Tejam Jankhola Vally, Kali Valley, Sarju Valley, Nainital-Nainital, Bhowali, Ramgarh, Fatehgarh, Above Malli Tal; Almora-Binsar, Almora, Lorakhet, Ranikhet to Chaubatia.

Ayurvedic drug properties :– It is emollient, aphrodisiac, rejuvenating and tonic and is beneficial in aggravated vata and pitta, burning sensation in the body, hyperdipsia, fever, cough, epilepsy, insanity, emanciation and general debility (Bhav Prakash, kai, Nirs, so, Ni, Ni, Ra)

Substitutes-Varahi Kand ((Tacca aspera Roxb.) salam panja (Dactylorhiza hatagirea) Mahabala (Sida acuta, seeds of Sida cordifolia).

Status-It is a rare species because grows in assocaiton with grasses and is being cut in early stages before seeds are mature.

Rdhi –(Habenaria intermedia D. Don)

Stem-Erect, 25-60cm high, terete, robust, leafy.

Leaves-Scattered usually 5-nerved, ovate-lanceolate acuminate, cordate at the base.

Raceme-2-6 flowered.

Flowers-5cm across white or greenish-white few, distant. Bracts leaf like lanceolate, acuminate, equal or more than ovary. Sepals persistent, 20-25mm long, green, spreading tips reflexed, upper one white inside. Petals white, 5-nerved. Lip 3-lobed, longer than sepals, green spur 5-6cm stout, longer than ovary more or less curved. Side lobes deeply fringed. Flowering time-July-August Characteristics Usable Drug Part-Tubers are round at the opposite end but tapering towards stem joint. Skin is dirty white, flesh white and is slightly bitter in taste.

Distribution-Himanchal Pradesh, Koti (Shimla) Summer Hill Indian Institute of Advance study, Kamana Hill), Rwanda and Kamarunag (Karsog), Rewalsar hills (Mandi), Shimla (Fagu), Dalhousie (Chamba), Kinnaur.

Jammu &Kashmir-Azmabad, Poonch, Pirpanjal Range.

Uttaranchal-Dehradun-Mussoorie (Jaberkhet), Camel back road, company bagh, Bhatta Fall, Kampty fall; Tehri (Nagtibba) Suakholi, Chamoli-on way to Kedarnath, Jangal chatti, way to valley of flowers, Gaurikund (Rambera); Utarrkashi-Tons Valley, Bhagirathi valley and way to Dodital.

Ayurvedic Medicinal Properties

Rdhi is Sheetvirya, pacifies vata, pitta, rakta doshas. It is useful in consumption and fevers. It increases kapha dosha and shukra dhatu. It is intellect promoting, aphrodisiac, rejuvenating, tonic and cures emaciation, epilepsy, cough, skin diseases, haematemesis and general debility.

Substitutes :-Varahi Kand (Tacca aspera Roxb.) Utangan seeds (Blepharis edulis Pers.) Bala (Sida cordifolia), Chiriya Musali (Asparagus filicinus Buch. -Ham.)

Jeevak —(Malaxis acuminata D. Don)

Syn. Microstylis wallichii Lindl.

Stem-5 to 25 cm, ribbed bearing pseudo bulbs

Leaves – Usually 3 may be more,, 5-10cm ovate-lanceolate, acute with prominent veins and light green.

Flowers – Shortly stalked about 10mm in diameter, yellowish-green with purple centre. Sepals oblong, 2 lateral rather shorter than the dorsal, margins recurved. Petals linear longer than sepals, margin recurved. Lip shied-like, slightly convex, tip notched or bilobulate, auricles straight and slightly over lapping.

Flowering Time-July-August.

Characteristics of Usable Drug Part

Pseudo bulbs are in pair and new formation looks like a garlic clove (hence called rasona kand vat). Colour is green white and these remain alive over long period. Flesh is bitterish in taste.

Distribution:-Himalaya, Khasihills (Meghalaya) Andaman Islands, Travencore, Mdhya Pradesh. In Himalaya 1850 m to 2300 m Himachal Pradesh to Arunachal Pradesh, Assam, Nagaland, Manipur, Mizoram, Tripura.

Himachal Pradesh:-Shimla-Glen, Boileaugunj, Elysium Hill in forests, way to Rani forest, way from Khajiar to Chmba, Chail, Hattoo, Narkanda.

Uttaranchal :-Dehradun-Camel back road, Below Mussoorie bypass road, above barlowgunj, chakrata, Jaunsar, Tehri (Magra); Pauri-Pode khal, Chamoli-Nagnath; Ukhimath, Gopeshwar, Pithoragarh-Sarju Valley, Berenag, Thal Kedar; Nainital, Bhowali, Ramagarh, Almora-Ranikhet, Between Ranikhet-Chaubatia.

Ayurvedic Medicinal Properties :-It is sheet virya and calms down vata, rakta and pitta doshas and is beneficial in burning sensation of the body, fever, and consumption. It increases kapha and Shukra dhatu. It is aphrodisiac and tonic. It cures haematemesis, aggravated vata and pitta doshas, seminal weakness, dipsia, emaciation, tuberculosis and general body weakness. It increases body flesh and is jeevniya.

Substitutes :-Vidari kand, Bahaman Safed (Centaurea behen Linn.), Guruchi (Tinospora cordifolia)

Rshbhak-(Malaxis muscifera (Lindl.)

Kuntze- Synonym Microstylis muscifera Lindl.

Stem – 3 to 25cm high with ovoid pseudo bulbs

Leaves-One or two (unequal) 3-10 x 2-4cm sessile, ovate to ovate-lanceolate obtuse, narrowed at base to sheathing petiole.

Inflorescence-10 to 25 cm. long.

Flowers :3-4 mm long, pale-yellow-green, Bracts lanceolate shorter than ovary sepals broadly lanceolate. Petals linear Shorter than sepals. Lip ovate abruptly pointed, margins thickened.

Flowering Time-July –August.

Characteristics of the usable drug

Part-Tubers round, shining white bearing stem giving shape of bullock horn having a similar curvature. The taste is slightly bitter with mucilaginous substance.

Distribution-Himalaya between 1800-3500m eastward to Sikkim.

Himachal Pradesh-Shimla (Mashobra, Fagu, Hattoo forests) Rahala forest, Dhanchoo, Sangla, chamba.

Jammu &Kashmir-Gulmarg, Datni, Leh.

Uttaranchal-Pithoragarh-Tejum Haya, Bakariudiyar, Ralam Valley,

Palangarh, Ralam, Almora-Dwali, Dehradun-Chakrata, Deoban Tehri-Masartal, Bokhills, Dhanolti, way to Nagtibba; Chamoli-Vasukital, Bajmora, Jumma Area, Dunagiri, Valley of flowers, Rambara, Hemkund; Uttarkashi-Jamuna Valley above village kharsil.

Ayurvedic Medicinal Properties-Tubers are efficacious cure for pitta, rakta, vata doshas. It is useful in phthisis, burning sensation in the body, fever and increases Kapha and shukra. It is styptic, aphrodisiac and tonic. It is an effective cure in vitiated pitta and vata, seminal weakness, dysentery, emaciation and general debility.

Substitutes:-Vida ri Kanda (Pueraria tuberosa DC.) Ba haman Lal

(Centaurium roxburghii (G. Don) Druce), Vansalochan.

Status:-Malaxis muscifera is also a rare species and at present its reasons are not clear.

Kakoli —(Roscoea alpina Royle, Roscoea procera Wall.)

Stem-6-20cm and 30-60cm, robust.

Leaves-2-6 lanceolate, 15x3 cm.

Flowers-Several lilak, purple or white, corolla tube much longer than the calyx, borne in a short stem with or without leaves, upper lobe (petal) rounded, hooded and narrower reflexed lateral petals. Lower staminode 5x3cm obscurly

3-lobed spreading, notched at the tip.

Flowering Time-July –August or June for R. alpina.

Characteristics of the usable drug part-Fingers replacing roots are thickened 3-4 and have sickle shape, white and flesh inside is also white, tastes sweet resembling shatavar.

Distribution-Western Himalaya 1000 to 2700m commonly found in these altitudes in Himachal Pradesh, Jammu and Uttaranchal (Joshi Math, Mussoorie) and in other all districts.

Ayurvedic Medicinal Properties-Root fingers are sweet sheetvirya, pacifies vata pitta, fever due to vitiated vata-pitta. It is beneficial in consumption, burning sensation in body, increases Kapha dosa and shukra. It is also an effective cure for pains due to pitta, vata, rakta dosha, thirst due to pitta, rakta pitta etc.

Substitutes-Aswagandha (Withania somnifera) Curculigo orchioides (Kali musali)

Kshirkakoli —(Lilium polyphyllum D. Don)

Stem-30 to 100cm high, erect.

Leaves-Sessile, alternate or nearly opposite or whorled, narrow lanceolate or linear 7cm-13cmx 5mm-12mm. Bracts leaf like whorled.

Flowers-Solitary, racemed or whorled stalked (3cm-10cm), Perianth 6cm-8cm long, green-white with purple dots inside. Stigma 3-lobed, capsule 2cm to 3cm.

Flowering Time-15June-15 July

Characteristics of Usable Drug Part-The bulb is a loose mass of fleshy scales white in colour and is sweetish bitter in taste.

Distribution-Himachal-Hattoo peak, Narkanda forests, Chail (Solan district), Sungari-Bahli on Rampur Road.

Jammu & Kashmir-Gulmarg, Liddar Valley.

Uttaranchal-Gangotri, Rainthal, Amardhar, Kedarnath, Madmaheshwar. It is a rare species and its populations are very small that is 10-15 plants.

Ayurvedic Medicinal Properties- It promotes appetite and pacifies vata, pitta, rakta dosas. It is efficacious in bleeding disorders, cardiac diseases, dyspnoea, cough, consumption and diseases of urine system and is vrsya (tonic). Bulbs are refrigerant, galactagogue, expectorant and aphrodisiac. They are useful in bronchitis, burning sensation, hyperdipsia, rheumatalgia and general weakness in the body.

Substitutes- Aswagandha (Withania somnifera Dunal), swet musali (Chlorophytum arundinaceum), Fritillaria roylei Hook. f., Fritillaria oxypetala Royle.

Comments on Lilum Polyphyllum Don-Sir Col. Henry Collett (1902) wrote Flora Simlensis and in frontispiece he gave a diagram of this plant species and also mentioned under the description of species in family Orchidaceae that it is common in Shimla woods. But a search of this plant species in forests in and around was futile because even a single plant specimen was not found. This is because of disturbance in natural habitat and changing ecological conditions. Similar experience was felt in some other habitats in Uttaranchal especially in Ponwali Kanta, Rainthal area. The species has become rare and need immediate action for its conservation.

Meda —(Polygonatum verticillatum Allioni)

Stem-30cm to 1. 20m, erect, angled, grooved and sometimes mottled. Leaves-in whorls of 4-8 sessile, linear, 10-20cm long and 5-13mm broad or lanceolate 8cm x 18mm, tips usually acute, sometimes obtuse or slightly enrolled to the midrib.

Raceme-whorled 2-3 flowered. Parianth-5mm white often greenish Berry-6-7mm in diameter green and red or orange on ripening.

Flowering &Fruiting Time-July-September

Characteristics of the Usable Drug Part- Plants bear rhizomes as under ground part which resemble ginger but comparatively much less thick except in very old (7-8 years) plants. The rhizomes are white or dull white in colour but flesh inside is white and is sweet in taste when dried.

Distribution- The species is widely distributed in temperate Himalaya between 1600m and 3500m.

Himachal Pradesh – Shimla,, Narkanda, Hattoo, Churdhar, Janjelli, Sikari Tibba, Kamarunagh.

Jammu & Kashmir- Trikuta Hills, Udhampur, Doda area.

Uttaranchal- Ponwalikanta, Tali, Amardhar, Ganganani dhar, Rainthal, Kedarnath, Gangotri, Madmaheshwar.

Ayurvedic Medicinal Properties- Meda rhizomes are sweet in taste sheetvirya, pacify pitta dosh and increase kapha and shukra dhatu. They are beneficial in phthisis, burning sensation in the body, and fever (Dhan. Ni.). They are emollient, aphrodisiac, tonic, galactagogue, and beneficial in aggravation of pitta, cough, ulcers, skin diseases, general debility and vulnerary.

Substitutes- Asparagus racemosus Dunal (Shatavari), Salam misri (Eulophia campestris Wall).

Mahameda —(Polygonatum cirrifolium Royle)

Stem- 30 to 130cm tall, terete, round or grooved, climbing by means of tendril like tips of the leaves and grow generally in association with bushes. leaves-are always in whorls of 3-6, sessile, linear, 5cm to 8cm long and 3-5mm broad, lower surface glaucus, the margins usually inrolled to the midrib.

Racemes- Whorled 2-4 flowered.

Parianth- 5mm white often greenish or slightly purple.

Berry- 6-7mm in diameter, green and on ripening Orange-Red.

Flowering & Fruiting Time –July-September

Characteristics of the usable Drug Part- The rhizomes generally look like ginger but less thick, white or dull white in colour and are sweet in taste on drying.

Distribution- Temperate Himalaya 1500m to 2700m

Himachal Pradesh- Shimla, Matiana, Narkanda.

Uttaranchal- Mussoorie, Chakrata, Gaurikund, Rambara, Harshal, Ganganani, Devban, Rainthal, Mandakini Ghati, Bhilangana Ghati, Ponwali, Kalimath.

Ayurvedic Medicinal Properties- According to Dhanwantri Nighantu, Mahameda is sweet in taste, sheet virya, increases Kapha and shukra dhatu and is beneficial in consumption burning sensation, and fever. Various Nighantus describe its properties as emollient aphrodisiac, galactagoue, tonic and useful invitiation of vata-pitta, strangury seminal weakness, anorexia and general body weakness.

Substitutes- Shatavari (Asparagus racemosus Willd.) Nagbala (S. Veronicaefolia Linn.) Shakaakul mishri (Polygonatum multiflorum (Linn.) All.), Paederia foetida Linn. (Prasarani).

Status- It is also a rare species because of early cutting before Seeds are mature and burning of grassy plots for removal of bushes.

Henbane: Qualities and Benefits

Family name: Solanaceae. black colored henbane Latin name: Hyoscyamus Niger Linn

Sanskrit: Prasik Yamani, Madakarani, Turushka

Hindi: Khurasani Ajwain Gujarati: Khurasani Ajmo Marathi: Khuasani Oba Bengali: Khurasani Yamani Telangi: Khurasani Vamu Dravidi: Kurishani Vanam Arabian: Teralbanj, Bajul French: Tukhme Bunj, Bunj Punjabi: Khurasani Ajwain

The plants of Henbane are found in the Garhwal regions of northern India and grow up to a height of 800 to 10, 000 feet. They are cultivated in

Saharanpur, Kolkata, Agra, Ajmer, Pune and government parks and fields.

Chemical Composition

The seeds have 25 to 30 per cent oil; the leaves and flowers have hiosimine and alkaline called hiosan along with atopin and scopin in little quantities. The biannual atropine plants grow in mud.

External Form

The plants are longer than the plants of thymol seeds, annual or biannual. The roots have fibres and round in shape, straight and strong. The leaves are broad and long, with sharp edges, green in colour. The branches also have fibres. The flowers grow in bunches in yellowish colors with violet stripes.

The fruits are small, there are two segments at a distance of half inch and each section has black coloured henbane with flat shape.

Qualities

1. It is dry, bitter and pungent, hot. It has alcoholic affect and causes anxiety. It cures kapha, respiratory problems, heart pain and sexual problems.
2. It is curative hence beneficial in case of piles, pain in the stomach early ejaculation, dreams, menses. painful discharge of menses and irregular menstrual cycle. It calms down the sexual desire as well.
3. Henbane has alcoholic tendency and causes urination. If taken in small doses it reduces the pace of heart beat at night and strengthens but excess quantity is harmful for the heart.
4. The weariness effect is seen on the brain, genital organs and intestines. Opium and thorn apple are similar medicines but opium causes constipation, whereas henbane is free from this quality. Thorn apple leads to drowsiness and illusions but this herb does not have any such effect hence henbane is considered to be a betzer medicine. It is the best medicine for sleepiness and getting rid off weariness.
5. It has an effect on the nervous system. It calms down the mind, gives good sleep.

Medicinal Use

Toothache: Grind henbane with leaves and keep it on the cavity to get rid off toothache.

Joint pain: Boil it in sesame oil. Massage the painful area to cure joint pain. sciatica pain and backache etc.

Ear pain: Boil henbane in sesame oil and our feu drops in the ear to cure ear pain.

Liver pain: Lep with this oil cures chronic liver er pain and chest pain.

Bleeding gums: Rinsing the mouth With the kwath (decoction) of henbane leaves stops bleeding from the gums.

Urinary Problems: The extract of henbane seeds is beneficial in case of stones, pain or burning sensation. It causes urination and thereby reduces the pain.

Anxiety:-Add 30 drops of henbane juice in 25ml of water and should be administered to patients at an interval of one hour. This is very effective in case of hysteria, lunacy and other vata related doshas.

Worms: The male having worms in the stomach should eat jaggery on empty stomach and then take henbane churna with stale water. The worms present in the intestines will come out through stools.

Uterus pain: Make a long stick with the henbane powder and insert it in the vagina.

Stomachache: Make a pill with jaggery and henbane and take to control stomachache. Alternatively add black salt in henbane churna and take it.

Add one gram dry ginger powder in two to four drops of henbane oil and eat it and drink hot aniseed extract over it, this controls stomachache immediately or add little amount of jaggery in its kwath and take it.

Cough, hiccups and vomiting

1. Keep henbane and sugar candy in a betel leaf and suck the juice to cure dry cough caused due to vata.
2. Keep the henbane seeds in mouth and suck the juice to stop hiccups caused after meals.
3. Grind the top portion of henbane and clove and lick with honey to cure vomiting.

Dysentery: Take equal quantities of henbane, ginger, tea and mochrasa, make a fine powder. Take 2 to 3 grams with water less curd, it stops dysentery.

Stones: Take 5 gm of henbane churna with 20 gm of radish juice to dissolve stones.

Worms: Grind the henbane or give its fumigation in the rectum of children to get rid off small white worms.

Leprosy: Take henbane churna with jaggery for seven days and maintain strict diet.

Piles: Make a poultice of henbane and give fomentation on the piles and with salt it calms down the urinary pain.

Fever due to indigestion: Swallow four henbane seeds with cold water without chewing it. It can also be taken with honey.

Wounds: Grind it with little jaggery and tie a poultice with rapeseed oil to heal the wounds quickly.

MEDICINAL PLANTS

- Conservation of natural resources and the capability to utilize them in sustained manner are essential for the well being and continued survival of man.
- Under the duress of over exploration and habitat degradation a number of wild plants are essentially facing a constant threat of

extinction.

- Out of the 60, 000 plant species that are listed as threatened of extinction, over 20, 000 (or more) are from India alone.
- The botanical survey of India has prepared a provisional list of threatened plants which includes a large number wild (or) wild relatives of food, horticultural, medicinal and aromatic plants.
- India is endowed with a unique wealth of biota which inlcude a large number of medicinal and aromatic plants.
- Many of these plants are rare and endemic and found only in wild sources.
- The population explosion coupled with the improved standard of living led to ruthless exploitation, resulting in the imminent danger of extinction of these plants.
- Most of these wild medicinal and aromatic plants are highly habitual specific, found only in forests and occupying highly specialized ecological niche with restricted distribution.
- There are neither biological informations nor adequate knowledge of casual factors that led to their rarity in the habital.
- There is however, now an urgent need to evolve a sound strategy for the management and conservation of these plants on a long term basis.
- To evolve suitable strategies for conservation (or) the domestication/ cultivation of medicinal plants, it is very essential to study the complete biological and ecological back ground of these species.
- Under domestication outside their normal ecological range (or) under the distributed eco-system conditions may of the wild medicinal and aromatic plants tend to behave differently.
- In some cases it becomes difficult to grow them (or) it may not even survive.
- In certain other cases if survives and grows but may not be producing the desired traits.
- A through understanding on their reproductive and growth biology as well as identification of the biological and ecological constraints leading to their reduced fitness, restricted distribution (or) even extinction etc., is therefore, necessary.
- An understanding of the biological and ecological back ground of the species in their normal habitat is also essential to understand their conservation biology as well as to predict their behaviour under artificial cultivation.

Strategies for conservation of medicinal plants:

- The conservation of the wild medicinal plants or any other such threatened species can be tackled by scientific techniques as well as social actions.

- There are basically two scientific techniques of conservation of genetic diversity of these plants.
- They are the in situ and ex situ method of conservation. In Situ conservation:
- It is only in nature that plant diversity at the genetic, species and eco-system level can be conserved on long-term basis.
- Unless plant populations are conserved in the wild, that is in natural habitats, in viable breeding populations, they run the risk of extinction.
- It is necessary to conserve in distinct, representative biogeographic zones inter and intraspecific genetic variation.

Current status:

- In Karnataka, Kerala and Tamil nadu and more recently in Maharashtra the forest department in collaboration with FRUHT (Foundation for Rural Revitalization of Local Health Tradition) have established a network of 33 "Medicinal Plants Conservation Areas" (MPCAs) across the entire altitudinal range of south India.
- Each of these reserves is around 200 ha in size. Regulation and wild collection:
- Regulating the harvest of medicinal plants from the wild for commercial purposes.
- Particularly those species whose harvest inevitably involves destructive collection.
- Local communities can develop a stake in sustainable harvesting of medicinal plants from the forest and village, district and state level co- operative are set up to manage collection, storage and marketing.

Current status:

- LAMP societies as they function at present neither benefit the primary tribal collectors nor provides adequate powers (or) accountability of the LAMPs with regard to protection and management of forests.
- The marketing function of LAMPs is also weak, so that collectors do not get remunerative prices through LAMP sales.

EX situ conservation

A. Ethno-medicinal plant gardens:

- Creation of a network of regional and sub-regional ethno-medicinal plant gardens which should contain accessions of all the medicinal plants known to the various ethnic communities in different regions of India.
- This chain of gardens will act as regional repositories of our cultural and ethno-medicinal history and embody the living traditions of our socity's knowledge of medicinal plants.

Current status:

- There are estimated to be around 50 such gardens in the country ranging from acre to 40 acres some of them were set up by an All India Health Network.
- More recently a network of 15 such gardens have been set up in 3 states of South India with the initiative of FRLHT. One of the gardens is located in TBGRI, (Tropical botanical garden research institute) Palode at Thiruvananthapuram.

B. Gene banks:

- While it is known that the largest proportion of local bio-diversity in all our eco-system is used for medicinal purposes, very little is known about their conservation status in the wild.
- What is likely is that a large number of medicinal plant species are under various degrees of threat.
- The precautionary principles would suggest that an immediate and country-wide exercise be taken up to deposit seeds of wild medicinal plants with a first priority to known Red listed species and endemic species.

Current status:

- The department of bio-technology, Government of India has recently taken the initiative to establish 3 gene banks in the country.
- One is with ICAR at the NBPGR (National Bureau of plant genetic Resources) Campus, the second is with CIMAPs, (Cental Institute of Medicinal and Aromatic plants) Lucknow and the third with TBFRI in Thiruvananthapuram.

C. Nursery network:

- The most urgent and primary task in order to ensure immediate availability of plants and planting materials to various user groups is to promote a nation wide network of medicinal plant nurseries, which will multiply all the regional specific plants that are used in the current practice of traditional medicine.

Current status:

- Planting material for 40 odd species of medicinal and aromatic plants is reportedly available in the ICAR and CSIR (CIMAP) network.
- In South India FRLHT has recently set up a network of 55 supply nurseries.

D. Cultivation:

- Figures projecting demand and trade in medicinal plant species globally indicate a step upward trend in the near future.
- One estimate puts the figure of world trade in medicinal plants and related products at US $ 5 trillion by A.D. 2050 (world bank report,

1996).

- The demand so far has been met mainly from wild sources.
- This can't go on for much longer; policy intervention is urgently needed to encourage and facilitate investments into commercial cultivation of medicinal plants.
- Cultivation of medicinal plants however, is inversely linked to prevalence of easy and cheap collection from the wild, lack of regulation in trade, cornering of the profits from wild collection by a vast network of traders and middlemen and absence of industry's interest in providing buy-back guarantees to growers.

Current status:

- In the Govt. sector agro-technology of 40 odd species has been developed by ICAR-Agricultural University System and CSIR (CIMAOs & RRL, Jammu and Jorhat).
- In recent years industries like Dabur, Zandu, Indian Herbs, Arya Vaidya Shala, and Arya Vaidya Pharmacy and others have made some symbolic efforts to initiate cultivation.
- Since 1984 NABARD (National Bank of Agricultural and Rural Development) has formulated schemes for financing cultivation and processing of medicinal plants.

E. Community based enterprises:

- The income generated by the traditional medicine industry benefits small section of the socity.
- A strong case exists for promotion of community level enterprises for value addition to medicinal plants through simple, on site techniques like drying, cleaning, crushing, powdering, grading, packaging etc.
- This will also increase the stake of rural communities in conservation and change the skewed nature of income distribution of the industry.

Current status:

- Three community based enterprises are known in south India, one in Gandhigram Trust, (Dindigul), Preemade development Society (Peermade) Kerala and the third by VGKK in B. R. Hills, Mysore.

MEDICINAL PLANTS IN SOUTH INDIA

In India about 7300 plant species are used in traditional health care systems such as Ayurveda, Siddha, Unani and folk healing practices. The booming of traditional medicine industry results in an increasing demand on medicinal plant products. 90% of the medicinal plants come from natural habitats. The declining availability of such plants and the fading of local traditional knowledge make the sustainable management of natural habitats a crucial environmental issue in South India, concerning biodiversity conservation and welfare of local communities.

In order to address these issues, this programme links up ecology and social sciences departments at IFP.

- Documentation of medicinal plants will be collected and organised in a database to understand their ecosystem, distribution and harvesting.
- Social sciences investigations will examine those environmentally related aspects as they pertain to the notion of space and to the local social and political dynamics.
- Spatial, social and political dynamics will be comprehended through the analysis of collection and marketing of medicinal plants, with a particular emphasis on the relationships between actors.
- This study on medicinal plants in South India is of interest for researchers and stakeholders to improve the conservation and forest management strategies.

MATERIALS AND METHODS

Surveys for building a regional database on medicinal plants, their uses and procurement will be conducted in three Southern Indian states (Karnataka, Kerala and Tamil Nadu). Data on the diversity, abundance and distribution of medicinal plant species in various forest types will be gathered using the existing floristic and ecological database of FIP and additional field missions. Iconographic data on traits of species and parts used in different healing methods will be incorporated into the database.

In the initial phase, the analysis of medicinal plants' collection and marketing will be carried out in the landscape unit identified by FIP in. Data on spatial, social, economical, historical and political aspects of the medicinal plant procurement and marketing will be integrated to a Geographical Information System.

Medicinal plants, since times immemorial, have been used in virtually all cultures as a source of medicine. The widespread use of herbal remedies and healthcare preparations, as those described in ancient texts such as the Vedas and the Bible, and obtained from commonly used traditional herbs and medicinal plants, has been traced to the occurrence of natural products with medicinal properties.

The use of traditional medicine and medicinal plants in most developing countries, as a normative basis for the maintenance of good health, has been widely observed (UNESCO, 1996). Furthermore, an increasing reliance on the use of medicinal plants in the industrialised societies has been traced to the extraction and development of several drugs and chemotherapeutics from these plants as well as from traditionally used rural herbal remedies (UNESCO, 1998). Moreover, in these societies, herbal remedies have become more popular in the treatment of minor ailments, and also on account of the increasing costs of personal health maintenance. Indeed, the market and public demand has been so great that there is a great risk that many medicinal plants today, face either extinction or loss of genetic diversity.

BACKGROUND

Medicine, in several developing countries, using local traditions and beliefs, is still the mainstay of health care. As defined by WHO, health is a state of complete physical, mental, and social well being and not merely the absence of disease or infirmity. The practise of traditional medicine is widespread in China, India, Japan, Pakistan, Sri Lanka and Thailand. In China about 40% of the total medicinal consumption is attributed to traditional tribal medicines. In Thailand, herbal medicines make use of legumes encountered in the Caesalpiniaceae, the Fabaceae, and the Mimosaceae. In the mid-90s, it is estimated that receipts of more than US$2. 5 billion have resulted from the sales of herbal medicines. And, in Japan, herbal medicinal preparations are more in demand than mainstream pharmaceutical products.

Africa is a rich source of medicinal plants. Perhaps, the best known species is Phytolacca dodecandra. Extracts of the plant, commonly known as endod, are used as an effective molluscicide to control schistosomiasis (Lemma, 1991). Other notable examples are Catharanthus roseus, which yields anti-tumour agents such as vinblastine and vincristine; and Ricinus communis, which yields the laxative—castor oil. In Botswana, Lesotho, Namibia and South Africa, Harpagophytum procumbens is produced as a crude drug for export. Similarly, Hibiscus sabdariffa is exported from Sudan and Egypt. Other exports are Pausinystalia yohimbe from Cameroon, Nigeria and Rwanda, which yields yohimbine; and Rauwolfia vomitoria, from Madagascar, Mozambique and Zaire, which is exploited to yield reserpine and ajmaline.

The use of medicinal plants like Eupatorium perfoliatum (bonest), Podophyllum peltatum (mayapple), and Panax quinquefolium (ginseng) in the USA has long been associated with the American Indians. These plants have also been appreciated and recognised for their aesthetic and ornamental value. In Central America medicinal plants have been widely used-by the Maya Indians in Mexico, the Miskitos and Sumus in Honduras and Nicaragua, the Pech, Lencas, and Xicaques in Honduras, the Pipiles in El Salvador, the Talamancas in Costa Rica, and the Guaymis and Kunas in Panama.

In Europe, some 1500 species of medicinal and aromatic plants are widely used in Albania, Bulgaria, Croatia, France, Germany, Hungary, Poland, Spain, Turkey, and the United Kingdom. The Maltese islands constitute an apt example where medicinal plants are widely used in every day life as part of folk medicinal remedies (Lanfranco, 1992).

Issues

Traditional and folklore medicine bequeathed from generation to generation is rich in domestic recipes and communal practice. Encompassing concepts and methods for the protection and restoration of health, traditional medicine has served as a fount of alternative medicine, new pharmaceuticals, and healthcare products. The best known examples of traditional medicine, differing in concept and protocol, are well-developed systems such as acupuncture and ayurvedic medicine that have been widely used to conserve human health in China and India.

Developed countries, in recent times, are turning to the use of traditional medicinal systems that involve the use of herbal drugs and remedies. About 1400 herbal preparations are used widely, according to a recent survey in Member States of the European Union. Herbal preparations are popular and are of significance in primary healthcare in Belgium, France, Germany and the Netherlands. Such popularity of healthcare plant-derived products has been traced to their increasing acceptance and use in the cosmetic industry as well as to increasing public costs in the daily maintenance of personal health and well being. Examples of such beauty-oriented therapeuticals are skin tissue regenerators, anti-wrinkling agents and anti-age creams. Most dermaceuticals are derived from algal extracts that are rich in minerals and the vitamin B group. Skincare products such as skin creams, skin tonics, etc. derived from medicinal plants are grouped together as dermaceuticals. Also, amongst the poor, cures and drugs, derived from plants, constitute the main source of healthcare products.

Gorman (1992) drew attention to the power of Chinese folk medicinal potions in treating maladies from eczema and malaria to respiratory disorders. In the quest for new medicines to treat old and emergent diseases such as malaria and AIDS, attention is now being given to discovering the active ingredients encountered in the treasury of over 5, 000 Chinese herbs, plants and roots that have been used routinely and traditionally. Quinghaosu and Chaihu are two such examples. Whereas the former, called artemisinin and obtained from Artemisia annua is expected to yield, in the coming millennium, a potent new class of antimalarials, the latter, obtained from Bupleurum chinense and used as a popular remedy for hepatitis is the focus of intense research by the Japanese pharmaceutical industry. More recently, the biochemistry of tianhuafen or cucumber is being studied in the USA to decipher the identity of compound Q, an extract used in China and credited with remedial and relief properties in AIDS sufferers.

Medicinal plants are an integral component of ethnoveterinary medicine. Farmers and pastoralists in several countries use medicinal plants in the maintenance and conservation of the healthcare of livestock. Intestinal disorders in cows, in Mexico, are treated with herbal extracts of Polakowskia tacacco. Dietary supplements such as vitamin A in poultry feeds in Uganda are supplied through enrichments of amaranth (Amaranthus sp.). It is estimated that medicinal plants, for several centuries, have been widely used as a primary source of prevention and control of livestock diseases. In fact, interest of such use in the veterinary sector has resulted primarily from the increasing cost of livestock maintenance and the introduction of new technology in the production of veterinary medicines and vaccines.

Mc Gee (1998), surveying the use of spice and their medicinal properties around the world, concluded that spices serve the adaptive purpose of reducing food-borne disease. In reviewing relevant texts ranging from the preservative properties of spices against food spoilage to the presence of antimicrobial substances that lay claim to the elimination of pathogenic organisms in food preparations, the case is made for a more objective analysis and study of the medicinal properties of spices in victu rather than in victo. A whole range of plant-derived dietary supplements, phytochemicals and pro-vitamins that assist in maintaining good health and combating disease are now being described as functional foods, nutriceuticals and nutraceuticals.

Despite the increasing use of medicinal plants, their future, seemingly, is being threatened by complacency concerning their conservation. Reserves of herbs and stocks of medicinal plants in developing countries are diminishing and in danger of extinction as a result of growing trade demands for cheaper healthcare products and new plant-based therapeutic markets in preference to more expensive target-specific drugs and biopharmaceuticals. Such concerns have stimulated positive legal and economic interest.

Issues concerning intellectual property rights, compensation for loss of finance-rich biodiversity resources, and the acquisition and safeguarding of traditional healthcare knowledge are no longer neglected. Bioprospecting of new drugs from medicinal plants and the exploitation of unprotected traditional knowledge in starting-up potentially new bioindustries are the focus of new monitoring measures. Such concerns that call for adherence to and observation of cultural and intellectual property rights have been addressed and enshrined in the Chiang-Mai and Kari-Oca Declarations. The first countries to seriously tackle these issues are China and India. Indeed, programmes dealing with medicinal plant conservation, cultivation, community involvement and sustainable development being initiated elsewhere, could benefit immensely from the Chinese and Indian experiences (World Bank, 1997).

Genetic biodiversity of traditional medicinal herbs and plants is continuously under the threat of extinction as a result of growth-exploitation, environment-unfriendly harvesting techniques, loss of growth habitats and unmonitored trade of medicinal plants.

Medicinal herbs, possessing penile potency properties and anti-cancer principles are the focus of smuggling to import markets in Germany, France, Switzerland, Japan, the U. K., and the U. S. A. The best known example, in recent times, is that of tetu lakda (Nothadoytes foetida). Commonly encountered in southern India and Sri Lanka, the herb is exploited as a source of anti-cancer drugs.

On the other hand, Adonis vernalis, extinct in Italy and the Netherlands, is an endangered species in Germany, Slovakia, Sweden and Switzerland. Fortunately, to safeguard against such practices and losses, guidelines and licensing concerning the use of such plants are provided for in the Convention on International Trade Endangered Species of Wild Flora and Fauna (CITES).

The industrial uses of medicinal plants are many. These range from traditional medicines, herbal teas, and health foods such as nutriceuticals to galenicals, phytopharmaceuticals and industrially produced pharmaceuticals. Furthermore, medicinal plants constitute a source of valuable foreign exchange for most developing countries, as they are a ready source of drugs such as quinine and reserpine; of galenicals like tinctures and of intermediates (e.g. diosgenin from Discorea sp.) in the production of semi-synthetic drugs. The world market for plant-derived chemicals – pharmaceuticals, fragrances, flavours, and colour ingredients, alone exceeds several billion dollars per year. Classic examples of phytochemicals in biology and medicine include taxol, vincristine, vinblastine, colchicine as well as the Chinese antimalarial-artemisinin, and the Indian ayurdevic drug-forkolin. Trade in medicinal plants is growing in volume and in exports. It is estimated that the global trade in medicinal plants is US$800 million per year.

The botanical market, inclusive of herbs and medicinal plants, in the USA, is estimated, at retail, at approximately US$1. 6 billion p. a. China with exports of over 120, 000 tonnes p. a., and India with some 32, 000 tonnes p. a. dominate the international markets. It is estimated that Europe, annually, imports about 400, 000 t of medicinal plants with an average market value of US$ 1 billion from Africa and Asia. A growing awareness of this new contributor to the foreign-exchange reserves of several national treasuries is beginning to emerge. To satisfy growing market demands, surveys are being conducted to unearth new plant sources of herbal remedies and medicines.

In several industrialised societies, plant-derived prescription drugs constitute an element in the maintenance of health. Medicinal plants are an integral component of research developments in the pharmaceutical industry. Such research focuses on the isolation and direct use of active medicinal constituents, or on the development of semi-synthetic drugs, or still again on the active screening of natural products to yield synthetic pharmacologically- active compounds. In Germany, for example, over 1500 plant species encountered in some 200 families and 800 genera have been processed into medicinal products. In South Africa, likewise, some 500 species are commercialised trade products. Today, Bulgaria, Germany and Poland are recognised as major exporters of plant-based medicinal products.

The development and commercialisation of medicinal plant-based bioindustries in the developing countries is dependent upon the availability of facilities and information concerning upstream and downstream bioprocessing, extraction, purification, and marketing of the industrial potential of medicinal plants. Absence of such infrastructure compounded by lack of governmental interest and financial support restricts the evolution of traditional herbal extracts into authenticated market products. Furthermore the absence of modernised socio-economic and public healthcare systems reinforces reliance of rural and lower-income urban populations on the use of traditional medicinal herbs and plants as complementary aids to routine pharmaceutical market products.

The prophylactic and therapeutic effects of plant foods and extracts in reducing cardiovascular disease has been reviewed (Walker, 1996). Non-nutrient phytochemicals are increasingly being recognised as potential health promoters in reducing the risks of cardiovascular disease and atherosclerosis. Prominent herbs identified were Achillea millefolium (yarrow), Allium sativum (garlic), Convallaria majalis (lily of the valley), Cratageus laevigata (hawthorn), Cynara scolymus (globe artichoke), Gingko biloba (gingko) and Viburnum opulus (cramp bark).

Saint-John's wort known as Johanniskrant in German for centuries has been used to treat people with mild and moderate depression without the side effects of Prozac. Widely sold in Germany and other European countries, and awaiting official approval by the US Food and Drug Administration, Saint-John's wort is being regarded as a serious rival to Prozac (Andrews, 1997).

Medicinal plants can make an important contribution to the WHO goal to ensure, by the year 2000, that all peoples, worldwide, will lead a sustainable socio-economic productive life. The Centre for Science and Technology of the Non-Aligned and other Developing Countries in India organised an international workshop on Tissue Culture of Economic Plants in April, 1994, as a means of using modern biotechnological techniques to nurture and conserve medicinal plants.

In late 1997, the World Bank, within the framework of the Global Environmental Facility, provided a US$ 4. 5 million grant for the Sri Lanka Conservation of Medicinal Plants Project which focuses on the conservation of medicinal plant populations, their habitats, and their sustainable use in Medicinal Plant Conservation Areas (MPCAs). Inventories with emphasis on the management, research and conservation of rare and endangered species of medicinal plants are the main programmes at MPCAs at Ritigala, Naula, Rajawaka, Kanneliya, and Bibile.

Aspects of policy and research concerning the cultivation of non-tropical and tropical medicinal plants and their genetic improvement; their conservation in botanical gardens; their storage in liquid nitrogen; their economic potential in international pharmaceutical trade; and their vulnerability to over-exploitation and extinction have been dealt with authoritatively. Moreover, such concerns and issues are addressed through a variety of programme activities and projects conducted, and promoted by several international, regional, and non-governmental organisations.

Concluding Remarks

Recent and renewed interest in medicinal plants coupled to developments in information technology has fuelled an explosion in the range and content of electronic information concerning medicinal plants as a re-emergent health aid. Bhat (1997) recently reviewed diverse sources of such information in traditional abstracting services as well as in a variety of online electronic databases. As a result of such developments, access to indigenous peoples and cultures concerning medicinal plants are greatly facilitated. Furthermore, the active participation of such natural custodians and practitioners of valuable knowledge is guaranteed in the generation of research focussing on screening programmes dealing with the isolation of bioactive principles and the development of new drugs.

IMPORTANCE OF MEDICINAL PLANTS

Important Medicinal Plants and their active constituents

Plant	Active principle	Pharmacological activity
1 Rauvolfia serpentina	Reserpine	Hypotensive
2 Catharanthus roseus	Ajmalicine	Vasodilator
	Vinblastine	Anticancer
	Vincristine	Anticancer
3 Cassia angustifolia, Cassia acutifolia	Sennosides	Laxative
4 Plantago ovata	Psyllium mucilage	laxative
5 Glycyrrhiza glabra	Glycyrrhizic acid	Antiinflammatory
6 Berberis sp.	Berberin	Antidiarrhoeal
7 Digitalis lanata	Digitoxin Lanatoside	Cardiotonic
8 Taxus baccata	Taxol	Anticancer
9 Podophyllum emodi Etoposide	Podophyllotoxin	
Tenoposide	Anticancer	
10 Datura species,		
Hyocymus musticus,		
Duboisia myoporoides	Hyoscine	
Syoscyamina		
Atropine	Parasympatholytic	
11 Artemisai annua	Artemisinin	Antimalarial
12 Mappia foetida	Camptothecine	Anticancer

Medicinal Plants used as Crude Extracts/Tinctures in Medicines

Botanical Name	Common Name
1 Belladonna	Atropa belladonna
2 Ipecac	Cephaelis ipecacuanha
3 Opium	Papaver somniferum

4 Henbane	Hyoscyamus niger
5 Stramonium	Datura stramonium
6 Liquorice	Glycyrrhiza glabra
7 Rhubarb	Rheum officinale
8 Podophyllum	Podophyllium emodi
9 Capscicum oleoresin	Capsicum annum
10 Digitalis	Digitalis lanata, Digitalis purpurea
11 Aloe	Aloe vera

Important Plant Products having great potential in Medicine

Plant Product	**Source**	**Pharmacological activity**
1 Valepotriates	Valeriana wallichii	Sedative, tranquilizer
2 Silymarin	Silybum marianum	Antihepatoxic
3 Podophyllotoxin (Etoposide/tenoposide)	Podophyllum emodi, P. pellatum	Anticancer
4 Taxol	Taxus baccata	Anticancer
5 Guggul saponins Cormmiphora wiightii	Hypolipidaemic	
6 Artemisinin	Artemisai annua	Antimalarial

Some important medicinal plants suggested for cultivation :

Botanical name of the plant	Common
Aegle marmalos	Bilva (Hindi); Maredu (Telugu)
Glycyrrhiza glabra	Mulethi (Hindi); Athimadhuramu (Telugu)
Gmelina arborea	Gambhiri (Hindi); Gummadi (Telugu)
Mesua ferrea	Nagkesara (Hindi); Keearamu (Telugu)
Piper longum	Pipli (Hindi); Pippali (Telugu)
Picrorhiza kurroa	Kutki (Hindi); Katukarogani (Telugu)
Phyllanthus niruri	Jar-amla (Hindi); Nelausiri (Telugu)
Saraca indica	Ashoka (Hindi); Asokachettu (Telugu)
Swertia chirayata	Chirayata (Hindi); Nilavemyu (Telugu)
Andrographis paniculata	Kalmegha (Hindi); Nelavemu (Telugu)
Terminalia arjuna	Arjuna (Hindi); Tellamaddi (Telugu)
Valeriana wallichii	Tagar (Hindi)
Tinospora cordifolia	Gulancha (Hindi); Thippatheega (Telugu)
Asparagus racemosus	Shatavar (Hindi); Pillitheegalu (Telugu)

Plumbago zeylanica	Chita (Hindi); Chitramulamu (Telugu)
Conuniphora wightii	Guggul (Hindi, Telugu)
Boerhaavia diffusa	Punarnava, Sant (Hindi, Telugu)
Withania somnifera	Ashwagandha (Hindi, Telugu)
Bacopa monnieri	Brahmi (Hindi, Telugu)

Systems of Medicine

- There are mainly 3 systems of medicine practised in the world today. They are :

Modern System or Allopathy

- This system was developed in the Western countries. In this system drugs (tablets, capsules, injections, tonics etc.) are manufactured using synthetic chemicals and/or chemicals derived from natural products like plants, animals, minerals etc. This system also uses modern equipment for diagnosis, analysis, surgery etc.
- Medicines or drugs of this system is often criticised for its treatment of the symptoms rather than the cause of the disease, harmful side effects of certain drugs and for being out of reach of common/poor people due to the high cost of drugs and treatment.
- This system is used in all the countries of the world today.

Alternative Medicine or Traditional System

- Different countries of the world developed independently their own traditional systems of medicine using locally available materials like minerals and products of plants and animals.
- The World Health Organisation is giving considerable importance to these alternate medicine (as they act as alternative to allopathy) systems to provide Primary Health Care to millions of people in the developing countries.
- China developed the Chinese system of medicine, which is practised in China, Singapore, Taiwan, Japan and other countries.
- In Indonesia, Jamu and in South Africa, Zulu systems of herbal medicine are practised. The Unani or Tibb system was developed in the Middle Eastern Arab countries and is practised in India and in many countries.
- In India, Ayurveda (developed in North India), Siddha (developed in Tamil Nadu) and Nagarjuna (developed in Andhra Pradesh) systems of medicine were developed. Ayurveda is practised in Sri Lanka, Pakistan and Bangladesh also. Herbo-mineral is another traditional system used in India and other neighbouring countries.
- Drugs (balms, oils, pills, tonics, paste etc) are manufactured and marketed in these systems. The major advantage of these systems is that they are within the reach of the people, particularly rural poor.

- These systems are claimed to be pollution free, eco-freindly and have minimal or no harmful side effects. Ayurveda claims to cure the cause of the disease rather than the symptoms and is wholistic in its approach.
- In this system a disease is conceived as an imbalance in the systems of the body and the treatment aims at restoring the balance in the various systems of the body.

Folk Medicine

- The medicinal systems followed by various tribals/aborigins of different countries is popularly known as folk or tribal medicine.
- In the system, the "medicine man" or the "doctor " of the tribe who has the knowledge of treating diseases, keeps this knowledge as a closely guarded secret and passes it to the next generation by word of mouth.
- No written texts on these systems are available and different tribes follow different time tested methods. The treatment is often associated with lengthy and mystic rituals, in addition to prescription of drugs (decoctions, pastes, powders, oils, ashed materials etc.).
- Mostly locally available natural materials are used for the preparation of drugs, which are not commercially made and marketed. Generally speaking, folk medicine can also be regarded as a traditional system of medicine.
- The basic aim of all the above systems of medicine is to alleviate the sufferings of human beings and their domesticated animals.
- The knowledge of the traditional systems is undergoing close scientific scrutiny and is being increasingly incorporated into the modern system.

Other Systems

- Yoga, Acupressure, Acupuncture, Reiki, Magneto therepy, Pyramid therapy, Flower therapy, Homeopathy, Nature Cure or Naturopathy etc. are some of the other systems of medicine practised in different parts of the world today.

Utilization of Medicinal Plants

- The utility of medicinal plants has four major segments:
  - o Medicinal plants utilised in indigenous or traditional systems of medicines (ISM) -Ayurveda, Siddha, Unani and Homeopathy systems of medicines.
  - o OTC (over the country, non-prescription) items/products involving plant parts, extracts galenicals etc.
  - o Essential oils
  - o Phyto-pharmaceuticals or plants used in modern systems of medicine.

Medicinal plants used in Traditional Systems of Medicine

- Traditional medicine is widespread through the world and it comprises of those practices based on beliefs that were in existence, often for hundreds of years, before the development and spread of modern scientific medicines and which are still in use today.
- As its name implies, it is the part of tradition of each country which employs practices that have been handed down from generation to generation. Its acceptance by a population is largely conditioned by cultural factors and much of traditional medicine, therefore, may not be easily transferable from one culture to another.
- An important feature of traditional therapy is the preference of practitioner for compound prescriptions over single substance/drug as it is being held that some constituents are effective only in the presence of others.
- This renders assessment of efficacy and eventually identification of active principles as required in international standards much difficult than for simple preparation.
- In India, earlier the medicines used in indigenous systems of medicines were generally prepared by the practicing physicians by themselves, but now this practice has been largely replaced by the establishment of organised indigenous drug industries.
- It is estimated that at present there are more than 1, 00, 000 licensed registered practitioners of Ayurveda, Siddha, Unani medicine or Homeopathy.
- As far as the Ayurveda system of medicine is concerned, it does not rule out any substances being used as potential source of medicine.
- Presently about 10 00 single drugs and 8000 compound drug formulations of recognised merit are in vogue.
- In fact reliable data on availability in different regions of country as well as supply and demand of medicinal plants used in production of indigenous medicines are not available.
- However, annual herbal drug market has been estimated around 2200 crores and is expected to reach up to 4000 crores by the year 2000.

Plants-parts, extracts and galenicals

- The direct utilisation of plant material is not only a feature of ISM in the developing world but also in developed countries like USA, UK, Germany etc., the various herbal formulations are sold on health food shops.
- Preparation of decoctions, tinctures, galenicals and total extracts of plants also form a part of many pharmacopoeias of the world.
- The current trend of medicinal plants based drug industry is to procedure standard extracts of plants as raw material.

Essential Oils from plants

- The essential oil industry was traditionally a cottage industry in India. Since 1947, a number of industrial companies have been established for large scale production of essential oils, oleoresins and perfumes.
- The essential oil from plants includes Ajowan oil, Eucalyptus oil, Geranium oil, Lavender oil, Palmarosa oil, Patchouli oil, Rose oil, Sandalwood oil, Turpentine oil and Vetiver oil.

Phyto-pharmaceuticals

- During the past decades, bulk production of plant based drugs has become an important segment of Indian pharmaceutical industry.
- Some of the phyto-pharmaceuticals which are produced in India at present include
  1. morphone,
  2. codeine,
  3. papaverine (Papaver somniferum),
  4. quinine,
  5. quinidine,
  6. cinchonine and cinchonidine (Cinchona sp., C. calisaya, C. ledgeriana, C. officinais and C. succirubra);
  7. hyoscine,
  8. hyoscyamine (Hyocyamus niger and H. muticus),
  9. colchicine (Gloriosa superbad, Colchicum luteum and Iphigenia stellata),
  10. cephaeline and emetin (Cephalis ipacacuanha),
  11. sennosides A & B (Cassia angustifolia and C. acutifolia),
  12. reserpine,
  13. rescinnamine,
  14. ajmalicine and ajmaline (Rauvolfia serpentina);
  15. vinblastine and vincristine,
  16. ajmalicine (raubacine) (Catharanthus roseus);
  17. guggul lipid (Commiphora wightii);
  18. taxol (Taxus baccata);
  19. artemisinin (Artemisai annua) etc.
- For all these segments of drug, perfumery, flavouring and cosmetic industries, mostly the higher plants are one of the raw materials and comes from the natural resources i.e. forests through forest contractors employing local or tribal people or from the drug farms maintained by the growers of aromatic and medicinal plants.

❒

Medicinal Plants as Alternative Medicine

Alternative medicine is defined as "any of various systems of healing or treating disease (as chiropractic, homeopathy, or faith healing) not included in the traditional medical curricula taught in the United States and Britain". Complementary medicine is defined as "any of the practices (as acupuncture) of alternative medicine accepted and utilized by mainstream medical practitioners". The term complementary and alternative medicine (CAM) is an umbrella term for both branches. CAM includes practices that incorporate spiritual, metaphysical, or religious underpinnings; non-evidence based practices, non-European medical traditions, or newly developed approaches to healing.

The list of therapies included under CAM changes gradually. If and when an unproven therapy is proven to be safe and effective, it becomes adopted into conventional health care and gradually ceases to be considered "alternative", since adoption and acceptance often take time. If a CAM therapy is proven dangerous and ineffective, it should cease to be advocated by CAM practitioners, although there are no clear instances of this happening.

Definitions

The National Centre for Complementary and Alternative Medicine defines complementary and alternative medicine as "a group of diverse medical and health care systems, practices, and products that are not presently considered to be part of conventional medicine". It also defines integrative medicine as "[combining] mainstream medical therapies and CAM therapies for which there is some high-quality scientific evidence of safety and effectiveness".

Ralph Snyderman and Andrew Weil state "integrative medicine is not synonymous with complementary and alternative medicine (CAM). It has a far larger meaning and mission in that it calls for restoration of the focus of physician relationship".

In a frequently-cited review, David M. Eisenberg used the term "unconventional medicine" to signify "medical interventions not taught widely at U.S. Medical Schools or generally available at U.S. Hospitals."

Criticisms of the Term

Some scientists reject the above classification and to varying degrees reject the term "alternative medicine" itself.

The following three commentators argue for classifying treatments based on the objectively verifiable criteria of the scientific method, not based on the changing curricula of various medical schools or social sphere of usage. They advocate a classification based on evidence-based medicine, i.e., scientifically proven evidence of efficacy (or lack thereof). According to them it is possible for a method to change categories (proven vs. nonproven) in either direction, based on increased knowledge of its effectiveness or lack thereof:

- Marcia Angell, former editor-in-chief of the New England Journal of Medicine, states that "...since many alternative remedies have recently found their way into the medical mainstream [there] cannot be two kinds of medicine - conventional and alternative. There is only medicine that has been adequately tested and medicine that has not, medicine that works and medicine that may or may not work. Once a treatment has been tested rigorously, it no longer matters whether it was considered alternative at the outset. If it is found to be reasonably safe and effective, it will be accepted."
- George D. Lundberg, former editor of the Journal of the American Medical Association (JAMA), and Phil B. Fontanarosa, Senior Editor of JAMA, state: "There is no alternative medicine. There is only scientifically proven, evidence-based medicine supported by solid data or unproven medicine, for which scientific evidence is lacking. Whether a therapeutic practice is 'Eastern' or 'Western,' is unconventional or mainstream, or involves mind-body techniques or molecular genetics is largely irrelevant except for historical purposes and cultural interest. As believers in science and evidence, we must focus on fundamental issues-namely, the patient, the target disease or condition, the proposed or practiced treatment, and the need for convincing data on safety and therapeutic efficacy."
- Richard Dawkins, Professor of the Public Understanding of Science at Oxford, defines alternative medicine as a "set of practices which cannot be tested, refuse to be tested, or consistently fail tests. If a healing technique is demonstrated to have curative properties in properly simply becomes medicine." He also states that "There is no alternative medicine. There is only medicine that works and medicine that doesn't work."

Other well-known proponents of evidence-based medicine, such as the Cochrane Collaboration and Edzard Ernst, Professor of Complementary Medicine at the University of Exeter, use the term "alternative medicine" but agree with the above commentators that all treatments, whether "mainstream" or "alternative", ought to be held to standards of the scientific method. Oxford University Press publishes a peer-reviewed journal entitled Evidence-based Complementary and Alternative Medicine (eCAM).

Regulation

Jurisdiction differs concerning which branches of alternative medicine are legal, which are regulated, and which (if any) are provided by a government-controlled health service or reimbursed by a private health medical insurance company.

A number of alternative medicine advocates disagree with the restrictions of government agencies that approve medical treatments (such as the American Food and Drug Administration) and the agencies' adherence to experimental evaluation methods. They claim that this impedes those seeking to bring useful and effective treatments and approaches to the public, and protest that their contributions and discoveries are unfairly dismissed, overlooked or suppressed. Alternative medicine providers often argue that health fraud should be dealt with appropriately when it occurs.

In India, which is the home of several alternative systems of medicines, Ayurveda, Siddha, Unani, and Homeopathy are licenced by the government, despite lack of reputable scientific evidence. Naturopathy will also be licensed soon because several Universities now offer bachelors degrees in it. Other activities connected with AM/CM, such as Panchakarma and massage therapy related to Ayurveda are also licenced by the government now.

Contemporary Use of Alternative Medicine

Edzard Ernst wrote in the Medical Journal of Australia that "about half the general population in developed countries use complementary and alternative medicine (CAM)." A survey released in May 2004 by the National Centre for Complementary and Alternative Medicine, part of the National Institutes of Health in the United States, found that in 2002, 36% of Americans used some form of alternative therapy in the past 12 months, 50% in a lifetime - a category that included yoga, meditation, herbal treatments and the Atkins diet. If prayer was counted as an alternative therapy, the figure rose to 62.1%. 25% of people who use CAM do so because medical professional suggested it. Another study suggests a similar figure of 40%. A British telephone survey by the BBC of 1209 adults in 1998 shows that around 20% of adults in Britain had used alternative medicine in the past 12 months.

The use of alternative medicine appears to be increasing, as a 1998 study showed that the use of alternative medicine had risen from 33.8% in 1990 to 42.1% in 1997. In the United Kingdom, a 2000 report ordered by the House of

Lords suggested that "...limited data seem to support the idea that CAM use in the United Kingdom is high and is increasing."

Support for Alternative Medicine

Alternative therapies provide some services not available from conventional medicine. Examples are patient empowerment, treatment methods that support the biopsychosocial model of health, palliative care and preventive health services that are not typically a part of conventional medicine.

Salient Features of Alternative Medicines

Efficacy: Advocates of alternative medicine hold that the various alternative treatment methods are effective in treating a wide range of major and minor medical conditions, and contend that recently published research (such as Michalsen, 2003, Gonsalkorale 2003, and Berga 2003) proves the effectiveness of specific alternative treatments. They assert that a PubMed search revealed over 370,000 research papers classified as alternative medicine published in Medline-recognized journals since 1966 in the National Library of Medicine database. See also Kleijnen 1991, and Linde 1997.

Advocates of alternative medicine hold that alternative medicine may provide health benefits through patient empowerment, by offering more choices to the public, including treatments that are simply not available in conventional medicine:

"Most Americans who consult alternative providers would probably jump at the chance to consult a physician who is well trained in scientifically based medicine and who is also open-minded and knowledgeable about the body's innate mechanisms of healing, the role of lifestyle factors in influencing health, and the appropriate uses of dietary supplements, herbs, and other forms of treatment, from osteopathic manipulation to Chinese and Ayurvedic medicine. In other words, they want competent help in navigating the confusing maze of therapeutic options that are available today, especially in those cases in which conventional approaches are relatively ineffective or harmful."

It must be added though that most practitioners do not hold a degree in official medicine or even have a solid understanding of scientific principles, as can be deduced from many of their publications. And providing more advocates of alternative medicine acknowledge that the placebo effect may play a role in the benefits that some receive from alternative therapies, they point out that this does not diminish their validity. Researchers who judge treatments using the scientific method are concerned by this viewpoint, since, according to standard controlled studies, it is an acknowledgement of the inefficacy of alternative treatments.

Danger Reduced when Used as a Complement to Conventional Medicine

A major objection to alternative medicine is that it may be done in place of conventional medical treatments. As long as alternative treatments are used alongside standard conventional medical treatments, most medical doctors find most forms of complementary medicine acceptable. Consistent with previous studies, the CDC recently reported that the majority of individuals in the United States (i.e., 54.9%) used CAM in conjunction with conventional medicine.

It would be ideal for patients to inform their medical doctor when they are using alternative medicine. Some alternative treatments may interact with orthodox medical treatments, and such potential conflicts should be explored in the interest of the patient. However, many conventional practitioners are biased or uninformed about alternatives, and the exhortations to disclose alternative treatments to one's doctor do not address the complexities involved. Patients are often reluctant to share this information with their medical doctors since they fear it will hurt their patient-doctor relationship.

The issue of alternative medicine interfering with conventional medical practices is minimized when it is only turned to after the conventional medicine path has been exhausted. Many patients believe alternative medicine can help in coping with chronic illnesses for which conventional medicine offers no cure and only management. It is becoming more common for a patient's own MD to suggest alternatives when they cannot offer a treatment.

There are also the patients who have made it a habit to turn to alternatives for non-threatening disorders that may only need medical intervention in rare recalcitrant cases. They typically utilize mainstream medicine for diagnosis and basic information, while turning to alternatives for what are believed to be health-enhancing measures.

Criticism of Alternative Medicine

Due to the wide range of therapies that are considered to be "alternative medicine" few criticisms apply across the board, except possibly that of not being scientifically supported or even testable. Criticisms directed at specific branches of alternative medicine range from the fairly minor (conventional treatment is believed to be more effective in a particular area) to incompatibility with the known laws of physics (for example, in homeopathy).

Critics argue that alternative medicine practitioners may not have an accredited medical degree or be licensed physicians or general practitioners and make sweeping claims without demonstrated expertise. This cannot always be considered a serious criticism, because unless a new system of medicine becomes established, it does not receive accreditation of any kind, except by its own professional organizations. This is the route homeopathy, ayurveda, siddha, unani, and naturopathy had to follow in those countries where it is now offered by accredited institutions. Proponents of the various forms of alternative medicine reject criticism as being founded in prejudice, financial self-interest, or ignorance. Refutations of criticism sometimes take the form of an appeal to nature.

Efficacy

Lack of proper testing: Evidence-based medicine (EBM) applies the scientific method to medical practice, and aims for the ideal that healthcare professionals should make "conscientious, explicit, and judicious use of current best evidence" in their everyday practice. Prof. Edzard Ernst is a notable proponent of applying EBM to CAM.

Although proponents of alternative medicine often cite the large number of studies which have been performed, critics point out the fact that there are no statistics on exactly how many of these studies were controlled, double-blind peer-reviewed experiments or how many produced results supporting alternative medicine or parts thereof.

They contend that many forms of alternative medicine are rejected by conventional medicine because the efficacy of the treatments has not been demonstrated through double-blind randomized controlled trials; this is not a moot point, since all conventional drugs reach the market only after such trials have proved their efficacy. One is led to wonder why whole categories of drugs or treatments should be excused from these routine tests. Also, some skeptics of alternative practices point out that a person may attribute symptomatic relief to an otherwise ineffective therapy due to the natural recovery from or the cyclical nature of an illness (the regression fallacy), the placebo effect, or the possibility that the person never originally had a true illness.

Problems with known tests and studies: Critics contend that observer bias and poor study design invalidate the results of many studies carried out by alternative medicine promoters.

Some argue that less research is carried out on alternative medicine because many alternative medicine techniques cannot be patented, and hence there is little financial incentive to study them. Drug research, by contrast, can be very lucrative, which has resulted in funding of trials by pharmaceutical companies. Many people, including conventional and alternative medical practitioners, contend that this funding has led to corruption of the scientific process for approval of drug usage, and that ghostwritten work has appeared in major peer-reviewed medical journals.

Increasing the funding for research of alternative medicine techniques was the purpose of the National Centre for Complementary and Alternative Medicine. NCCAM and its predecessor, the Office of Alternative Medicine, have spent more than $200 million on such research since 1991. The German Federal Institute for Drugs and Medical Devices Commission E has studied many herbal remedies for efficacy.

Safety

Critics contend that some people have been hurt or killed directly from the various practices or indirectly by failed diagnoses or the subsequent avoidance of conventional medicine which they believe is truly efficacious.

Alternative medicine critics agree with its proponents that people should be free to choose whatever method of healthcare they want, but stipulate that people must be informed as to the safety and efficacy of whatever method they choose. People who choose alternative medicine may think they are choosing a safe, effective medicine, while they may only be getting quack remedies. Grapefruit seed extract is an example of quackery when multiple studies demonstrate its universal antimicrobial effect is due to synthetic antimicrobial contamination.

Introduction to Alternative Medicine

We have made great strides in developing western medicine in the last century. Countless diseases were eliminated or controlled through advances in immunology, parasitology, and the discovery of antibiotic drugs and vitamins; the advances in surgery made possible by antiseptics and anesthesia; and the discovery of insulin and human growth hormones. From pacemakers to birth control plus, from kidney transplants to artificial hearts, America has an international reputation for making medical breakthroughs. This, however has come at a cost. Modern medicine has raised expectations of people on the capabilities of the medicine. We have stopped taking an active part in our own healing. We trust the doctor to take care of us. Doctors, on the other hand, are very busy.

They spent more time filling up insurance forms, documenting case histories to ward of any potential malpractice suits or for meeting the "quality assurance requirements", peer reviews and other formalities that takes away the time available to practice medicine. Health care administration is reviewing the "productivity" of physicians and the only yardstick they can use to measure the performance of a doctor is how many patients he or she has seen or what is the "billable hours".

Among all these high technology shuffle, a fundamental factor that distinguished the healing profession from the time of Hypocrites has changed. Hypocrites viewed the treatment of disease as a dual process. One part was represented by systematic medicine; the other part was the full activation of the patient's own healing system. In the centuries since the great physician taught his students under the sycamore tree on the Greek island of Kos, there has been a shift away from the concept of the patient as the centre of the healing process. The physician has come increasingly to the fore as the dominant force.

The family doctor of a century ago was really a holistic doctor. He knew three generations of the family, and he knew that the mother's diabetes got worse when the teenager acted up. He saw the big picture. That's something conventional medicine has definitely lost. Family physicians, with their waiting rooms full of patients, claim that they simply do not have the time to give their full attention to patients as people, and that even if they had, many of them would be surprised, even irritated, if questioned about, say, their diet or their love life. Patients come to their doctors for tonics or tranquilizers, not for analysis.

Conventional medicine offers little for those suffering from back pain, arthritis, the effects of stress, and other chronic ailments such as cancer and AIDS. High-tech medicine is very expensive. It can also be dangerous. Its methods are potent and invasive, and it is frequently harmful. This tendency is nowhere more evident than in the amount of drug toxicity caused by modern prescribing practices. Adverse drug reactions are now so common that most patients will experience one sooner or later. The problem is that most pharmaceutical drugs are too strong.

The landscape is changing, though. Many have turning to ancient healing arts for an answer. Stone Age cave dwellers dug for medicinal plants, and the healing repertoire of the Egyptians included herbal remedies for crocodile bites. The Ayurvedic texts of ancient India are replete with magical treatments, botanical drugs, and charms designed to vanquish demons. Ayurvedic text written 5000 years ago, contain references to hardening of the arteries and recommended healing herbs to combat the problem.

The Chinese, who discovered smallpox immunization a thousand years before Europeans did, saw man as a mirror of the universe, infused with qi, vital energy that courses through channels in the body. Surgery began in prehistoric times: ancient Peruvians cut holes in the skulls of the living to provide disease with an avenue of escape.

In much of the world, Western medicine is too expensive, is unavailable, or is presented in a way that is inconsistent with traditional beliefs. There is an increasing sense that certain ancient and esoteric healing practices, long ignored by Western science, may in fact represent profound insights into the very nature of well-being.

Worldwide, only an estimated 10 percent to 30 percent of human health care is delivered by conventional, biomedically oriented practitioners. The remaining 70 percent to 90 percent ranges from self-care according to folk principles to care given in an organized health care system based on an alternative tradition or practice. The World Health Organization (WHO) estimates that 4 billion people, 80 percent of the world population, presently use herbal medicine for some aspect of primary health care.

Alternative Medicine: Definitions

What is Alternative Medicine? : Alternative medicine is any form of practice that is outside the realm of conventional modern medicine. It covers a broad range of healing philosophies, approaches, and therapies. Most of these treatments and health care practices are not taught widely in medical schools. Examples are naturopathy, chiropractic, ayurveda, homeopathy and acupuncture. (A complete listing of alternative medical practices are given later.)

What is Complementary Medicine?: If alternative medicine or therapy is used alone or instead of conventional medicine, it is called "alternative" medicine. If the treatment or therapy is done along with or in addition to conventional medicine, it is referred to as "Complementary Medicine" as the two practices complements each other. For example, many Chinese hospitals use acupuncture to reduce the pain during the surgery instead of anesthetics. This is complementary medicine. Later, we refer to the use of sesame oil as a complementary treatment for cancer. Dean Ornish uses life style changes to combat heart disease. These are all examples of complementary medicine.

What is Holistic Medicine?: Many of the alternative practices pay attention to the mental, emotional, and spiritual aspects of health, in addition to the physical body. Therapies like hypnosis and visualization claims to be able to change physical conditions through purely mental interventions. They believe that our bodies are remarkably resilient machines, capable, with some occasional prodding or intervention, of healing themselves. The name "holistic medicine" came from this unification of the mind and the body. Holistic practitioners treat the "whole person" as opposed to the individual organs of the body where symptoms occur. The importance of self care and preventing illness are stressed by holistic practitioners.

What is Natural Medicine?: Any therapy that relies on the body's own healing powers may be considered natural medicine. These include herbal remedies, diet and water therapies.

How Popular is Alternative Medicine?: According to a study in the Jan. 28, 1993, New England Journal of Medicine, 1 in 3 patients used alternative therapy in 1990. More than 80 percent of those who use alternative therapies used conventional medicine at the same time, but did not tell their doctors about the alternative treatments. In 1990, Americans made an estimated 425 million visits to alternative health practitioners-more than they made to primary care physicians.

In 1992, the National Institutes of Health in Bethesda, Maryland, established the Office of Alternative Medicine, which devotes more than $3 million a year to exploring unconventional healing techniques such as meditation, massage, vitamin therapy and herbal therapy.

In 1993, Americans spent an estimated $1.5 billion on herbal remedies, including teas and supplements. While that's a lot less than the $13.3 billion spent on over-the-counter drugs, it's more than ten times the amount we spend on over-the-counter sleeping pills from grocery stores and drugstores.

As mentioned before, worldwide, only an estimated 10 percent to 30 percent of human health care is delivered by conventional, biomedically oriented practitioners. The remaining 70 percent to 90 percent ranges from self-care according to folk principles to care given in an organized health care system based on an alternative tradition or practice.

The World Health Organization (WHO) estimates that 4 billion people, 80 percent of the world population, presently use herbal medicine for some aspect of primary health care. Herbal medicine is a major component in all indigenous peoples' traditional medicine and a common element in Ayurvedic, homeopathic, naturopathic, traditional oriental, and Native American Indian medicine.

As more and more people are being attracted to alternative medicine, the willingness to consider alternative therapies is also beginning to spread to the health insurance industry. A few large carriers have started to experiment with covering alternative treatments. A pilot programme at Mutual of Omaha, for instance, covers the Dean Ornish cardiac rehabilitation programme, and Blue Cross of Washington has a policy that covers naturopathy and homeopathy.

American Western Life Insurance Company of Foster City, California covers naturopathic treatments, including Ayurveda, homeopathy, nutritional counselling, massage and physical therapy. The company maintains a full-time Wellness Line, staffed by trained naturopathic doctors who answer clients' health care questions. Premiums for the Wellness plan are about 20 percent lower than for the company's traditional plans, says Lisa WolfKlaln, an American Western vice-president who oversees the Wellness plan, "because we believe very strongly that if people do take care of themselves, if they take preventive measures, it's going to save us all a lot of money in the long run."

DNA MICROARRAYS IN HERBAL DRUG RESEARCH

Understanding the functions of genes is a major post-genomics challenge. Strategies like proteomics, transcriptomics, metabolomics are implemented to assign the role of genes in molecular networks. The gene expression profile of a cell determines its phenotype, function and response to the environment. The complement of genes expressed by a cell is very dynamic and responds rapidly to external stimuli. Therefore, analysis of gene expression becomes necessary for providing clues about regulatory mechanisms, biochemical pathways and broader cellular function. Conventional strategies for expression profiling such as northern blot, reverse northern blot, reverse transcriptase- polymerase chain reaction (RT-PCR), nuclease protection, enzyme-linked immunosorbent assay (ELISA), western blot, in situ hybridization and immunohistochemistry are optimized for single gene analysis. Although, it is possible to modify at least some of these techniques for multiplexing, the procedure becomes increasingly technically cumbersome.

For genome wide expression analysis it is necessary to develop technologies having high degree of automation, since in any living organism thousands of genes and their products function in a complicated and orchestrated way. DNA microarrays were developed in response to the need for a high-throughput, efficient and comprehensive strategy that can simultaneously measure all the genes, or a large defined subset, encoded by a genome. Several different methodologies including differential display PCR, northern blots, quantitative

PCR, serial analysis of gene expression (SAGE) and TIGR Orthologous Gene Alignments (TOGA) are used alongside microarrays as research tools.

With an initial focus in the post-genomic era on tracking gene expression changes for target identification, microarray applications soon widened to span the entire drug discovery pipeline. DNA microarrays are being used to study the transcriptional profile in various physiological and pathological conditions, leading to the mining of novel genes and molecular markers for diagnosis, prediction or prognosis of those specific states.

Success in the DNA microarray field has led to protein array development. Protein microarrays are mainly applied to protein function studies, screening the production of antibodies and recombinant proteins, discovery of proteins implicated in disease or those that are potential drug targets, rapid detection or diagnosis of disease screening for protein-protein, DNA-protein and enzyme- substrate interactions. High-density human protein arrays are undermined by the incomplete knowledge of full-length human gene clones and the vast idiosyncrasies of proteins with respect to stability and structure. Although protein microarrays may not have reached the stage of maturity of DNA microarrays, recent developments have shown that many of the barriers holding back the technology can be overcome.

Recently cell-based arrays employing matrices of living cells engineered to express select proteins have rapidly emerged as versatile tools for the high-throughput analysis of gene function. Such arrays can facilitate genome-scale studies on different aspects of protein function, including biochemical activities, gene disruption phenotypes and protein-protein interactions. Another version of living arrays called transfection microarray has been demonstrated as an alternative to protein microarrays for the identification of drug targets, and as an expression cloning system for the discovery of gene products that alter cellular physiology. A siRNA transfected cell microarray has been developed to facilitate large-scale, high-throughput functional genomics studies using RNAi. Chemical microarrays, which are arrays of small organic compounds, represent a novel approach towards analysis of chemical libraries. They are widely used to analyze the interaction of proteins with organic compounds in a miniaturized and high-throughput fashion. Several modified technologies spanning wide range of macromolecular microarrays to cell arrays have opened new horizons in molecular and physiological systems.

The DNA Microarray

DNA micro array is an orderly arrrangement of thousands of oligonucleotides or identified sequenced genes printed on an impermeable solid support, usually glass, silicon chips or nylon membrane. A number of terms such as DNA arrays, gene chips and biochips are often used to describe these devices. The DNA microarray field is a combination of several technologies, including automated DNA sequencing, DNA amplification by PCR, oligonucleotide synthesis, nucleic acid labeling chemistries and bio-informatics. Two most common types of DNA microarrays include one in which the DNA (in the form of a single stranded short oligonucleotide) is synthesized in situ using photolithographic or other techniques and another where the DNA (usually in the form of a cDNA or full-length ORF) is post-synthetically attached to a solid support.

Depending on the kind of probe (immobilized DNA) used to generate the array and, ultimately, the information that is derived from it, DNA microarrays are used for different applications. As a definition in the context of microarrays, a 'probe' is the (partial) genomic sequence of a gene deposited and fixed on the Microarray, whereas the 'target' is the biological sample material.

Although there are many protocols and types of microarray experiments, the basic steps involved in any microarray experiment are isolating RNA or mRNA from appropriate biological samples; applying a fluorescent tag to the RNA or cDNA copy of it; hybridizing the labelled RNA or cDNA (target) to a microarray (probe) for a period of time after which the excess is washed off; scanning the microarray under laser light and data analysis using appropriate software.

Natural product research is often based on ethnobotanical information and many of the drugs used today were employed in indigenous societies. One of the aims of ethnopharmaceutical research is better understanding of the pharmacological effects of different medicinal plants traditionally used in healthcare. Plants are regarded as a promising source of novel therapeutic agents due to their higher structural diversity as compared to standard synthetic chemistry. Plants have applications in the development of therapeutic agents: as a source of bioactive compounds for possible use as drugs. There are three approaches to natural product-based drug discovery: screening of crude extracts; screening of pre-fractionated extracts; screening of pure compounds.

In the past decade there has been a paradigm shift from single-target drugs to multi-target drugs. Multi-target approaches are directed toward activation of defence, protective and repair mechanisms of the body rather than destruction of the damage-causing agent. This may be achieved by the use of a combination of drugs as in AIDS, cancer, atherosclerosis or use of single compounds that affect many targets simultaneously, e.g. Gleevec™, salicylate, metformin, Pemetrexed (Alimta) and a multi-targeted antifolate. The concept of multi-targeted therapy exists in traditional medical treatments that employ multi-component extracts of natural products. With the exception of pure substances, botanical derivatives obtained from medicinal plants usually contain several classes of compounds, which simultaneously act on multiple targets. However, very few herbal medicinal products have documentation comparable to synthetic drugs. Preparation of highly standardized herbal products with respect to chemical composition and biological activity is complicated due to the myriad range of chemicals. This also makes it difficult to precisely predict the molecular targets, mechanism of action and side effects of such products.

Use of validated analytical methods to quantify specific chemical markers remains the key point to obtain chemically standardized extracts. However many minor components with potential biological effects remain neglected from quantitative analysis of chemical markers. In the past years the development of assays on the level of molecules (receptor binding and enzyme inhibition) opened complete new perspectives for plant-based products as source of new drugs.

Advances in high-throughput experimentation have resulted in massive databases of genomic, proteomic and chemical data which in combination with efficient separation methods and powerful spectrometric methods for identification and structure elucidation can be used for identification of active compounds. In addition, the past two decades has witnessed a number of citations that describe a diverse range of molecular mechanisms that govern cellular behaviour. A systems biology approach that integrates such large and diverse sources of information together will serve to make useful biological predictions about the pharmacological effects of natural products.

DNA microarrays may provide a suitable high-throughput platform for research and development of drugs from natural products. In natural products a broad repertoire of chemical entities act together on multiple targets that makes it necessary to study the changes in expression of multiple genes simultaneously. Novel technologies such as SAGE and DNA microarrays allow rapid and detailed analysis of thousands of transcripts, providing a revolutionary approach to the investigation of gene expression.

In this review, we discuss the applications of DNA microarray technology in herbal drug research and development with suitable examples.

There are three main applications of DNA microarrays: first, in pharmacodynamics for discovery of new diagnostic and prognostic indicators and bio-markers of therapeutic response; elucidation of molecular mechanism of action of a herb, its formulations or its phytochemical components and identification and validation of new molecular targets for herbal drug development. Second, in pharmacogenomics for prediction of potential side-effects of the herbal drug during preclinical activity and safety studies; identification of genes involved in conferring drug sensitivity or resistance and prediction of patients most likely to benefit from the drug and use in general pharmacogenomic studies. Third, in pharmacognosy for correct botanical identification and authentication of crude plant materials as part of standardization and quality control. These applications are described here with some examples.

Herbal products are usually whole herbs, their formulations or extracts consisting of several bioactive compounds. With the increased demand for scientifically validated and standardized herbal product there is a need for better understanding of the molecular mechanisms underlying their biological activity. Although, the physiological actions of many herbal drugs are being studied at the molecular level, it remains unclear what are the targets of individual phytochemical components of herbs and how these molecules contribute to biological activities. Examples of the applications of microarray-based gene expression studies in elucidating molecular mechanism of action of pure compounds, different phytochemical groups and herbal extracts are discussed here.

The molecular pathways underlying diverse biological activity of the triterpenoid compounds isolated from the tropical medicinal plant Centella asiatica when studied with gene microarrays showed that Centella triterpenes evoke a gene-expression response consistent with their prevailing medical uses in the treatment of connective tissue disorders such as wound healing and microangiopathy.

The identification of genes modulated by these compounds provides the basis for a molecular understanding of Centella's bioactivity, and opportunities for the quantitative correlation of this activity with clinical effectiveness at a molecular level. Similarly, the antiproliferative activity of Coptidis rhizoma, a medicinal herb, and its major component berberine was investigated in human pancreatic cancer cell lines.

Gene expression patterns associated with sensitivities to each agent were analyzed with oligonucleotide arrays that comprised approximately 11,000 genes. It was possible to identify common and distinct genes related to anti-proliferative activities of purified berberine and C. rhizoma.

Involvement of genes in apoptosis inducing activity of alkaloids from Chinese medicinal herb Tripterygium hypoglaucum (levl.) Hutch (Celastraceae) root was examined using cDNA microarrays containing 3000 human genes derived from a leukocyte cDNA library. Induction of apoptosis by Tripterygium hypoglaucum alkaloids was found to be through c-myc and NF-kappa B signaling pathways.

Gene expression pattern of inferior colliculus from DBA/2J mice with audiogenic seizure and those treated with Qingyangshenylycosides, a traditional Chinese medicine, were examined. Gene expression analysis using Agilent oligo microarray showed that total of 134 genes were either up- or down-regulated during audiogenic seizure. Qingyang-shenylycosides prevented many of the audiogenic seizure induced gene expression changes.

Nevertheless, some of the audiogenic seizure induced genes were further enhanced or reversed by Qingyangshenylycosides treatment. The data provided important information regarding the molecular mechanisms of audiogenic seizure and the mechanism of action of Qingyangshenylycosides.

Oligonucleotide microarrays consisting of 87 probes representing 87 human cardiovascular disease-related genes were used to investigate the molecular mechanisms of saponins from the rhizome of Anemarrhena asphodeloides Bunge. Gene expression patterns in saponin treated and untreated human umbilical vein endothelial cells were analyzed. The results suggest that saponins may have beneficial effect on cardiovascular diseases by modulating the function of vein endothelial cells.

A gene chip, (Rat Genome U34A) was used to elucidate the gene regulatory pattern of Epimedium flavonoids in immune homeostasis remodeling in the aged rats. Expression pattern characterized by up-regulation of apoptosis promoting gene expression and down-regulation of apoptosis inhibiting genes expression, is the important gene background of immuno-homeostasis imbalance in aged. Epimedium flavonoids reverse these abnormal changes to reconstruct a beneficial equilibrium of gene expression and thus to further remodel the immuno-homeostasis in the aged.

Mechanism of herbal glycoside recipes retrieving deficient ability of spatial learning memory in mice suffering from cerebral ischemia/repurfusion was studied using DNA micoarray system. Gene expression pattern was analyzed in the groups that showed increased ability of spatial learning. A 18-fold increase in expression was observed for many genes (38-46) including genes in cell cycle regulation, signal transduction, nerve system transcription factors, DNA-binding protein, etc. Nine genes related to retrieving deficient ability of spatial learning memory when treated with glycoside recipes were found in this study.

Chronic cocaine use is known to elicit changes in the pattern of gene expression within the brain. The hippocampus plays a critical role in learning and memory and may also play a role in mediating behaviours associated with cocaine abuse. To profile the gene expression response of the hippocampus to chronic cocaine treatment, cDNA hybridization arrays were used to illuminate cocaine-regulated genes in rats treated non-contingently with a binge model of cocaine.

Similarly, using DNA microarray analysis gene expression changes with chronic morphine and antagonist-precipitated withdrawal in two brain regions involved in behavioural effects of morphine in both mice and rats, were characterized Si-Jun-Zi decoction (SJZD), a traditional Chinese herbal prescription, has been used clinically for treating patients with disorders of the digestive system. Previous studies indicated that the polysaccharides of SJZD are the active components contributing towards its pharmacological effects in improving gastro-intestinal function a nd immunity. SJZD polysaccharide was found to have protective effect and enhanced re-epithelialization on wounded IEC-6 cells.

To elucidate the modulatory effect of polysaccharides of SJZD on wounded IEC-6 cells at the molecular level, an oligonucleotide microarray was employed to study differential gene expression of treated IEC-6 cells and the candidate genes were validated by RT-PCR. There was increased expression of genes coding for ion channels and transporters, which are critical to cell migration and restoration of wounded intestinal cells, suggesting a possible mechanism for re-epithelialization.

Clinical trials on antimicrotubule agents, docetaxel and estramustine combination treatment have suggested improved antitumor activity in hormone-refractory prostate cancer. However, the molecular mechanisms involved in the combination treatment with docetaxel and estramustine have not been fully elucidated. In order to establish such molecular mechanisms in both hormone insensitive and sensitive prostate cancer cells, gene expression profiles of docetaxel- and estramustine-treated prostate cancer cells were obtained by using Affymetrix Human Genome U133A Array. Clustering analysis based on biological function showed that docetaxel and estramustine combination treatment down-regulated some genes that are known to regulate cell proliferation, transcription, translation, and oncogenesis.

In contrast, docetaxel and estramustine combination treatment up-regulated some genes related to induction of apoptosis, cell cycle arrest, and tumor suppression. Docetaxel and estramustine also showed differential effects on gene expression between mono- and combination treatment. Combination treatment with docetaxel and estramustine caused alternations of a large number of genes, many of which may contribute to the molecular mechanisms by which docetaxel and estramustine inhibit the growth of prostate cancer cells. These results provide novel molecular targets of docetaxel and estramustine combination treatment in prostate cancer cells.

Extracts

High-density oligonucleotide microarrays have been used for pioneer studies on the multiple gene expression effects exhibited by Ginkgo biloba leaf extract EGb 761, changing traditional pharmacology and medicine concepts. EGb 761 has been known to have neuroprotective effects ranging from molecular and cellular, to animal and human studies, however, the mechanisms remain unclear. DNA microarray based analyses has largely helped in identifying its targets and mechanism of action. High-density oligonucleotide microarrays were used to define the transcriptional effects in the cortex and hippocampus of mice whose diets were supplemented with the herbal extract.

This study reveals that diets supplemented with Ginkgo biloba extract have notable neuromodulatory effects in vivo and illustrates the utility of genome-wide expression monitoring to investigate the biological actions of complex extracts. Further, DNA microarray analyses revealed that transcription of multiple apoptosis-related genes is either up- or down-regulated in cells treated with EGb 761. These results suggest that inhibition of apoptotic machinery may, at least in part, mediate multiple neuroprotective effects of EGb 761. Mechanism of cytostatic action of EGb 761 was elucidated with the help of DNA microarray and the genes important for tumour growth were identified.

Ginkgo extract and one of its terpenoid constituents, ginkgolide B, inhibited the proliferation of a highly aggressive human breast cancer cell line and xenografts of this cell line in nude mice. cDNA microarray analyses have shown that exposure of human breast cancer cells to a Ginkgo extract altered the expression of genes that are involved in the regulation of cell proliferation, cell differentiation or apoptosis, and that exposure of human bladder cancer cells to a Ginkgo extract produced an adaptive transcriptional response that augments antioxidant status and inhibits DNA damage.

A human genome screen for TNF?-inducible genes was used to identify the genetic basis of the anti-inflammatory effects of standardized Boswellia serrata extract, 5-Loxin in microvascular endothelial cells. Acutely, TNF?-induced 522 genes; of which 113 genes were clearly sensitive to 5-Loxin treatment. Such genes directly related to inflammation, cell adhesion, and proteolysis. The robust 5-Loxin -sensitive candidate genes were then subjected to further processing which led to the recognition of the primary 5-Loxin -sensitive TNF?-inducible pathways. One mechanism by which TNF?, causes inflammation is by potently inducing the expression of adhesion molecule VCAM-1. 5-Loxin was found to completely inhibit VCAM-1 expression.

Water-extract of Paeoniae Radix has inhibitory effect on the growth of both HepG2 and Hep3B cell lines. Using cDNA microarray technology and RT-PCR analysis the drug targets of Paeoniae Radix in inhibition of tumour cells growth were elucidated.

Several studies have indicated that extracts of S. barbata have growth inhibitory effects on a number of human cancers. However, the mechanism underlying the antitumor activity was unclear. cDNA microarray analysis showed that 16 genes, involved in DNA damage, cell cycle control, nucleic acid binding and protein phosphorylation, underwent more than 5-fold change. These data indicated that these processes are involved in S. barbata-mediated killing of cancer cells.

The effect of Syzygium aromaticum (L.) Merrill and Perry (clove) extract on tissues that regulate glucose metabolism was studied by analysis of gene expression using DNA microarray. The data showed that the extract acts like insulin in hepatocytes and hepatoma cells by reducing phosphoenolpyruvate carboxykinase and glucose 6-phosphatase gene expression. Much like insulin, clove-mediated repression was reversed by PI3 K inhibitors and N- acetylcysteine. Moreover, clove and insulin were found to regulate the expression of many of the same genes in a similar manner. These results indicate a potential role for compounds derived from clove as insulin-mimetic agents.

A cDNA microarray study demonstrated significant inhibition of inducible endothelial CD36 expression, a novel cardioregulatory gene, by IH636 grape seed proanthocyanidin extract.

Both the prototypic tricyclic antidepressant imipramine (IMI) and the extract of St John's wort (SJW) can be effective in the treatment of major depressive disorder. Affymetrix chips were used to study hypothalamic gene expression in rats treated with SJW or IMI to test the hypothesis that chronic antidepressant treatment by various classes of drugs results in shared patterns of gene expression that may underlie their therapeutic effects. SJW treatment differentially regulated 66 genes and expression sequence tags (ESTs) and IMI treatment differentially regulated 74 genes and ESTs. Six common transcripts in response to both treatments were found. Both treatments also affected different genes that are part of the same cell function processes, such as glycolytic pathways and synaptic function. The data support the hypothesis that chronic antidepressant treatment by drugs of various classes may result in a common, final pathway of changes in gene expression in a discrete brain region.

Recently, a rapid throughput screening system involving gene expression analysis was developed in order to investigate the potential of bioactive chemicals contained in natural health products as effective drug therapy, in particular the ability of these chemicals to alleviate the inflammatory response in human airway epithelial cells. The pharmacogenomic activities of Anoectochilus formosanus extract as a crude phytocompound mixture were compared to those conferred by the single-compound drug, plumbagin in MCF-7 cancer cells. This study offers evidence to support the search for fractionated medicinal herb extracts or phytocompound mixtures, in addition to single-compound drugs, as defined therapeutic agents. DNA microarray can be used for activity-guided fractionation of herbal extracts in order to determine active principles.

DNA MICROARRAYS IN PHARMACOGENOMICS

Pharmacogenomics is the study of genes and the gene products (proteins) essential for pharmacological or toxicological responses to pharmaceutical agents. Oligonucleotide-based DNA chip technology or cDNA microarray can be used to analyze gene expression profiles that are induced or repressed by xenobiotics.

An attempt has been made to develop microarray genotyping system for multiplex analysis of a panel of single nucleotide polymorphisms (SNPs) in genes encoding proteins involved in blood pressure regulation, and to apply this system in a pilot study demonstrating its feasibility in the pharmacogenetics of anti-hypertensive drug response. DNA microarray techniques might prove to be a reliable basis for predicting response (or lack of response) of individuals to herbal drugs. Technologies designed to characterize genes and their products on a discovery scale are now having an impact on many areas of biology, including toxicology. Toxicogenomics is the sub-discipline that merges genomics with toxicology. In toxicology research, gene expression profiling facilitates mechanism-based research on toxicant action by comparing results for an experimental compound with a database. Recently several studies have demonstrated the utility of microarray analysis for studying genome-wide effects of xenobiotics and the rapid identification of toxic hazards for novel drug candidates.

An example of such a platform is ToxBlot II, a custom microarray containing cDNAs representing 12564 human genes chosen on the basis of their potential relevance to a broad range of toxicities. ToxBlot II allows the simultaneous expression profiling of genes representing entire cellular pathways, facilitating a very detailed investigation of potential mechanisms of toxicity. cDNA microarray analysis was used to study the expression level of genes in oral fibroblast cell lines in response to exposure to ripe areca nut extract. The results showed up-regulation of IL-6 expression and down-regulation of PDGFR, APP-1 and KGF-1 expressions in multiple cell lines assayed. The down-regulation of KGF-1 expression in oral fibroblast cell lines potentially impairs the proliferation of overlying keratinocytes, which could partially explain the frequent epithelial atrophy observed in chronic areca chewers in vivo.

This study established a novel toxicogenomic database for areca nut extract. cDNA microarray analysis was also used to analyze the mRNA expression patterns of 1177 genes in ten oral cancer patients with betel quid chewing history. This study provides pilot data for understanding the pathogenesis of oral cancer in countries like Taiwan where betel quid chewing is prevalent.

Recent studies have highlighted that concurrent use of herbs may mimic, magnify, or oppose the effect of drugs. DNA microarray can be used for studying herb-drug interactions, and the mechanisms underlying these interactions.

Several botanical constituents in PC-SPES, a botanical preparation, inhibit tumour growth through cell cycle arrest and apoptosis. LNCaP prostate carcinoma cells were treated with PC-SPES, and changes in gene expression were determined by complementary DNA (cDNA) microarray hybridization and northern blot analyses. mRNA levels of? -tubulin decreased sevenfold. The results show that PC-SPES may interfere with microtubule polymerization.

This activity has implications for the clinical management of patients with advanced prostate cancer who may be taking PC-SPES concurrently with microtubule-modulating chemotherapeutic agents, such as paclitaxel. cDNA microarray analysis was used to identify gene expression changes in LNCaP prostate carcinoma cells exposed to PC-SPES and estrogenic agents including diethylstilbestrol. Transcripts encoding cell cycle-regulatory proteins,? - and? -tubulins, and the androgen receptor were down-regulated by PC-SPES. A comparison of gene expression profiles resulting from these treatments indicates that PCSP ES exhibits activities distinct from those attributa ble to diethylstilbestrol and suggests that alterations in specific genes involved in modulating the cell cycle, cell structure, and androgen response may be responsible for PC-SPES-mediated cytotoxicity.

DNA Microarray in Pharmacognosy

Use of authentic herbal materials is the first step to ensure quality, safety and efficacy of herbal medicines. DNA polymorphism-based assays have been developed for the identification of herbal medicines. In this approach, small amounts of DNA are amplified by the polymerase chain reaction and the reaction products are analyzed by gel electrophoresis, sequencing, or hybridization with species-specific probes. Recently, microarrays have been applied for the DNA sequence-based identification of medicinal plants. To utilize DNA microarrays for identification and authentication of herbal material, it is necessary to identify a distinct DNA sequence that is unique to each species of medicinal plant. The DNA sequence information is then used to synthesize a corresponding probe on a silicon-based gene chip. These probes are capable of detecting complementary target DNA sequences if present in the test sample being analyzed.

Oligonucleotide probes specific for polymorphisms in the D2 and D3 regions of 26S rDNA gene of several Fritillaria species were designed and printed on the poly-lysine coated slides to prepare a DNA chip. Differentiation of the various Fritillaria species was accomplished based on hybridization of fluorescent labelled PCR products with the DNA chip. The results demonstrated the reliability of using DNA chips to identify different species of Fritillaria, and that the DNA chip technology can provide a rapid, high throughput tool for genotyping and plant species authentication.

Similarly, using fluorescence-labelled ITS2 sequences as probes, distinctive signals were obtained for the five medicinal Dendrobium species listed in the Chinese Pharmacopoeia. The established microarray was able to detect the presence of D. nobile in a Chinese medicinal formulation containing nine herbal components.

A silicon-based DNA microarray using species-specific oligonucleotide probes is designed and fabricated to identify multiple toxic traditional Chinese medicinal plant species by parallel genotyping. Chip-based authentication of medicinal plants may be useful as economical, precise tool for quality control and safety monitoring of herbal pharmaceuticals and neutraceuticals. Identification of herbal materials, which commonly consist of dried or processed parts, is difficult. This is particularly true for similar looking herbal materials that can often vary greatly in their medicinal properties and market value. DNA microarray based technology can provide an efficient, accurate and chea per means of testing the a uthenticity of hundreds of samples simultaneously while conventional chemical methodologies usually take several days for verification. Chip-based authentication of medicinal plants can be useful as a tool for quality control and safety monitoring of herbal pharmaceuticals and neutraceuticals and will significantly add to the medical potential and commercial profitability of herbal products.

This application of DNA microarrays will not only benefit the herbal drug industry but can also facilitate the identification of herbal products by regulatory authorities. An international initiative, the Consortium for the Barcode of Life (CBOL) is devoted to developing DNA barcoding as a tool for correct taxonomic identification of species, including medicinal plants. DNA microarrays can provide a suitable technology platform for such an initiative.

Perspective

Traditionally, the pharmaceutical industry has focused on modifying one gene or protein at a time as the basis for identifying new drugs. The quest for a molecule to modify a single key factor in a disease process may not provide a solution for many complex diseases where multiple cell types and/or multiple pathways contribute to disease. Herbal extracts or mixtures represent combinatorial chemistry of nature with vast repertoire of chemical entities that have a complex effect on numerous cellular components and functions.

They have great potential in the multi-target approach to diseases. However, potential of herbal drugs as defined therapeutic agents is undermined by the difficulty in standardization, pharmacodynamics and pharmacokinetics of these multi-component mixtures. Microarray analysis of gene expression can be useful for elucidating the molecular mechanisms and networks underlying the complex pharmacological function of herbal extracts and mixtures. Studying the patterns of gene expression at many stages during the treatment process can reveal mechanism from a modern genetic perspective and will help to identify bio-markers of adverse or favourable response. A positive correlation between the transcriptional response induced by an herbal drug and a database profile of an existing therapeutic agent can provide insight into target specificity, mechanism of action, as well as facilitate analysis of pathways downstream of the target.

It will also help in identification of novel therapeutic applications of a herbal drug. DNA microarrays can also be used for activity-guided fractionation of herbal extracts thereby helping in narrowing down upon the active principle producing the desired effect. Microarrays have applications in the entire drug discovery pipeline to improve selection of biological targets and lead compounds. Correlation of gene expression data of herbal drug candidates with clinical outcome or bio-markers of response in biological system will facilitate selection of best candidate for drug development. In the area of pharmacogenomics, DNA microarrays will facilitate development of individually optimized drugs based on differential gene expression patterns. Genetic polymorphism studies can be done to classify individuals according to their drug metabolizing capacities or response to disease. SNP screening of patients undergoing treatment with a particular herbal drug and correlating these data with recovery profile would help to understand which individuals or groups are likely to be benefited by the drug.

Microarray analysis of gene expression has become a suitable approach for the biological effects of drugs and other chemicals. Gene expression profile screens focused on genes that are relevant to toxicity can be useful for prediction of potential herbal drug side effects during pre-clinical development and toxicology studies. They can also be applied for studying herb-drug interactions and their underlying mechanisms.

Medicinal plants are an integral part of TM/CAM such as Ayurvedic, Chinese, Native American and many other traditional systems of medicine. Clinical experiences, observations or documented data becomes a starting point for traditional knowledge based drug development. Although the clinical existence of traditional medicine spans several generations, it may be hazardous to extrapolate from such uses to current practice, since herbs and or their formulations used may be very different from the commercial herbal products available today.

Many questions remain concerning quality, efficacy, safety, bioavailability and mechanisms of action of even the most widely used herbs. These questions can be answered by rigorous application of scientific principles in high quality basic and clinical research. There is a need for scientific validation of safety, efficacy, therapeutic claims, bioavailability and mechanism of action of these medicines that are being used in the population since centuries. Microarray based approach can facilitate high throughput, fast track evidence-based herbal drug development following Reverse Pharmacology path. Phytomics, a technology platform for characterization of herbal compositions wherein, Herbal Bio Response Arrays (HBR Arrays) are used to determine bioactive constituents and biological activities of an herbal composition has recently been developed and patented.

Further, CAM disciplines owing to their holistic nature may be impacting gene expression and signaling pathways. Application of such novel expression analysis tools may help to understand and characterize the genes and signaling pathways involved in CAM modalities.

DNA microarrays have the potential for application in different phases of herbal drug discovery and development. This includes quality control and standardization of the herbal drugs, identification and validation of new targets, the profiling of on-target and off-target effects during the optimization of new therapeutic agents, understanding molecular mechanisms of action, structure-activity relationships and the prediction of side-effects, and the discovery of diagnostic, prognostic, and pharmacodynamic bio-markers.

At present the major practical applicability of DNA microarrays remains in SNP mapping, genotyping and pharmacogenetics. In recent years, array-based sequencing (minisequencing/resequencing arrays) that combines target hybridization with enzymatic primer extension reactions has emerged as a powerful means to scan for all possible DNA sequence variations.

Highly multiplexed microarray systems offering potential for mutation analysis and genome-wide SNP mapping have been developed. DNA microarrays are a effective new strategy for global gene expression profiling, but reliable detection of expression changes and understanding the functional relevance of these expression profiles is a challenge. Other problems in microarray experiments include non-reproducibility, difficulty in statistical analysis and comparability of data from different experiments.

Inconsistencies in data may arise due to low specificity of cDNA probes, discrepancy in fold-change calculations, variations in laboratories, technicians, probe labeling, biochemical reactions, scanners, lasers etc. Also the sensitivity and specificity of DNA microarrays depends on the nucleotide composition of the target and probe. Repetitive sequence elements and highly structured nucleic acids can greatly decrease the sensitivity of hybridization based analysis.

In its current stage, a microarray experiment needs to be validated by independent confirmation of results by laboratory-based analysis and in silico comparison with information available in literature and expression databases. Although DNA microarrays have huge potential for pharmacodynamics and toxigenomics applications, these are still in exploratory stage and need validation by other biological experiments. Bio-informatics and statistical tools have a major role to play in the microarray field, whereby data from multiple experiments can be integrated to answer complex biological questions.

Another factor limiting microarray application is the cost of the technology. The challenge today is to provide standardized, sensitive, reproducible microarray platforms, databases and visualization methods for expression profiles that are also affordable to scientists. With the development of new, uniform and more sophisticated experimental designs, data management systems statistical tools and algorithms for data analysis DNA microarrays can be optimally used in herbal drug research.

In spite of the huge potential offered by microarray technology, the importance of in vitro biological assays, cell-line studies and in vivo animal studies cannot be ignored. A comprehensive strategy integrating information from diverse scientific experiments and technologies will lead to molecular evidence-based herbal medicine.

MEDICINAL PLANTS IN AYURVEDA

Ayurveda is India's traditional, natural system of medicine that has been practiced for more than 5,000 years. Ayurveda is a Sanskrit word that literally translated means "science of life" or "practices of longevity." Ayurveda was the system of health care conceived and developed by the seers (rishis) and natural scientists through centuries of observations, experiments, discussions, and meditations. For several thousand years their teachings were passed on orally from teacher to student; about the fifth to sixth century BC, elaborately detailed texts were written in Sanskrit, the ancient language of India. For many years Ayurveda flourished and was used by rich and poor alike in India and Southeast Asia.

Manuscript page from Atharva-Veda, earliest Indian text (approx. 1500 BC) with much medical information, one of several Vedas (meaning "knowledge"), upon which Ayurvedic medical practice is based on. Ayurvedic manuals were written by Charaka, Sushruta, and Vagbhata that give detailed descriptions of the various practices. Charaka listed 500 hundred remedies and Sushruta over 700 vegetable medicines.

Ayurveda emphasizes prevention of disease, rejuvenation of our body systems, and extension of life span. The profound premise and promise of Ayurveda is that through certain practices, not only can we prevent heart disease and make our headaches go away, but we can also better understand ourselves and the world around us, live a long healthy life in balance and harmony, achieve our fullest potential, and express our true inner nature on a daily basis.

Ayurveda provides an integrated approach to preventing and treating illness through lifestyle interventions and natural therapies. It is based on the view that the elements, forces, and principles that comprise all of nature - and that holds it together and make it function are also seen in human beings.

In Ayurveda, the mind (or consciousness) and the body (or physical mass) not only influence each other—they are each other. Together they form the mind-body. The universal consciousness is an intelligent, aware ocean of energy that gives rise to the physical world we perceive through our five senses. Ayurvedic philosophy and practices link us to every aspect of ourselves and remind us that we are in union with every aspect of nature, each other, and the entire universe.

There can be no mental health without physical health, and vice versa. In Ayurveda, symptoms and diseases that could be categorized as mental thoughts or feelings are just as important as symptoms and diseases of the physical body. Both are due to imbalances within a person, and both are treated by restoring the natural balance mentally and physically. In Ayurveda your whole life and lifestyle must be in harmony before you can enjoy true well being. Lifestyle interventions are a major Ayurvedic preventive and therapeutic approach.

In India, Ayurvedic practitioners receive state-recognized, institutionalized training in parallel to their physician counterparts. The research base is growing concerning the physiological effects of meditative techniques and yoga postures in Indian medical literature and Western psychological literature. Published studies have documented reductions in cardiovascular disease risk factors, including blood pressure, cholesterol, and reaction to stress, in individuals who practice Ayurvedic methods.

Laboratory and clinical studies on Ayurvedic herbal preparations and other therapies have shown them to have a range of potentially beneficial effects for preventing and treating certain cancers, treating infectious disease, treating diabetes, promoting health, and treating aging. Mechanisms underlying these effects may include free-radical scavenging effects, immune system modulation, brain neurotransmitter modulation, and hormonal effects.

Basis for Ayurvedic Philosophy

Ayurveda is applicable to every living thing, as implied by its name, the science of life. Vedic sciences attribute life to more things than we normally do - the things such as air, wind, fire, the earth, planets, stars, etc. are all thought to possess conscience like living beings.

The basic premise of Ayurveda is that the entire cosmos or universe is part of one singular absolute. Everything that exists in the vast external universe (macrocosm), also appears in the internal cosmos of the human body (microcosm). The human body consisting of 50-100 million cells, when healthy, is in harmony, self-perpetuating and self-correcting just as the universe is. The ancient Ayurveda text, Charaka, says, "Man is the epitome of the universe. Within man, there is as much diversity as in the world outside. Similarly, the outside world is as diverse as human beings themselves." In other words, all human beings are a living microcosm of the universe and the universe is a living macrocosm of the human beings.

Siddha

Directorate of Indian Medicine and Homoeopathy: Siddha System is one of the ancient traditional systems of medicine in India. Siddhars the spiritual scientists of Tamil land are the founding fathers of this scientific system.

According to Siddha System the human body is the replica of the universe so are the food and drugs irrespective of their origin. Siddha system believes that all objects in the universe including human body are composed of five basic primordial elements, namely earth, water, fire, air and space. The human body is a conglomeration of three humours and seven physical components. The Food is considered to be basic building material of human body, which gets processed into humours, tissues and wastes. The equilibrium of humours, body tissues and waste products is considered as health and its disturbance or imbalance leads to disease or pathologic state.

This system also deals with the concept of immortality and salvation in this life. The exponents of this system consider that achievement of this state is possible by regulated diet, medicine and processing of mind by yogic or spiritual exercises like meditation and yoga.

Siddhars described 96 principles as the constituents of Human Being. They include Physical, Physiological, Mental and Intellectual components of a person. They are nothing but the manifestations of the " Five Basic Elements".

Disease: Disease is a condition in which there is imbalance in the "Five Elements, which alters the "Three Humours" which is also reflected in the seven physical constituents. The change disturbs the equilibrium and cause disease.

The basic concept of Siddha system of medicine is "Food is Medicine—Medicine is Food"

Saint Thiruvalluvar says:

"Miginum Kuraiyinum Noi Seyyum Noolor Vali Mudhala Enniya Moondru" "Wind, bile and phlegm three cause disease so Doctors deem it more or less"

Diagnosis: "Noi Naadi Noi Mudhal Naadi Athu thanikkum Vaai Naadi Vayppa Seyal"

"Test disease, its causes and cure and apply remedy that is sure" — Thiruvalluvar.

It is always essential to identify the cause for any disease to be accepted as a "Scientific method" The Diagnostic methodology in Siddha Treatment is unique as it is made purely on the basis of the "Clinical Acumen" of the Physician. He examines the Tongue, complexion, speech, eyes, palpation in a patient and he also examines the urine and stools. The diagnosis is then confirmed by the "Pulse Diagnosis". The above approach is collectively known as "Eight types of examinations". However, the Siddha Physician now also accepts the modern diagnostic methods for the purpose of diagonosis.

Treatment : The following line of treatment have been in practice in Siddha medicine.

- Using medicines like Choornam, Kudineer, Vadagam etc. made of herbs.
- Surgical methods like incision, excision, heat application, blood letting and leech application etc.
- Physiotherapy - Thokkanam and Varma, the Siddha way of Touch therapy, Medicated Oil application, Fomentation, herbal steam bath etc.
- Using medicines like Parpam, Chenduram, Chuxnam etc. made of minerals especially of metals.

Materia Medica: Siddhars, with their clarified and inituitive intellect resulting from their yogic powers explored the nature and exploited the natural resources for the sake of humanity. They documented their findings about the characteristics of plants, metals, minerals and animal products. They documented all their findings in the form of poems for the use of posterity. Knowledge was transmitted from Guru to disciples. Their boundless knowledge on the properties of drugs, purification, processing, heat application, fixing dosage, toxicity, antidote and clinical application is astonishing the modern scientific world.

Significance: The Siddha System is capable of treating all types of chronic diseases especially arthritis, skin problems urinary tract disorders, infertility, degenerative disorders like osteo arthritis, Senile Dementia, disease of the liver, medicinally treatable Spinal disorders ,general debility ,diarrhoea and intractable allergic disorders. Aringnar Anna Govt. Hospital of Indian Medicine, Arumbakkam, being the premier institute in Tamil Nadu for Indian Medicine and Homoeopathy treats both outpatient and inpatient.

Ayurveda

Directorate of Indian Medicine and Homoeopathy: Ayurveda is an ancient system of medicine, which originated in northern India antiquity of which dates back to the period of vedas and this is said to be born from Atharva Veda. This knowledge has been gathered due to constant observation of nature for long years by men since the advent of civilization and cannot be attributed to any individual or a group of individuals by any stretch of imagination. Ayurveda is basically based on the predominance of three humours namely Vatha, Pittha and Kapha in the human body. Balanced state of these doshas denotes health and their imbalance produces disease.

Preceptors like Charaka, Susrutha have been benevolent enough to compile these invaluable treasure troves of knowledge to be passed on to posterity. The fact that Ayurveda has stood the test of time bears ample testimony to its efficacy till date.

It comprises of eight branches namely.

1. Kaya Chikitsa (General Medicine)
2. Kaumara Bhruthya (Paediatrics)
3. Bhutha Vidhya (Psychiatry)
4. Salakya (ENT and Ophthalmology and dentistry)
5. Shalya (Surgery)
6. Agada Tantra (Toxicology)
7. Rasayana (Rejuvenation Therapy)
8. Vajeekarana (Aphrodisiac therapy)

Pancha karma one of the areas of specialization, which has earned public acclaim in recent times, is also a part of the above branches. It enjoys popularity because of its being a hands on therapy and is very relaxing to the fatigued body and tired mind.

Unani

Unani system of Medicine has originated in Greece. It was further enriched and developed by Arabs and Persians. Hippocrates explained that the disease was a normal process and its symptoms were the reaction of the body to the disease. The chief function of the physician was to aid the natural forces of the body. He held that there exists in the body four humours that keep up the balance of it. He also laid emphasis on diet, drugs of plants, animal and mineral origin for curing the disease.

The Unani system of Medicine is based on the Humoural theory. Humoural pathology which presupposes the presence of four humours namely - Blood (Dam), Phlegm (Balgham), Yellow bile (Safra) and Black bile (Sauda) in the body. The temperament of persons is expressed accordingly by the words Sa ng ui ne , P hl eg ma ti c, Ch ol er ic a n d Me la nc hol ic a cc ord in g to t he preponderance of them in the body. Everybody has got unique humoural constitution which represents the healthy state of humoural balance of the body. The Unani medicine plays a vital role when the individual experiences the humoural imbalance.

The correct diet and digestion can bring back the humoural balance. Its main emphasis is on diagnosis of a disease through Nabz (Pulse), Baul (Urine), Baraz (stool) etc. It has laid down six essential prerequisites for the prevention of disease. They are known as 'Asbab-e-sitte Zarooriya' viz. air, drinks and foods; bodily movement and repose; psychic movement and repose; sleep and wakefulness; excretion and retention.

The modes of treatment are as follows:-

(i) Ilaj bid-Tadbeer (Regimental therapy)
(ii) Ilaj bid Ghiza (Dieto Therapy)
(iii) Ilaj bid Dawa (Pharmaco Therapy)
(iv) Jarahat (Surgery)

The regimental therapy includes venesection, cupping, sweating, diuresis, bath (Hammam), massage, cauterization, purging, vomiting, exercise and leeching etc. Dieto therapy aims at treating certain ailments by administration of specific diets, whereas pharmaco therapy deals with use of naturally occuring drugs, mostly herbals though drugs of animals and mineral origin are also used.

Diagnosis and Treatment: The unani system of diagnosis of diseases and treatment restoring health, revolves round the concept of temperament or 'Mizaj'. The humours also have specific temperament. Changes in temperament are related to changes in the balance of humours. Any change in temperament brings about a change in the health of the individual. Thus imbalance of the harmony of humours and temperament along with failure of one or more parts of the body to eliminate pathogentic waste causes disease.

The Government recognized the merit of Unani system and attempts were made to develop it as a viable system of medicine for National Health care. The Unani drugs are cost effective, safe and widely accepted by the people of India. Therefore, the Tamil Nadu Government have established a Unani Medical College and Unani dispensaries.

Homoeopathy

Definition: "Homoeopathy is a system of treatment of the diseased by drugs usually prescribed in minute doses, that in a healthy person would produce symptoms like those of disease."

Origin: The Homoeopathy way of healing was devised by the Great German physician Dr. Christian Frederick Samuel Hahnemann in the late 18th Century. He came across an old idea of the efficacy of 'Cinchona bark' in treating intermittent fever due to its toxic effect on the stomach and conducted experiments upon himself in order to get the truth. He deduced from the experiment that Cinchona was used as a remedy for intermittent fever and it could produce symptoms similar to those of intermittent fever in healthy people, if taken for a specific period of time. The law of 'Similia Similibus Curentur' or 'let likes be treated by the likes' thus forms the basis of treatment under the Homoeopathic method of drug therapy employed to cure the natural suffering of person by the administration of drugs which have been experimentally proved to possess the power of producing similar artificial suffering or symptoms of diseases in healthy human being.

Basic Concepts : In Homoeopathy the main emphasis is on the remedial agents in illness and in health. It is a low cost system using only the non-toxic drugs. It has established a reputation for successful treatment of acute and chronic illness and in certain disease for which there is no or less treatment in other systems. Dr. Samuel Hanemann, who was the founder of this system enunciated the basic concepts and its principles in "Organon the Art of Healing" in the year 1810.

Due to various reasons like cost-effectiveness and non-toxic nature of its drugs, no side effects of easy in take. Homoeopathy is getting a very high recognition and acceptance from the people. Having its origin in the modern scientific age, it has the benefit of basing its theory and concept on demonstrable scientific principles and procedures.

It is based on the following cardinal principles:

1. The law of Similars
2. The law of Single Remedy
3. The law of Minimum Dose
4. Doctrine of Drug proving
5. Doctrine of dynamisation
6. Doctrine of vital force
7. Doctrine of Chronic disease

Among this, the most fundamental is the 'law of Similars'. This law states that the symptoms experienced by the sick person are reactions of the body which it mobilizes in order to counteract a morbid influence, be it a specific stress such as bacteria or viruses, or a non-specific stress such as climatic changes, environmental pollution, mental and emotional disturbances etc.

Among the seven, first three are having more therapeautic importance and value.

Health and Disease in Homoeopathy: This system assumes that any disease symptoms, syndrome is the reaction of the defence mechanism of human body against the disease-causing agent. The symptoms are the means through which the body tries to regain its lost balance. According to it, the symptoms syndrome in a disease is not the disease per se but the reaction of the defense mechanism mobilized by the body in order to counteract a morbific influence existing in the body and causing the loss of balance of the healthy body. Thus the disequilibrium in the normal functioning of the organs of body implies sickness.

Diagnosis and Treatment: In Homoeopathy patients are diagnosed (their individual symptoms) but not their disease. As there is specific medicine for specific disease, unless the diseases are diagnosed, they cannot be treated, in other systems of medicine, where as in Homoeopathy, medicine are proved in healthy individuals are their symptoms are recorded.

In order to treat the diseased individual their symptoms are to be matched with the patients' symptoms. Therefore, importance is given to the symptomatology than the diagnosis. By treating in this way, the natural defence mechanism (Immunity) of the individual is strengthened and recurrence of the disease is curtailed.

In deciding the treatment, the Homoeopathic practitioner follows the well-known principles of 'Similia Similibus Curentur'. In simple terms it means let the similar substance which can produce specific symptoms in a healthy individual cure those similar symptoms in a sick individual, although the symptoms have arisen from another cause i.e. Bacteria, virus etc.,

The cure is based on the assumption that the patient is extremely sensitive to that particular remedy and only to that remedy which can produce his/her symptomatology. Homoeopathy has a definite and effective treatment for some disease such as Diabetes, Arthritis, Bronchial Asthma, Epilepsy, Skin Eruption, Allergic conditions and Mental or Emotional disorders. Even, some surgical disease gets cured in Homoeopathy with out undergoing surgery.

Thus the sick person after taking treatment not only gets cured of his disease, but simultaneously regains a perfect state of health.

Advent of Homoeopathy in India

Homoeopathic system of treatment was first introduced in India in 1839 by Dr. J. M. Honigberger. During his visit to India, he cured Maharaja Ranjit Singh of Punjab. The Homoeopathic system of treatment spread successfully among all sections of the people. This system of treatment is economical and the medicines have no side effects.

HOME REMEDIES - SIDDHA, AYURVEDA & UNANI

Siddha

Fever: For ordinary fever and intermittent fever the following decoction may be administered:-

Preparation: Take Nilavembu (Chiratta) leaves two handful add 2 glass of water boil and reduce to 50ml. and filter.

Dose: 1/2 glass 2 times or 3 times a day

If fever is accompanied with bodyache, 2 piece of Arathai (Galanga the lesser), one teaspoon of MILAGU (pepper) and 2 piece of CHUKKU (Dry Ginger) may be added for the above preparation. But the quantity of water to be increased proportionately.

If cough is present with fever, 10 Nos of Adathodai leaves (ADATHODA VASICA) may be added with the preparation.

Cough

(a) Take three leaves of Adathodai (ADATHODA VASICA) cut them into small pieces, and put the pieces into a vessel, add two teaspoon full of honey and fry the content until some pleasant smell comes. At that stage add the following coarsely powdered Athimathuram (Jamaica liquorice) 1 piece Thippli (Piper longum) 1 pinch Thalisapathri (Flucourtia calaphracta) 1/2 gm., Chitharathai (galanga the lesser) 3 piece then add 4 glasses of water and boil, reduce to 1/2 glass. Dose: 1/2 glass two times a day.

(b) Take 2 glasses of water. Add the following drugs, Adathodai leaves (Adathoda Vasica) three numbers, Kandankathiri leaves (Solanum Xanthocarpum) five numbers. Thulasi (holy basil) leaves five numbers Thoothuvalai (Trilobatum) leaves ten numbers and 3 gms., of Athimathuram (Jamaica liquorice) after roughly powdering them boil and reduce into 1/2 glass.
Dose: 1/2 glass two times a day with honey.

(c) 10 gms., of the root of Thoothuvalai (Trilobatum), grind with Cow's milk and to be taken in the morning.

(d) Adathodai leaves juice 30 ml. (ADATHODA VASICA), Finely powdered Milagu (pepper) 6 gms., Perugayam (asafoetida) 1 gm. mixed all and take in the morning and evening.

(e) For Chronic cough, it will give relief when 2 gms., of chooranam (powder) which is made out of equal quantity of Kadukkai (Chebulic myrobolan, Ink nut) and "Thippli" (Piper longum) is administered in honey twice daily.

Ayurveda

Pyrexia (Fever)

1. Decoction of Parpataka herb (parpadakapul) 1/4 tumbler relieves pyrexia.
2. Tinospora (Seenthikodi) decoction with some black pepper powder will relieve chronic fevers -1/4 tumbler & 1/4 tea spoon respectively.
3. Sacred basil leaf (tulasi) juice and Leucus (tumbai) leaf juice along with some black pepper will cure periodic fevers—two teaspoon each and 1/4 tea spoon respectively.

Coughs

1. Take the decoction of Adhatoda roots with some honey and powder of long pepper-1/4 tumbler with 1/4 tea spoon and one teaspoon honey.
2. Ginger juice with honey is also a good remedy—1/2 teaspoon juice with one teaspoon honey.
3. Take about 1 pinch of Chebulic myrobalan (Kadukkai) powder with some honey or equal quantity of liquor ice root powder (Athimadhuram). It cures cough with inflamed throat.
4. Leucus Leaf (tumbai) juice with honey is useful in whooping cough 1/2 teaspoonful with 1/2 teaspoon honey.

Diarrhoea

1. Take the pulp of Bael fruit (bilva) along with some sugar to relieve Diarrhoeas accompanied by stomach ache—1 tea spoon.
2. Mix equal volumes of yellow wood sorrel leaf (puliyarai) juice and butter milk and boil. Add 1/4 tea spoon of Ajowan (omam) powder. It cures diarrhoeas and dysentery 2 teaspoon.
3. Take powdered nut gall (masikkai) and mix with some honey 1/4 tea spoon. Three doses will cure diarrhoes and dysentery in children.
4. Take Nutmeg (Jadikkai) and tender mango leaves in equal parts by weight and make decoction. This is to be given with honey 2 teaspoon.
5. Powder of nut grass tubers (korai Kizhangu) and Aswagand tubers (amukara kizhangu) in equal quantity is given with honey—1 teaspoon.
6. Long pepper (arisitippili) ground with milk is to be given for three days to treat chronic dysentery—1/2 tea spoon.

Emesis (Vomiting)

1. Take powdered coriander (daniya) or cardamom (elakkai) with tender coconut water —1/2 tea spoon..
2. Give some quantity of coriander powder with rice washed water and sugar candy to cure morning sickness— 1 tea spoon in 1/4 tumbler

Constipation

1. Take castor (amanakku) root decoction with cow's milk and sugar in the morning in empty stomach—Each 1/4 tumbler.
2. Grind castor root with some butter into fine paste, Apply a little on the tongue of infants to relieve constipation—1pinch.

Emaciation and Weakness: Take equal 2 tea spoon powder of Aswagant roots with some milk and sugar or with gingelly oil. Regular in take will remove fatigue and weakness and it is an anabolic.

Tooth Ache

1. Use long pepper powder with some guggulu glu for brushing and cleaning the teeth.
2. Grind Fenugreek seeds (vendayam) with egg albumin into a fine paste and apply on the cheek (2 tea spoon.).
3. Gargle with ginger juice mixed with honey
4. Gargle with a decoction of drum stick root juice and Mustard 1/2 tumbler. (2 tea spoon Mustard).

Head Ache

1. Grind cleaning nut (tetrankotai) in egg albumin and apply externally.

COFFEE

Coffee is prepared by roasting and then grinding up the ingredients, or sometimes by decoction. It is normally stored as a powder or as granules. This is dropped directly into the hot water. Some preparations dissolve completely, while others remain partly solid, giving the drink a gritty texture.

Where the coffee remains gritty, it must be left to infuse before drinking. To avoid the gritty texture, a machine such as a coffee percolator or French press may be used.

Generic Western Coffee is the roasted seeds of either Coffea arabica or Coffea canephora. Its properties are similar to the generic tea plant Camelia Sinensis, but it has about twice as much caffeine, a richer, mellower taste, and different additives. The roasting process eliminates caffeine, and (like tea) the darker the coffee, the less caffeine it contains. When coffee is scarce, people often drink coffee substitutes.

Herbal teas include many of the coffee substitutes, and others; but they are used here for a wide range of properties, rather than merely to simulate the taste of coffee.

Herbal Tinctures

Steeping a medicinal plant in alcohol extracts the alcohol-soluble principles into a liquid form that can be stored for long periods. Different concentrations of alcohol are used to extract different constituents of the plants. For example; resins require high alcohol content and sugars usually require low alcohol content for optimal extraction. There are many schools of thought about tincture making. In the traditional view an herb is either steeped once (single maceration) or more than once. In a double maceration the mark (or used plant material) is removed and replaced by a new batch (using the same alcohol) thus increasing the strength of the tincture. Sometimes the mark is then ashed (burnt until ash) and added back in which increase the amount of some minerals in the tincture.

In the scientific model tincture strengths are measured by a ratio of herb to alcohol (1:5 and 1:2 are the most common where the 1:2 is the stronger tincture). Many tinctures use a combination of vegetable glycerine and alcohol to extract which changes the compounds that are extracted. Herbalists often mix several herbal tinctures to form an individualized prescription for each patient.

Plant tinctures are also the basis for many homeopathic medicines. Herbal medicine and homeopathic medicine should not be confused with one another as they are very different. For a step by step instruction on how to make & use herbal tinctures visit the article series, Be Your Own Herbal Expert- How to Make Tinctures.

Fluid Extracts

Fluid extracts are stronger than herbal tinctures, and can be preserved with alcohol or glycerin. They are just highly concentrated tinctures, made by distilling off some of the alcohol used in the tincture process. The final result is a liquid plant compound that can be 40 times more potent than a tincture.

Note: glycerates are herbal extracts that use glycerin as the sole extractant. They are very different and often have completely different medicinal properties than alcohol extracts. Tinctures or fluid extracts that are alcohol free should have the alcohol removed after the extraction process and replaced with glycerin which then acts just as the preservative.

Solid Extracts

Solid extracts are made from tinctures just like fluid extracts, but the entire solvent is separated from the plant compound, leaving a soft paste-like solid exract or a dry solid extract that is often as much as 400 times more potent than tinctures. Solid extracts can be diluted back to either fluid extracts or tinctures.

Many solid extracts are made in the way that apple butter is made, by simply cooking the plant material and water slowly over low heat until it forms a paste. Sometimes these are sold with a preservative added (glycerine is the most common), and sometimes they need to be refrigerated when they are opened (like apple butter).

Herbal Poultices

Poultices are a solid, vegetable fat-based mixture used externally. They have the shortest life span of any herbal remedy and must be made fresh for every use.

Poultices can be made with water or just fresh ground herb. They are applied topically often in conjunction with a heat source (hot water bottle or heating pad). They are used mostly (but not exclusively) for a localized injury (sprains, strains, scrapes, burns, bruises or cuts). They are excellent for hiking injuries (where there are usually plants and not pharmacies), but can be used for many other things.

Powdered Herbs and Tablets

Herbs that are dried and (usually) certain parts are separated out then ground to a powder fine consistency. Powdered matter can then be compressed or put in an empty capsule to form a tablet. Most tablets these days are made from some form of concentrated extract and not just plain herbal powders. This method is optimal for foul tasting herbs, highly concentrated forms and for travelling.

Powders are also used simply in their powdered form. Many Chinese medicine practitioners use powdered herbs as a base for making teas. Powdered herbs are also used topically as powders where dry skin is advantageous (some diaper rashes respond bettered to powdered herbs than ointments).

Herbal Ointments

An ointment or salve is a semi-solid preparation made to be applied to the skin. Depending on the purpose for which it is designed and its method of preparation, the texture can vary from very greasy to a thick paste.

Most ointments use vegetable oils (olive and almond are common) in conjunction with a thickener like bees wax. The herbs are often extracted in the oils for months before they are ready to be made into an ointment. The herb is then removed from the oil and it is slowly heated with bees wax to form the desired consistency. Vitamin E and essential oils are often used to preserve the salve or ointment.

The simplest ointments use petroleum jelly as a base. In traditional ointments, a combination of carrier oils is used that helps them to be absorbed through the skin, plus hardening agents to create the desired texture.

Essential Oils

Extraction of volatile liquid plant materials and other aromatic compounds from plants gives essential oils. These plant oils may be used internally in some forms of herbal medicine as well as in aromatherapy and generally for their perfume, although their medicinal use as a natural treatment (alternative medicine) has proved highly efficacious in the treatment of headache and muscle pain, joint pain and certain skin diseases.

Herbal Supplements

Herbal supplements tend to be commercial products in tablet or capsule form manufactured and marketed by the health food industry for sale in retail outlets to the general public, although there are some types that are sold only to healthcare practitioners for prescription. Herbal supplements are often standardized to contain stated levels of active phytochemicals. Standardization can be done in a number of different ways. Many companies extract the supposedly active constituents and add them back into a base like rice fiber.

This is no longer an herbal preparation as the whole herb is no longer present. Some companies follow the same procedure but add the extracted constituent to whole powdered herb. Some companies simply concentrate their whole herb until the desired constituent concentration is reached.

Many herbalists do not agree with the extraction/standardization of active ingredients, preferring instead to use the whole plant.

Examples of Herbal Medicine

The following text needs to be harmonized with text in the article List of medicinal herbs. There are hundreds of herbal remedies. An experienced practitioner can offer a comprehensive holistic approach to health. Examples of some commonly used herbal medicines:

- Artichoke and several other plants reduced total serum cholesterol levels in preliminary studies.

- Black cohosh and other plants that contain phytoestrogens (plant molecules with estrogen activity) have some benefits for treatment of symptoms resulting from menopause.
- Echinacea extracts limit the length of colds in some clinical trials, although some studies have found it to have no effect at lower dosages than are normally given by herbalists.
- Garlic lowers total cholesterol levels, mildly reduces blood pressure, reduces platelet aggregation, and has antibacterial properties. It also has strong anti-viral and anti-fungal properties.
- Grapefruit seed extract as a natural antimicrobial has minimal effectiveness as an anti-bacterial, anti-parasitic, and anti-fungal herb.
- Nigella sativa (Black cumin) is a general medicinal plant used for diverse ailments such as cough, pulmonary infections, asthma, influenza, allergy, hypertension and stomach ache. The seeds are considered carminative, stimulant, diuretic and galactogogue. It is often taken with honey. Seed powder or oil is externally applied for eruptions of skin.
- Pawpaw used for insecticidal purposes (killing lice, worms), as well as cancer treatment and viral infections.
- Peppermint tea for problems with the digestive tract, including irritable bowel syndrome and nausea.
- Rauvolfia Serpentina, used extensively in India for sleeplessness, anxiety, and high blood pressure. The first proven allopathic medicine for high blood pressure was extracted from this herb.
- St. John's wort, has yielded positive results, proving more effective than a placebo for the treatment of mild to moderate depression in some clinical trials.
- Valerian root can be used to treat insomnia.
- Lemon juice or apple cider vinegar can be used to treat acne.
- Green tea can heal scars faster.
- Lemon grass can lower cholesterol.
- Honey can be a solution for cholesterol.

Risks and Benefits

A common misconception about herbalism and the use of "natural" products in general, is that "natural" equals safe. However many plants have chemical defence mechanisms against predators that can have adverse or lethal effects on humans. Examples are poison hemlock and nightshade, which can be deadly, although they are not sold as herbs. Herbs can also have undesirable side-effects just as pharmaceutical products can. These problems are exacerbated by lack of control over dosage and purity. Furthermore, if given in conjunction with drugs, there is danger of 'summation', where the herb and the drug have similar actions and add together to make an 'overdose'. In animals, there are other dangers. There may be residues in food from farm animals (e.g. eggs, milk, meat) or danger of 'doping' in competition animals. The latter may also apply to human athletes.

There is a danger that herbal remedies will be used in place of other medical treatments which have been scientifically tested for safety and efficacy, resulting in the development or worsening of a medical condition which could have been better prevented or treated. There is also a danger that an herbal remedy may itself cause harm which is unanticipated due to a lack of a full understanding of its composition and biochemical effects. In the UK, the profession's governing bodies such as The College of Phytotherapy Practitioners and The National Institute of Medical Herbalists offer membership, education and certification. A qualified Herbalist will have studied for four years and passed exams in botanical and medical subjects. He or she will be expected to have the required knowledge to prescribe and dispense herbs tailored to the individual, taking into account their medical history and any other medication.

Effectiveness

As noted above, there have been scientific studies which show that certain plant products can cure or prevent certain diseases. The gold standard for pharmaceutical testing is repeated, large-scale, randomized, double-blind tests. Some plant products or pharmaceutical drugs derived from them are incorporated into mainstream medicine. To recoup the considerable costs of testing to the regulatory standards, the substances are patented by pharmaceutical companies and sold for high profit. Pharmaceutical firms argue that the regulations protect public safety. Cynics point out that they have a secondary effect of setting a high financial barrier to competition.

Most herbal traditions have accumulated knowledge without modern scientific controls to distinguish between the placebo effect, the body's natural ability to heal itself, and the actual benefits of the herbs themselves.

Many herbs have shown positive results in in-vitro, animal model or small-scale clinical tests. The few randomized, double-blind tests that receive attention in mainstream medical publications are often questioned on methodological grounds or interpretation. Studies tend to carry more weight if they are performed in the same country as the medical scientists evaluating them. Likewise, studies published in wide circulation magazines such as JAMA receive more consideration than those published in specialized herbal journals.

Fortunately there is now much scientific research into the action and effectiveness of herbal remedies and many are justifying their traditional use. High quality trials involving proper controls and double blind methods are being increasingly carried out, with many useful results.

Herbalists tend to use parts of plants, such as the roots or leaves but not isolate particular phytochemicals. They argue that the synergy of the combined substances enhances the efficacy and dilutes toxicity. Western medicine on the other hand prefers single ingredients on the grounds that dosage can be more easily quantified. Dosage is in general an outstanding issue for herbal treatments: while most conventional medicines are heavily tested to determine the most effective and safest dosages (especially in relation to things like body weight, drug interactions, etc.), there are few established dosage standards for various herbal treatments on the market. Furthermore, herbal medicines taken in whole form cannot generally guarantee a consistent dosage or drug quality (since certain samples may contain more or less of a given active ingredient).

The issue of regulation is an area of continuing controversy in the EU and USA. On one end of the spectrum, some herbalists and consumers maintain that traditional remedies that have a long history of use do not require the level of safety testing as xenobiotics or single ingredients in an artificially concentrated form. On the other hand, others are in favour of legally enforced quality standards, safety testing and prescription by a qualified practitioner.

Some professional herbalist organizations have made statements calling for a category of regulation for herbal products. Yet others agree with the need for more quality testing but believe it can be managed through reputation without government intervention. Clearly the full debate involves issues of politics, economics and the role of government that are beyond the scope of this article.

Name Confusion

The common names of herbs (folk taxonomy) may not reflect differences in scientific taxonomy, and the same (or a very similar) common name might group together different plant species with different effects. For example, in 1993 in Belgium, in a formula created by medical doctors including some TCM herbs for weight loss, one herb (Stephania tetrandra) was swapped for another (Aristolochia fangchi) whose name in Chinese was extremely similar but which contained higher levels of a renal toxin, aristolochic acid; this quid pro quo resulted in 105 cases of kidney damage.

Note that neither herb used in a TCMcontext would be used for weight loss or given for long periods of time. In Chinese medicine these herbs are used for certain forms of acute arthritis and edema.

Standards and Quality Control

The legal status of herbal ingredients varies by country. For example, Ayurvedic herbal products may contain levels of heavy metals that are considered unsafe in the U.S., but heavy metals are considered therapeutic in Ayurvedic medicine. In the United States, most herbal remedies are regulated as dietary supplements. Many herbs for home use could also be grown in a small home garden.

In the UK, herbal remedies that are bought over the counter are regulated as supplements,as in the US. However, herbal remedies prescribed and dispensed by a qualified Medical Herbalist, after a personal consultation, are regulated as medicines. A Medical Herbalist can prescribe some herbs which are not available over the counter, covered by Schedule III of the Medicines Act, for example. Forthcoming changes to laws regulating Herbal products in the UK, are intended to ensure the quality of herbal products used. Most Medical Herbalists will be using herbal products from a supplier who already meets these standards.

Medical Interaction

In consultation with a physician, usage of herbal remedies should be clarified, as some herbal remedies have the potential to cause adverse drug interactions when used in combination with various prescription and over-the-counter pharmaceuticals. Dangerously low blood pressure may result from the combination of an herbal remedy that lowers blood pressure together with prescription medicine that has the same effect. In particular, many herbs should be avoided during pregnancy. However, most herbal books alert the reader to necessary precautions.

Not all physicians may be familiar with the effects of different types of herbal medicine, but general practitioners should be able to refer patients to a specialist, or investigate the medical literature on their behalf. A qualified Medical Herbalist, however, will be familiar with most commonly used medical drugs and their modes of action and therefore will only prescribe herbal remedies which will not interfere with these.

MEDICINAL PLANTS AND PHYTOMEDICINES

The past decade has witnessed a tremendous resurgence in the interest and use of medicinal plant products, especially in North America. Surveys of plant medicinal usage by the American public have shown an increase from just about 3% of the population in 1991 to over 37% in 1998 (Brevoort, 1998).

The North American market for sales of plant medicinals has climbed to about $3 billion/year (Glaser, 1999). Once the domain of health-food and specialty stores, phytomedicines have clearly re-emerged into the mainstream as evidenced by their availability for sale at a wide range of retail outlets, the extent of their advertisement in the popular media, and the recent entrance of several major pharmaceutical companies into the business of producing phytomedicinal products (Brevoort, 1998; Glaser, 1999). No doubt a major contributing factor to this great increase in phytomedicinal use in the United States has been the passing of federal legislation in 1994 (Dietary Supplement Health and Education Act or "DSHEA") that facilitated the production and marketing of phytomedicinal products (Brevoort, 1998).

The past decade has also witnessed intense interest in "nutraceuticals" (or "functional foods") in which phytochemical constituents can have long-term health promoting or medicinal qualities. Although the distinction between medicinal plants and nutraceuticals can sometimes be vague, a primary characteristic of the latter is that nutraceuticals have a nutritional role in the diet and the benefits to health may arise from long-term use as foods (i.e.

chemoprevention) (Korver, 1998). In contrast, many medicinal plants exert specific medicinal actions without serving a nutritional role in the human diet and may be used in response to specific health problems over short- or long-term intervals.

For many of the medicinal plants of current interest, a primary focus of research to date has been in the areas of phytochemistry, pharmacognosy, and horticulture. In the area of phytochemistry, medicinal plants have been characterized for their possible bioactive compounds, which have been separated and subjected to detailed structural analysis. Research in the pharmacognosy of medicinal plants has also involved assays of bio-activity, identification of potential modes of action, and target sites for active phytomedicinal compounds. Horticultural research on medicinal plants has focused on developing the capacity for optimal growth in cultivation.

This has been especially pertinent as many medicinal plants are still harvested in the wild, and conditions for growth in cultivation have not been optimized. Wild harvesting of medicinal plants can be problematic in terms of biodiversity loss, potential variation in medicinal plant quality, and occasionally, improper plant identification with potential tragic consequences.

From the perspective of plant physiology, extensive opportunities exist for basic research on medicinal plants and the study of their phytomedicinal chemical production. This review presents a discussion on some fundamental aspects of phytomedicinal chemical production by plant cells with an overview of several medicinal plants that have received considerable use and attention over the past decade.

PRODUCTS INVOLVED IN PLANT ECOPHYSIOLOGY

The beneficial medicinal effects of plant materials typically result from the combinations of secondary products present in the plant. That the medicinal actions of plants are unique to particular plant species or groups is consistent with this concept as the combinations of secondary products in a particular plant are often taxonomically distinct (Wink, 1999). This is in contrast to primary products, such as carbohydrates, lipids, proteins, heme, chlorophyll, and nucleic acids, which are common to all plants and are involved in the primary metabolic processes of building and maintaining plant cells (Kaufman et al., 1999; Wink, 1999).

Although plant secondary products have historically been defined as chemicals that do not appear to have a vital biochemical role in the process of building and maintaining plant cells, recent research has shown a pivotal role of these chemicals in the ecophysiology of plants. Accordingly, secondary products have both a defensive role against herbivory, pathogen attack, and inter-plant competition and an attractant role toward beneficial organisms such as pollinators or symbionts (Kaufman et al., 1999; Wink and Schimmer, 1999). Plant secondary products also have protective actions in relation to abiotic stresses such as those associated with changes in temperature, water status, light levels, UV exposure, and mineral nutrients (Kaufman et al., 1999). Furthermore, recent work has indicated potential roles of secondary products at the cellular level as plant growth regulators, modulators of gene expression, and in signal transduction (Kaufman et al., 1999).

Although secondary products can have a variety of functions in plants, it is likely that their ecological function may have some bearing on potential medicinal effects for humans. For example, secondary products involved in plant defense through cytotoxicity toward microbial pathogens could prove useful as antimicrobial medicines in humans, if not too toxic. Likewise, secondary products involved in defense against herbivores through neurotoxin activity could have beneficial effects in humans (i.e. as antidepressants, sedatives, muscle relaxants, or anesthetics) through their action on the central nervous system.

To promote the ecological survival of plants, structures of secondary products have evolved to interact with molecular targets affecting the cells, tissues, and physiological functions in competing microorganisms, plants, and animals. In this respect, some plant secondary products may exert their action by resembling endogenous metabolites, ligands, hormones, signal transduction molecules, or neurotransmitters and thus have beneficial medicinal effects on humans due to similarities in their potential target sites (e.g. central nervous system, endocrine system, etc.) (Kaufman et al., 1999). As noted by Wink (1999), the development of structural similarity between plant secondary products and the endogenous substances of other organisms could be termed "evolutionary molecular modeling."

THE BENEFITS OF PHYTOMEDICINES

In contrast to synthetic pharmaceuticals based upon single chemicals, many phytomedicines exert their beneficial effects through the additive or synergistic action of several chemical compounds acting at single or multiple target sites associated with a physiological process. As pointed out by Tyler (1999), this synergistic or additive pharmacological effect can be beneficial by eliminating the problematic side effects associated with the predominance of a single xenobiotic compound in the body. In this respect, Kaufman et al. (1999) extensively documented how synergistic interactions underlie the effectiveness of a number of phytomedicines. This theme of multiple chemicals acting in an additive or synergistic manner likely has its origin in the functional role of secondary products in promoting plant survival. For example, in the role of secondary products as defense chemicals, a mixture of chemicals having additive or synergistic effects at multiple target sites would not only ensure effectiveness against a wide range of herbivores or pathogens but would also decrease the chances of these organisms developing resistance or adaptive responses (Kaufman et al., 1999; Wink, 1999).

A PERSPECTIVE ON FIVE MEDICINAL PLANTS

Of the vast number of medicinal plants used in Western and non-Western medical approaches, a small number have received considerable interest and use in North America over the past few years. What follows is an overview of five medicinal plants of current interest focusing on their biochemical characteristics and pharmacological actions of their plant secondary product chemicals.

Ginseng

The name "ginseng" often leads to some confusion due to its use for different plants with different phytochemical constituents. True ginsengs are plants in the genus Panax from which Asian ginseng (Panax ginseng) and American ginseng (Panax quinquefolium) have received the most interest for phytomedicinal use (Bruneton, 1995; Schulz et al., 1998; Attele et al., 1999).

These plants are low-growing perennial shade plants that generate a bulky storage root that is used medicinally. However, Eleutherococcus senticosis, a completely different plant not even in the genus Panax, is sometimes referred to as Russian or Siberian "ginseng." Roots from this shrubby tree, native to regions of Siberia and Northern China, were studied in the former Soviet Union as a substitute for Asian ginseng (Bruneton, 1995; Schulz et al., 1998).

Interest in the use of ginseng and Eleutherococcus sp. comes from their purported "adaptogen" or "tonic" activities. Such activities are thought to increase the body's capacity to tolerate external stresses, leading to increased physical or mental performance (Schulz et al., 1998).

Although an extensive literature documenting adaptogenic effects in laboratory animal systems exists, results from human clinical studies are conflicting and variable (Schulz et al., 1998; Attele et al., 1999; Huang, 1999; World Health Organization, 1999). However, there is evidence that extracts of ginseng and Eleutherococcus sp. can have an immunostimulatory effect in humans, and this may contribute to the adaptogen or tonic effects of these plants (Schulz et al., 1998; World Health Organization, 1999; Blumenthal et al., 2000).

The major secondary products present in ginseng roots are an array of triterpene saponins, collectively called ginsenosides (Dewick, 1997; Huang, 1999). The ginsenosides are glycosylated derivatives of two major aglycones, panaxadiol and panaxatriol (Bruneton, 1995; Dewick, 1997). At present, 30 ginsenosides have been identified of which the ginsenosides, Rb1, Rb2, Rc, Rd, Re, Rf, Rg1, and Rg2 are considered to be the most relevant for pharmacological activity (Bruneton, 1995; Dewick, 1997; World Health Organization, 1999). Different ginseng species have different proportions of ginsenosides in root tissue, and this may relate to reported differences in the pharmacological properties of these plant materials (Attele et al., 1999). Moreover, within a particular ginseng species, levels of particular ginsenosides can also be affected by environmental factors such as soil mineral nutrient supply (Li and Mazza,

1999). From laboratory studies, it has been suggested that the pharmacological target sites for these compounds involve the hypothalamus-pituitary-adrenal axis due to the observed effects upon serum levels of adrenocorticotropic hormone and corticosterone (Huang, 1999). However, it should also be noted that the overall effects of the ginsenosides can be quite complex due to their potential for multiple actions even within a single tissue (Attele et al., 1999).

Although extracts of Eleutherococcus sp. roots have been reported to have similar effects as the ginsenosides in animal systems, the active constituents may be quite different (Dewick, 1997). In Eleutherococcus sp., the active constituents are thought to be lignan-glycosides (eleutheroside E) or phenylpropane glycosides (eleutheroside B) (Bruneton, 1995; Dewick, 1997). However, the pharmacological action of these compounds remains unclear, and little information is available on their biosynthetic pathway (Dewick, 1997 and refs. therein).

St. John's Wort

The use of St. John's wort (Hypericum perforatum) for depression has its origins in the medical traditions of Europe well before the 1600s (Upton, 1998). In Germany, St. John's wort is currently one of the most widely used prescription medications for depression and is also extensively used in the United States as a non-prescription botanical supplement (Schulz et al., 1998; Upton, 1998). For the botanical medicine, the aerial portion of the plant is harvested and dried just after flowering, and then an alcohol/water extract is produced (Schulz et al., 1998; Upton, 1998 and refs. therein; Blumenthal et al., 2000).

Naphthodianthrones such as hypericin and pseudohypericin are predominant components in St. John's wort extracts, and most St. John's wort phytomedicines are currently standardized according to their hypericin content (Schulz et al., 1998; Upton, 1998). These chemicals are localized in dark glandular structures mainly located on the margins of St. John's wort leaves and flower petals and appear to serve in the defense against insect herbivory (Fornasiero et al., 1998). Although there is some evidence that biosynthesis of St. John's wort naphthodianthrones involves the polyketide pathway, few details are known (Dewick, 1997; Nahrstedt and Butterwick, 1997 and refs. therein).

The production of napthodianthrones in St. John's wort can be influenced by environmental factors such as light and soil mineral nutrients (Upton, 1998). There is strong evidence that hypericin and pseudohypericin contribute to the antidepressant action of St. John's wort, but it is unclear if this is associated with its activity as a monoamine oxidase inhibitor (Nahrstedt and Butterwick, 1997; Upton, 1998). Inhibition of monoamine oxidase is one mechanism by which some antidepressants operate to increase levels of neurotransmitters such as serotonin, norepinephrine, or dopamine (Schulz et al., 1998).

The prenylated phloroglucinol derivative, hyperforin, can also be a predominant component in extracts of the flowers and leaves of St. John's wort, and there is recent evidence that this phytochemical contributes to the plant's antidepressant action (Schulz et al., 1998). In human clinical studies, the hyperforin content in St. John's wort extracts correlated with the level of antidepressant action (Laakman et al., 1998).

This chemical appears to block synaptic re-uptake of serotonin, dopamine, and norepinephrine (Chatterjee et al., 1998). Blocking neurotransmitter re- uptake elevates their synaptic concentration. This represents another mechanism by which synthetic antidepressants may operate (Schulz et al., 1998). Whereas hyperforin also has antibacterial activity (Upton, 1998), it is uncertain as to whether or not this compound is effective in defense functions for the plant.

Ginkgo (Ginkgo biloba)

Ginkgo is the last living relative of a primitive family of gymnosperms (Ginkgoaceae); all other species exist only as fossils (Bruneton, 1995). Ginkgo trees are used as ornamentals worldwide due to their hardiness and appearance. Although the therapeutic use of ginkgo dates back about 2,000 years in traditional Chinese medicine, most medical applications only involved use of the seeds (Huang, 1999).

However, the phytomedicine used today is based upon acetone extraction of the fan-shaped leaves and a further purification of active constituents (Schulz et al., 1998). Clinical studies have supported the effectiveness of ginkgo in improving peripheral and cerebrovascular circulation (Dewick, 1997; Schulz et al., 1998; Huang, 1999; Blumenthal et al., 2000). A major use of ginkgo is in the management of cognitive decline associated with disturbances in brain blood circulation (i.e. vascular insufficiency dementia) that can occur in the elderly (Schulz et al., 1998 and refs. therein; Blumenthal et al., 2000). In addition, ginkgo extracts are useful in the treatment of tinnitus, vertigo, and for improving circulation in the legs (Schulz et al., 1998 and refs. therein). However, it should be noted that the effectiveness of ginkgo extracts in improving the cognitive performance of young healthy individuals is less certain.

The active constituents present in extracts of ginkgo leaves have been shown to be a mixture of terpene lactones and flavonoids (Bruneton, 1995; Dewick, 1997). Most commercial preparations of ginkgo are leaf extracts standardized to approximately 5% to 7% terpene lactones and 22% to 27% flavonoids (Dewick, 1997; World Health Organization, 1999; Blumenthal et al., 2000).

The prominent terpene lactones in ginkgo extracts are ginkgolides A, B, C, J, M, and bilobalide. Although the ginkgolides are considered to be diterpenes, and bilobalide is considered to be a sesquiterpene, the latter compound most likely represents a product of ginkgolide metabolism (Dewick, 1997). Studies by Cartayrade et al. (1997) have shown that although ginkgo leaves represent sites of ginkgolide (and bilobalide) accumulation, biosynthesis of these compounds takes place in the roots.

Moreover, these authors demonstrated that for ginkgolides A to C, biosynthesis occurs in a sequential manner (ginkgolide A ginkgolide B ginkgolide C) through successive addition of hydroxyl groups (Cartayrade et al., 1997).

Pharmacological studies have demonstrated that the ginkgolides (especially ginkgolide B) represent potent antagonists of platelet activating factor, a bioregulatory molecule involved in blood platelet activation and inflammatory processes (Dewick, 1997; Schulz et al., 1998; Huang, 1999). The flavonoids present in ginkgo extracts exist primarily as glycosylated derivatives of kaempferol and quercetin (Bruneton, 1995; Dewick, 1997; World Health Organization, 1999; Blumenthal et al., 2000). These flavonoid glycosides have been shown to be extremely effective free-radical scavengers (Dewick, 1997; Schulz et al., 1998; Huang, 1999). It is believed that the collective action of these components leads to a reduction in damage and improved functioning of the blood vessels (Schulz et al., 1998; Huang, 1999; World Health Organization, 1999).

Kava

The use of Kava originated in the "Oceana" island communities encompassed by Polynesia, Melanesia, and Micronesia (Singh and Blumenthal, 1997). In these cultures "Kava" (also known as "Kava-Kava," "Ava," and "Awa") refers to an intoxicating beverage used in rituals and ceremonies, which is produced from the mashed rhizome and roots of the woody shrub, Piper methysticum. However, Kava is now used as the common name for P. methysticum as well as the phytomedicine produced from root/rhizome extracts. Worldwide, Kava is receiving considerable attention for its use as a treatment for anxiety, nervous tension, agitation, and/or insomnia. Clinical studies have shown an effectiveness of Kava that is comparable with sedatives such as benzodiazapines but without the development of either physical or psychological dependency (Singh and Blumenthal, 1997; Schulz et al., 1998).

From intensive chemical and pharmacological studies conducted on Kava root/rhizome extracts over the past century, several key active constituents have been identified (Bruneton, 1995; Singh and Blumenthal, 1997). The pharmacological activity of this plant appears to be associated with a family of styrylpyrones called "kavapyrones" (or "kavalactones") that have effects on several neurotransmitter systems including those involving Gln, GABA, dopamine, and serotonin (Schulz et al., 1998).

Whereas the kavapyrones shown in represent the predominant pharmacologically active components in Kava root extracts, a total of 18 have been identified at present (He et al., 1997). These remaining kavapyrones appear to be derivatives of either kawain, yangonin, or dihydromethysticin (Bruneton, 1995; He et al., 1997). Although details regarding kavapyrone biosynthesis are still lacking, evidence from other systems such as Equisetum arvense gametophytes suggest that styrylpyrones may arise from a triketide produced by successive condensation of two malonyl-coenzyme A (CoA) molecules with a phenylpropanoid CoA-ester (Schroder, 1997 and references therein).

This is similar to reactions catalyzed by chalcone synthase except that two, rather than three, successive condensations involving malonyl CoA are involved. Recent studies have shown that kavapyrone levels in Kava roots are influenced by environmental factors. In cultivated Kava plants, kavapyrone levels appear to increase with irrigation and mineral nutrient supplementation and decrease with shading (Lebot et al., 1999). Moreover, varietal differences in Kava also appear to have a role in determining the overall level of kavapyrone production (Lebot et al., 1999).

It is quite interesting that Kava plants are sterile and plantation production involves propagation from stem cuttings (Singh and Blumenthal, 1997). From genetic studies, it has been suggested that Kava likely represents a sterile relative of Piper wichmannii (native to New Guinea), which became distributed across the South Pacific islands with human migration and through somatic mutation became sterile (Lebot et al., 1999 and references therein). Kava's sterility combined with its limited growth habitat range (South Pacific Tropics), time required for growth before root harvest (approximately 8 years), and high world demand have raised concerns about potential over harvesting. Although attempts have been made to grow Kava in tissue culture for propagation and possible in vitro phytochemical production, little success has been achieved (Taylor and Taufa, 1998).

Echinacea sp.

Although there are 11 species in the genus Echinacea, this term is typically used to describe a phytomedicine produced from the aerial portion of Echinacea purpurea cv Purple Coneflower, roots of Echinacea pallida cv Pale-Purple Coneflower, roots of Echinacea angustifolia cv Narrow-Leaf Coneflower, or a combination of these materials (World Health Organization, 1999; Blumenthal et al., 2000).

These plants are herbaceous perennials native to North America, and were originally used in Native American herbal traditions for wound healing, infections, and rattlesnake bite (Bruneton, 1995). Use of this phytomedicine was subsequently introduced to Europe in the early 1900s, and current interest lies in its use for colds, flu-like infections, and upper-respiratory infections (Schulz et al., 1998; World Health Organization, 1999).

The most well-studied and effective versions of this phytomedicine involve the expressed juice of the aerial portion of E. purpurea and an alcohol extract of E. angustifolia roots (World Health Organization, 1999). A number of studies suggest that Echinacea sp.-based phytomedicines may be beneficial in reducing the symptoms and perhaps duration of upper-respiratory infections

(Schulz et al., 1998 and references therein; World Health Organization, 1999).

Pharmacological studies (>350 to date) have provided strong evidence for effects of Echinacea sp extracts in modulating immune system capacity including stimulation of the phagocytic activity of human lymphocytes, stimulation of fibroblasts for new tissue production, increased respiration, and elevated mobility of leukocytes (Schulz et al., 1998; World Health Organization, 1999). Extracts of Echinacea sp. also appear to inhibit both tissue and bacterial hyaluronidase, and this action is thought to aid in localization of infection, preventing its spread to other regions of the body (World Health Organization, 1999 and refs. therein).

The immunostimulatory activity of Echinacea sp. preparations appears to result from the combined effects of a complex array of constituents: (a) a series of alkylamides as isobutylamides; (b) caffeic acid derivatives (cichoric acid, cynarin, echinacoside); (c) a series of polyalkynes (polyacetylenes); (d) a series of polyalkenes; and (e) high-Mr polysaccharides including heteroxylans (35,000 approximate Mr) and arabinorhamnogalactans (45,000 approximate Mr) (Bruneton, 1995; Schulz et al., 1998; World Health Organization, 1999). Pharmacological studies have shown effects of the alkylamides, polyalkynes, and caffeic acid derivatives in stimulating white blood cell phagocytosis (World Health Organization, 1999 and refs. therein; Blumenthal et al., 2000).

The high-Mr polysaccharide components also appear active in stimulating phagocytosis as well as promoting production of interferon (World Health Organization, 1999 and references therein). Furthermore, through their inhibitory effect on 5-lipoxygenase, the alkylamide constituents may provide anti-inflammatory activity. Although details regarding the biosynthetic pathways of these active constituents are unknown, the hydrocarbon portion of alkylamides and polyalkynes most likely represent desaturation products of long-chain fatty acids (e.g. oleic acid) shortened through -oxidation (for discussion of these processes, see Dewick, 1997). Chicoric acid, cynarin, and echinacoside most likely arise as conjugated products of caffeic acid generated through the shikimic acid pathway. Although factors influencing the biosynthetic pathways of these chemicals are unknown, it has been shown that the phytomedicinal content of Echinacea sp. can be affected by environmental conditions (soil nitrogen and potassium) and the developmental state of the plant (El-Gengaihi et al., 1998).

Currently, many Echinacea sp. phytomedicines are standardized according to their echinacoside content because this caffeic acid derivative is a marker chemical unique to Echinacea sp. However, such standardization does not consider the complex chemical interactions and possible synergistic effects necessary for the beneficial affects of this phytomedicine on humans.

CONCLUSIONS AND OUTLOOK

For the plant physiologist, work on medicinal plants opens up a wide range of research possibilities, and plant physiological studies would indeed have a major role to play in this burgeoning field. With only a few exceptions, many widely used medicinal plants have not received the extensive plant physiological characterization received by food crops or model plant systems. Although active phytochemicals may have been identified, in general, many pathways for the biosynthesis of specific medicinal compounds and the factors (biotic and abiotic) regulating their production remain unclear.

At present, a major concern with the use of phytomedicines regards the maintenance of consistent medicinal quality in botanical medicines (Matthews et al., 1999). Whereas the focus has tended to be on quality control in herbal manufacturing practices, variation in phytomedicinal content due to environmental effects upon secondary plant metabolism in the plant material could represent a significant factor. It is clear that understanding how environmental factors affect phytomedicinal production will be of great importance toward optimizing field growth conditions for maximal recovery of phytomedicinal chemicals.

In most cases, it is also unknown as to the extent to which levels of phytomedicinal chemical production by medicinal plants are determined by genetic potential versus environmental modulation. Here, the use of molecular markers (i.e. RFLP, random-amplified polymorphic DNA, and amplified fragment length polymorphism) in the characterization of medicinal plant populations for levels of phytomedicinal chemical production could prove useful for the analysis of traits and in selective breeding.

The use of molecular approaches and biotechnology could also have wide application and promise especially with regard to such topics as the modification of phytomedicinal chemical pathways. Production of medicinal chemicals in plants may be modified by overexpression, antisense expression, or cosupression of biosynthetic genes. Transgenic genes could also be introduced to modify existing pathways.

Mutational alterations and analysis could also be performed to dissect out basic components of metabolic pathways. The application of molecular approaches with medicinal plants would also benefit from the development of cell, tissue, and organ culture systems for in vitro growth and regeneration of medicinal plants. In addition, such tissue culture systems could also prove useful for large-scale biotechnological production of medicinal plant phytochemicals.

Overall, metabolic engineering could be useful for modifying or enhancing synthesis of valuable therapeutic agents present in medicinal plants. However, as the beneficial actions of medicinal plants can be related to combinations of phytochemicals acting collectively or synergistically, alteration of single phytochemical components could potentially affect the efficacy of a phytomedicine. In this respect, any work on modification of the phytomedicinal chemical composition of a medicinal plant through molecular methods would need to be conducted in conjunction with pharmacological studies on drug effectiveness.

Quality Control for India's Herbal Drugs

Ashwagandha (Withania somnifera) is often described as the Indian equivalent of ginseng - the Chinese medicinal plant that has captured a huge chunk of the global market. Yet the Indian herb is not a commercial success. One of the reasons for this is the lack of standards, which has led to a wide variation in the chemical composition of ashwagandha-based drugs. The discrepancy, detected during a recent study, occurs in herbal products of even reputable companies.

These drugs are portrayed as potent healers with a wide range of benefits like improving memory, cognition, stamina, vigour and resistance to diseases, as well as relieving tension and depression.

But experts feel that in view of the latest findings, a huge question mark hangs on the efficacy of these medicines.

The study was published in the February 2004 issue of Current Science, a journal brought out by the Indian Institute of Science, Bangalore. Entitled

'Phytochemical variability in commercial herbal products and preparations of Withania somnifera ', it was conducted by three institutes of the Council of Scientific and Industrial Research (CSIR) - the Central Institute of Medicinal and Aromatic Plants (çimap) and National Botanical Research Institute, both in Lucknow, and the Regional Research Laboratory in Jammu.

During the study, the amount of withaferin a - one of the withanolides of ashwagandha - was analysed in 10 products being sold in the market. Withanolides are secondary chemicals produced by the plant. The scientists assumed withaferin a to be an indicator of the presence of ashwagandha. They found that the amount of the chemical per gramme of ashwagandha varied from 100 per cent to merely 0.9 per cent. In nine of the products, the quantity was less than 50 per cent.

The research highlights these inconsistencies to underscore the importance of standardising herbal products. It also points out that the anomaly can only be corrected through stringent legislation, which doesn't exist in the country at present. Several factors like sources of raw materials, harvest and Post Harvest conditions, and processing and manufacturing techniques have to be regulated for controlling the quality of herbal products. But the Drugs and Cosmetics Act, 1940, which governs the herbal medicine industry, only lays emphasis on making drugs in clean factories and testing raw materials for genuineness.

G. S. Lavekar, director, Central Council for Research in Ayurveda and Siddha, under the Union ministry of health and family welfare, says: "Parameters such as chemical and biological markers should be set so that an acceptable range can be established for chemical constituents."

R. S. Sangwan of cimap, a member of the study team, suggests that ashwagandha should be marketed as a single plant product and not a traditional medicine where a combination of plants is used. While modern scientists are in favour of identifying active ingredients in herbal products and using them as medicines, conventional practitioners believe that such isolates cease to be traditional medicines.

The report has evoked a mixed response from the industry. Some companies are of the opinion that the laws should be strengthened. At the same time, there are others who claim their products are up to the mark. Paranjay Sharma, president of Shree Baidyanath Ayurved Bhawan Private Limited, says a manufacturer can only be penalised if standards exist. He feels quality control should be introduced in the production process at the raw material stage itself. Significantly, the good manufacturing practices that are stipulated currently do not deal with this aspect.

S. K. Mitra of Himalaya Drug Company says his company uses chemical indicators to ensure that even products in different batches conform to a uniform standard. Further, it conducts trials on humans to ensure the efficacy of the drugs. A senior representative of another manufacturer implicated in the study asserts: "The researchers did not find the withanolide because it could have been masked by other chemicals present in the product." Sharad Goel, spokesperson for Dabur, says: "We believe that the researchers should have estimated total withanolides, which is a widely accepted biological benchmark, for the purpose of comparing different products available in the market."

❐

Aromatic Plants

The aromatic plants possess odoriferous and volatile substances which occur as essential oils, gum exudate, balsam and oleoresin in one or more parts, viz. root, wood, bark, foliage, flower and fruit. The chemical nature of these aromatic substances may be due to a variety of complex the chemical compounds. Many of these aromatics are powerful germicides and have anti-bacterial properties, but the bulk of the produce finds use in perfumery and the food-flavouring industries. Amongst the two, the per-fumeru and allied industries consume much larger amounts of the natural fragrant material. According to the UN Word Statistics (1972), the annual world trade (excluding countries in eastern Europe) in essential oils and perfummery aromatics for 1969 was of the order of Rs 2250 million; also, a large quantity of the aromatic material of plant origin is utilized in cosmetics, toiletries and allied industries.

Our current volume of foreign trade in the perfumery material, essential oils and aromatic compounds is around Rs 65 million and this amount accounts for 1. 6 per cent of the world trade. Some sixty-two types of essential oils come to the international market with a large and consistent demand. However, our treatment of the aromatic plants is confined to a few more important essential-oil crops grown in the country.

The methods employed to obtain aromatic substances from plants are classified into distillation, enfleurage, maceration, expression and solvent extraction. Expect in the case of flowers crops, such as jasmine and kewara in which the fragrant constituents are likely to be decomposed or destroyed, the essential oils are mostly obtained by distilling the produce; in fact, steam distillation is the oldest method of separation of essential oils. The perfumery material is filled in a large-galvanizediron still over a perforated netal grid. Water is filled in the still below the level of the grid so that it generates a low-pressure steam on heating to pass through the material. The water vapours carry with it the essential oil of the perfumery material. These vapours are passed through a condenser and collected in a vessel where the oil is ecanted with a separating-funnel.

A simple field distillation unit could be fabricated by a skilled blacksmith. For more efficient and quick distillation of the produce; " steam distillation" units are employed. These units are built on the same principle except that live steam at 40-100 1b pressure per inch is injected into the filling-still through perforated coils and the distillation is completed in a shorter period. It has the advantages of handling a larger quantity of the material, besides improving upon the recovery of the essential oil.

As stated earlier, the solvent-extraction method is employed for the extractors are of two types, viz. stationary and rotatory types, and low- bowling solvents, like petroleum either, alcohol or benzen, are used for extracting the odoriferous principles. The stationary type extractors consists of vertical cylinders provided with type extractors consists of vertical cylinders provided with perforated metal grids arranged horizontally around a central vertical shaft. The flower crop is charged over the grids which come into constant with the solvent periodically and the essential oil is removed in successive washings. The rotatory type consists of an iron drum which rotates on a horizontal axis. The interior of the drum is divided with a perforated metal partition of holding floers and the solvent is filled in the lower part of the extractor. While the drum moves, the solvent seeps through the perforations and drips back, so that the essential oil is washed out to the solvent. This extract is than distilled in a vacuum still at a low temperature to recover the disolvant. The floral concentrate, thus obtained, also contains some waxes and plant pigments which are removed by treating with warm alcohol. The filtered solution, so obtained, is either used as such, or is concentrated in vaccum into a viscous oil.

LEMON GRASS (Cymbopogon flexuosus Stapf.). It is a stemless perennial grass, found wild in the southern states of India. The leaves yield an aromatic oil, containing 75-85 per cent citral. The oil is used in soaps, cosmetics and disinfectants and is a raw material for manufacturing ions and vitamin A. The crop is grown on about 390, 000 ha in Kerals and about 90 per cent of the produce is exported, earning about Rs 10 million in foreign exchange annually.

The crop is grown mainly as a rain-fed crop on poor marginal lands. It is a hardy drought-resistant plant and is grown under a wided range of climatic conditions. Two types are recognized : (1) the red-stemmed grass is the true lemon-grass and a selection 'OD-19' made at the Lemon Grass Research Station, Oodakkali (Kerala) is recommended for high yield, (2) the white-stemmed (var. albscens) yields oil or low citral content. The crop is best propagated through seed raised in nurseries; 10kg of the seed produces enough seedlings for planting a hectare. About 2-month-old seedlings are planted in rows, 40 to 15x 10 cm apart, during rains and the first harvest is ready after 90 days. In Kerala, 3 harvests are obtained in the first year and 4 to 5 harvests during each of the 3 to 5 succeeding years; the crop is cut after every 60 to 65 days, except during the dry season. The fields are mannered liberally with ash and spent grass (obtained after the distillation of the oil); farmers seldom apply inorganic fertilizers. The herbage contains 0. 35% oil on fresh-weight basis. The grass yield ranges from 18 to 25 tonnes per hectare, giving 60-72 kg of oil.

CITRONELLA GRASS (Cymobopogon winteriaruns Jowitt). It is a stemless perennial grass. The oil is mainly used in soaps, Cosmetics, deodorants and mosquito-repellent creams. It is a recent introduction into India and its cultivation. mainly in the lower hills of Assam, in Karnataka and southern Gujrat, covers about 2, 000 hectares. A part of out requirement is still met by imports,

Java citronella is grown up to 1, 000 m above sea level on well-drained sandy-loanto clayey-loamy soils with pH varying from 5 to 7. 5 As a rainfed crop, it is propagated by using rooted slips, and is planted during the rainy season in rows, 60 to 45 cm x 45 to 30 cm apart, depending on the rate of growth and the soil fetility. Usually, the leafy portion is removed at planting during the monsoon season and the plants begin to tiller in 30 days after planting.

A healthy one-year-old clump yields 60 to 80 slips. The crop needs a large quantity of nitrogenous fertilizers, When grown on medium soils, it is given 60 kg of P, 40 kg of K and 20 kg of N per ha at planting, supplemented with 80 to 100 kg of N per hectare annually as top-dressing in 3 to 4 split doses.

The crop is irrigated after every 10-15 days during the dry season and the first harvest is count 20 cm above the ground after 90 days of planting; usually 3 cuttings are obtained annually (4 under Assam conditions) for 3 to 5 year after planting.

CELERY (Apium graveolens Linn). Celery is a native of the Mediterranean region, introduced into India during late nineteenth century. India is now the principal grower (of the annual type) and exports large quantities of celery seeds (worth 17. 5 millions to the American and European markets. About 8000 ha is put under this crop, mainly in the Amritsar, Gurdaspur and Jallundhar districts of the Punjab State and to a smaller extent in the Saharanpur district of Uttar Pradesh. The clery seed is used in ground form as a dry seasoning powder and for the extraction of an oleoresin used to flavour a large variety of canned food products. The celery seed oil commands a larger market mainly in the confectionery industry. Whereas the bulk of celery seed is exported, a few local firms also produce its essential oil and olioresin on a small scale.

Celery is an erect, branchin herb, about 100 cm tall. it is a rabi crop which remains for 2 months in the nursery and for another 4 to 4 1/2 months in the field. Nursery is raised during early November. The seed-rate used is 2 kg. per hectare. The nursery-beds are kept moist and free from weeds through periodic irrigation followed by interculture. The seedlings grow up to 10 cm tall by the end of December and are ready for transplanting. The seedlings are usually planted 45 cm x 20 cm apart in early January in well-prepared fields, to which 30-50 tonnes of farmyard manure per ha is added during the preparatory tillage. On medium soils, about 80 Kg N, 40 Kg of P and 20 Kg of K per ha is applied to the crop; half of N along with the entire quantity of P and K is given to the rows at the time of planting and the remaining N is given as a top-dressing after one month. The crop requires 10-12 irrigations, each about 5 cm deep. Once established the crop requires 3 to 4 hoeings to keep down weeds. The plants bear flowers in umbels during early March and the fruits mature in late April. The Crop is harvested when about 80 per cent of the umbels begin to turn light brown. The harvested crop as stacked in the field for few days and is then threshed to obtain the seeds. The average grain yield ranges from 10 to 12 quintals per ha.

The celery (seed) on distillation yields to 2. 1 to 2. 3% of an essential oil containing selinene, d-limonene and sesquiterpenes. Oleoresin is prepared by using the method of the solvent extraction of the seeds. The seeds yields glycoside opiin. The crop remains remarkably free from pests and diseases.

Rose geranium (Pelargonium graveolens L'Herit) Pelargonium is a native of the hilly tracts of Cape Colony (South Africa). The highly aromatic 'Rose Geranium' is a hybrid (P. graveolens x P. radens), introduced by two Frenchmen- Earnest Sen and J. Priors in Yercaud in the Sheraroy Hills (Salem district) in Tamilnadu. It is now grown in a limited areas around Bangalore, Yercaud and in the Nilgiri Hills. The major world supplies of the oil come from Malagasy Republic. The oil of geranium has a refreshingly delicate rose-like aroma containing 66-78 per cent of alcohols calculated as geraniol. As such also, it itself is a perfume; it blends well with a wide range of floral and oriental perfumes. It is used for scenting oinments, pharmaceutical and tobacco products. It is suitable in a slightly alkaline medium and, therefore, it is widely used in the manufacture of high-grade soaps and cosmetic products. Our total annual production of the oil is around 12 tonnes and, therefore, a sizeable quantity of the oil is annually imported.

Two plant types of 'Rose Geranium' are recognized in India, Viz. the Algeriaan type from the slender plants, with dark pink flowers. It is less suitable for humid conditions; the other is Bourbin type which produces more leafy growth and bears light pink flowers. It is a perennial crop and about two to three harvests of leaves are taken annually in the second and third years. It can be grown as a catch crop in newly planted orchards.

'Rose Geranium' flourishes well in deep well-drained, preferably sandy loam to clayey-loam soils. It grows luxuriantly in a mild subtropical climate; locality receiving excessive heat in summer or very low temperatures in winter are unsuitable. The 'Rose Geranium' can withstand drought but its yield is reduced. It is raised in nursery during early spring from 8-15 cm long stem cutting each with 2 to 4 nodes. Sandy beds are preferred for the nursery to avoid excessive moisture which damages the young sprouts. Under a favourable day temperature of 10 to 15 degree Centigrade, about 80 per cent cuttings sproute in 3 weeks and are ready for field planting at 50 x 100 cm spacing with the onset of the monsoon rains in May-June. The field are brought to a fine tilth, are mixed with 45 tonnes of farmyard manure per hectare. In the Nilgiris the crop is given a basal application of a fertilizer mixture, containing 35, 45 and 17 kg of N, P and K per hectare; therefore, another 35 kg of N may be applied in two split applications annually. Initially, the crop is given 1 to 2 hoeings and weedings and the rows close up. The pruning of branches after the rains helps to induce bushy growth. The crop is irrigated at intervals of 10 to 15 days during summer depending upon the soils texture and the atmospheric humidity. Too moist or continued dry conditions lowers the crop yield. Generally, the first crop is obtained 6 to 8 months after planting and the average oil yields 8 kg; two or three crop are received in subsequent years, yielding 8 to 18 kg. of oil per hectare. In countries, e.g. Algeria and Malagasy Republic, the oil yields is reported to range from 30 to 35 kg. per hectare. The fresh leaves contain 0. 12 to 0. 2% (w/w) volatile oil and semi-dry or even dry leaves can be distilled. The oil improves in odour on ageing.

Fusarium sp. serious damages the geranium crop; the diseases is favoured by continued misty weather and excess soils moisture. The removal of diseased parts arrests the spread of the diseases and the spraying of the crop with 5% Bordeaux mixture periodically is recommended to control the diseases. However, when the roots are attacked, the plant dies and such infected plants should be pulled out along with the adhering soils and burnet.

PATCHOULI (Pogostemon cablin Benth) Patchouli is a native of humid Indo-Malayan tropics. The plant is small bushy herb which yields fragrant leaves containing a very sweet smelling oil. It is grown in small pockets mainly in Karnataka and Tamil Nadu. The oil of Patchouli is used to manufacture soap, cosmetics and incense and for imparting lasting oriental perfumery notes to many fancy products.

Two plants types of Patchouli are mainly recognized, viz. Jahore type which yields a poor leafy growth but produces a superior quality of oil; the other is Singapore type that gives more foliage and, therefore, more oil. It is a perennial crop, remaining in the field for about 3 years and gives 2 to 3 crops of leaves annually. It is a good catch crop for young orchards and can be raised as an intercrop in plantations where the over head shade is not heavy.

Patchouli requires deep, well-drained, fertile, slightly acidic soils, rich in humus; its growth is luxuriant in regions experiencing mild summer (24-280C), and a good rainfall ranging from 150 to 300 cm. Its sursery is raised in shade by planting 10-12 cm-long cuttings at 10 x 10 cm spacing during the rainy season and the beds are kept continuously moist. Under favourable conditions, about 85-90 per cent cutting per forth roots in a fortnight and they are ready for planting in the field in six to eight weeks at 90 x 90 cm spacing. The crop requires a liberal amount of organic matter and fertilizers; usually 10-12 tonnes of farmyard manure with 100 kg of P per ha is incorporated into the soil at the planting time, followed by 80 to 100 kg of N per hectare to the crop annually as top dressing in two split applications. The first crop is ready for harvesting in the next 4 to 6 months as indicated by the browning of the lower leaves, and the herbage is cut 10-25 cm below the apex in the morning hours. Usually, one or two growing branches are left unplucked to ensure a better growth of the succeeding harvest. The harvested leaves are dried in thin layers in sgade for 3-4 days and they develop their characteristic odour. Mature stalks are removed before distillation. Ageing improves the odour and the dry HA-77 leaves are therefore stored for a few months before distillation. A good crop stand yields about 2 tonnes of dry leaves (with 3 to 3. 5% oil) per annum, yielding about 50-60 kg of oil per hectare.

Golden nematode (Meloidogyne incognito) seriously damages this crop. No effective measure to control the nematode are known.

VETIVER OR KHUS (Vetiveria zizanioides (Linn Nash). Khus is a tall perennial grass found wild in the drier tracts of western India. Its spongy, much-branched fine root lets contain a fragrant oil, which is a perfume by itself. The dry aromatic roots are made into curtains, mats, fans, etc. to emit scented cool aroma when moistened. The oil is used as a valuable fixative for blending perfumes and socmetics. A large bulk of the oil is produced by distilling the wild-growing plants found in Bharatpur (Rajasthan), Musanagar, Biswan and Nawabganj etc. in western Uttar Pradesh. The cultivation of khus is scattered over small areas in the Trichur, Palghat, Kozikode, Wynad and Trivandrum district of Kerala, in the Tirunelvelly, Madhrai and Coimbatore districts of Tamil Nadu and in the kurnool and East Godavari districts of Andhra Pradesh.

In southern states, khus is grown as a rainfed crop in well-drained sandy-loam soils in moderately humid localities which received 100-200 cm of rainfall annually. However, a luxuriant growth of healthier roots is obtained from plants growing under warm and damp conditions on rich, partially inundated, masrshy land (Bharatpur). The field are laid out into beds of convenient size and 15-20 cm-long rooted slips are planted. With the onset of the monsoon rains on both the sides of the ridges, made 45 cm apart. The planting of 2 to 3 slips is done in spring in pits when the crop is raised under irrigation. The crop is given 10-12 tonnes of farmyard manure or compost at planting, supplemented with ash and groundnutcake or ammonium sulphate, one month after planting to stimulate growth.

Khus is a 12 to 18 month crop and the roots are dug out during dry months before autumn. The aerial parts are first cut at a height of 15 to 20 cm and are removed, the clumps are then dug out and beaten. The soil is further dug out up to a depth of one metre to remove the remaining rootlets. The roots are light to yellowish brown containing usually 0. 6 to 0. 8 per cent of dark brown viscous, persistently fragrant oil. The yield is 3 to 5 tonnes of fresh root, yielding about 20 kg of oil per hectare.

JASMINE. Among the perfume yielding jasmines, juhi (Jasminum curiculatum Vahl) and chameli (J officinale Linn) are commonly used for producing attars which sell at fancy prices. Jasmine ' concrete' and absolutes' are used to impart a gentle pleasing aroma to innumerable high-grade preparations. In the Western countries, Spanish (alsocalled French) jasmine (J. officinale Linn var grandiflorum Bailey) is largely cultivated; it has 7 to 11 leaflets and the flower bud has a dull creamy to punish spot on the posterior most petal. A high yelding clone of the Spanish jasmine has been recently developed at the Tamil Nadu Agricultural University, Coimbatore.

It blooms from March to December and is reported to yield about 12 tonnes of fresh flowers per hectare annually against 1. 6 to 3 tonnes of flowers obtained from the Spanish jasmine in India. The crop remains in the field for 10 to 15 years.

The jasmines prefer well drained, rich sandy-loam to clayey-loam soils and remain in loom longer in a mild climate; the var. grandiflorum is more sensitive to fros. It is raised from 20 cm long stem cutting prepared from near mature wood and planted in deep pits at 1. 5 x 1 m spacing during the rainy season. The growing plants are pruned during January February and July to induce lateral branching and flowering, and are given farmyard manure liberally. The plantation needs fortnightly irrigation during dry months. Picking is done during the early morning hours and the percentage recovery of the concrete ranges from 0. 24 to 0. 38 by using the solvent extraction method. Fresh flowers lose their fragrance soon, and it is essential that the solvent extraction apparatus as available at the site where the jasmine plantation is raised for perfumery aromatics.

KEWARA (Pandanus odoratissimus Linn) Kewara is a large indigenous shrub, 3 to 6 m tall, bearing white or creamy dioecious flowers including its enclosing spathe contains a fragrant oil. The kewara attar and kewara water are commonly used at ceremonial functions in perfuming aerated waters, other drinks and confectionery products. Most of the cultivation is confined to the Ganjam district (400 ha) in Orissa where it is drains and ponds. The plant thrives in clayey loam soil in the tropical climate, usually receiving heavy rainfall.

Kewara is propagated from shoots, branches and leaves which readily from roots during the rainy season. It bears flowers in the fourth or fifth year and has an economic life of 20 years. The crops needs no special care, except periodic pruning. Thc flowers are borne from June to September. A plant may produce 15 to 40 flowers in a season. A flower takes 15 days to mature and grows grammes. The blossom contains 0. 1 to 0. 3 per cent oil. The attar is mosly produced over sandalwood oil or paraffin base.

MODERN EVIDENCE FOR THE ANTISEPTIC POWERS OF ESSENTIAL OILS

Towards the end of the 19th century, the first acknowledged research to prove the antiseptic properties of essential oils was that undertaken by Chamberland. This was followed early in the 20th century by Cavel's research into the individual effects of 35 essential oils on microbial cultures in sewage. The most effective oil in terms of the quantity required to render inactive 1000 ml of culture was found to be thyme (0.7 ml). Two other well-known oils showing high efficacy were sweet orange (1.2 ml, 3rd) and peppermint (2.5 ml, 9th). The antiseptic power of several oils has now been proved to be many times greater than that of phenol. Certain essential oils have also been shown to be effective against different bacteria, e.g lemon, which is one of the best in its antiseptic and bactericidal properties, neutralizing both the typhus bacillus and Staphylococcus aureus in a matter of minutes. Cinnamon kills the typhus bacillus even when diluted to 1 part in 300.

Professor Griffon, a member of the French Academy of Pharmacy, made up a blend of seven essential oils (cinnamon, clove, lavender, peppermint, pine, rosemary and thyme) to study their antiseptic effect on the surrounding air when sprayed from an aerosol; all the staphylococci and moulds present were destroyed after 30 minutes.

The bacteriological approach of aromatherapy is an extremely complex field of the utmost interest, opening the way to the ecological understanding and management of the different colonies and flora that live in cohabitation—or at war—within us. Allopathic medicine has begun to realise that the misuse of antibiotics leads to numerous side-effects and sometimes results in chronic disastrous conditions (i.e. systemic candidosis) that could have been avoided if medical aromatherapy had been implemented in due time.

Today, the properties of herb volatile oils are researched in many centres throughout the world.

WIDE-RANGING APPLICATION

Essential oils can be put to a multitude of uses both in general practice and in hospitals, as this quote from Dr. J. Valnet illustrates: The doctor who is familiar with essential oils can use them to treat a whole range of infections—pulmonary, hepatic, intestinal, urinary, uterine, rhinopharyngeal and cutaneous (infected wounds and suppurating dermatoses). The use of these oils usually produces satisfactory results, provided they have been prescribed wisely and that, in the case of certain long-standing complaints, the treatment is followed for a long enough period. Aromatic therapy can neutralise enteritis, colitis and putrid fermentations, and can relieve chronic bronchitis and pulmonary tuberculosis. The colon bacillus cannot resist essential oils.

Orthodox medicine currently uses plant material to help cure diseases which previously had a high death rate. Twenty years ago, four out of every five children with leukaemia lost their lives; nowadays four out of five are returned to health with the aid of vincristine and vinblastine, derivatives of the rosy periwinkle—a plant used for hundreds of years by tribal healers as a medicine. The snakeroot plant from India is now used in the Western world to treat hypertension; digitalis, for heart conditions, is produced from the humble foxglove and the well-known rhododendron is used in the treatment of fatigue. 'Plants are an intrinsic part of natural medicine, and not even the most orthodox doctor can get by without them; indeed they represent the link between the natural and the orthodox, the traditional and the ultra-new'.

Phytotherapy is the name increasingly given to the use of the whole, or part, of the plant for medicinal purposes. Aromatherapy and aromatology (similar to aromatherapy but including intensive and internal uses) are branches of this, utilizing only the essential oils produced by distillation and citrus oils produced by expression. These are simple to use and administer, yet can compete with the steroids and antibiotics used in allopathic medicine today without the body's defence mechanism becoming exhausted or tolerance developing to them.

The basic reason which accounts for the diversity of conception and application of aromatherapy lies in the very nature of the aromatic substance. Lending itself to easy cutaneous penetration, being endowed with the capacity to influence the mind through its powerful impact upon the olfactive sense, and owing multiple and strong pharmacological properties to its highly active molecular components, it was natural for the aromatic substance to find developments in so many areas.

POWERFUL HEALING AGENTS

Many plant extracts used in the production of conventional medicines are, like the foxglove, poisonous and therefore exceptionally low doses are employed. Some essential oils are also toxic when used incorrectly and the most powerful of these are not normally available to aroma therapists. Essential oils are concentrated and intensely energetic in their effects, so very little is needed (even of those in general use) for successful treatment—dilutions generally being in the range 0.05-3 percent, depending on the oil used. Apart from the difference in the intensity of the aroma, no apparent benefit is gained from higher concentrations, particularly where the problem is an emotional one, although neat oils are used in certain medical conditions and aromatology.

THEIR MODE OF ACTION

It cannot yet be proved exactly how they work, but research and extensive anecdotal evidence exists to prove that they do work. In the distant past, essences have been used to heal wounds, inhibit the decay of flesh (as in mummification) and reduce the spread of infection (as in the time of the Black Death)—all without anyone knowing how they worked, just as the humble aspirin was in use for many years before anyone knew its mode of action.

Bios is the Greek word for life and essential oils may be classed as probiotic (for life), as opposed to antibiotic (against life). To illustrate this point, antibiotics kill not only harmful bacteria, but also the beneficial flora that we need to keep us healthy, leaving the body in a weakened state. Carefully selected essential oils kill only the bacteria inimical to the successful functioning of the body. Some essential oils also possess antiviral and fungicidal qualities. 'A serious condition obviously authorises the use of antibiotics, and in high doses; but one should be aware that the price of a cure may be a permanent disability'.

USER-FRIENDLY

Natural, whole essential oils can be used on living tissue with minimal unwanted effects (unlike some synthetic drugs, however successful these may be against their intended targets). Also, the human body accustoms itself to the effects of chemical synthetics, leading to escalating doses. This has not been found to be the case with essential oils, which retain their effectiveness killing off the unwanted bacteria.

QUANTITIES OF ESSENTIAL OILS USED

Tens of thousands of tonnes of essential oils are used by the food and perfume industries with the food industry being the largest user. It is important to realise that the total amount of essential oil used by the aromatherapy profession is extremely small compared with these industries, and this contributes to the difficulties of obtaining high quality, pure, natural oils Some oils which could be beneficial when used in aromatherapy are not generally supplied by distillers because they are not required by the giant users. Fortunately, however, a small number of independent distillers produce essential oils solely for aromatherapy use, although such products tend to be more expensive.

ECONOMY OF USE

Compared with the very high price of drugs (perhaps due to the tremendous research and development costs) essential oils are extremely inexpensive—a factor which should interest those in charge of public health funds. Not only that, they are pleasant to use for both patient and career. In many hospitals and hospices they are used not only to improve the quality of a patient's life but in waiting rooms to relieve the anxiety of relatives and friends. More specifically, they can be used in place of secondary drugs, which might be prescribed to counteract iatrogenic effects of the primary drugs being taken. They have been found to aid relaxation effectively, both pre- and post-operatively, to regenerate tissue in cases of severe burns and inflammation, and to relieve pain in cases of rheumatoid arthritis. They have helped to improve the quality of life for the terminally ill, and they have also found important uses in maternity care.

AREAS OF USE

Essential oils are used extensively by aroma therapists and aromatologists to improve or uplift a patient's state of mind. The effect of the attitude of mind on a person's health is being recognized more and more and essential oils can play an important part here. Florence Nightingale said 'what nursing has to do... is to put the patient in the best condition for nature to act upon him', reinforcing the ancient tag medicus cura, natura sanat—the doctor treats, nature cures.

By far the majority of essential oil users are outside the medical profession, some people using them merely on instruction from one of the many books written for the general public on the subject. They are simple to use and it should come as a relief to GPs that minor everyday ailments such as a sore throat or a winter cold, and even some more serious problems like bronchitis, sinusitis and rheumatism, can be treated in the home easily and successfully, leaving the doctor 's time free for the cases requiring expert knowledge.

All this is achievable by anyone, without professional medical skills. However, in France (from where aromatherapy was introduced to the UK) doctors prescribe essential oils for internal use in capsules or in drops diluted in alcohol, or in suppositories and pessaries. They are used externally in dressings, fumigations, inhalations, ointments and in foot, hand or complete baths. The original concept of aromatherapy in England, as introduced by Mme Maury, was to use the essential oils in massage only— suitably diluted in a fixed vegetable oil. This unfortunately led to the belief that this is all there is to aromatherapy, and the authors are actively trying to correct this image. It needs the medical profession not only to take an interest but also to use its professional skills to utilize these precious commodities to their fullest capabilities in order to bring the benefits of this aromatic therapy to the hospitals of the world in the 21st century.

The subject of aromatherapy involves pharmacy and farming, botany and bodies, medicine and chemistry, toxicity and safety—all so intertwined and interconnected that it is scarcely possible to disentangle the ramifications for the purpose of setting them down without some repetition and much cross-referral.

SOME IMPORTANT GRASS AS AROMATIC PLANT

Lemon Grass (Cymbopogon Flexuosus Stapf.)

It is a stemless perennial grass, found wild in the southern states of India. The leaves yield an aromatic oil, containing 75-85 per cent citral. The oil is used in soaps, cosmetics and disinfectants and is a raw material for manufacturing ions and vitamin A. The crop is grown on about 390,000 ha in Kerals and about 90 per cent of the produce is exported, earning about Rs. 10 million in foreign exchange annually.

The crop is grown mainly as a rain-fed crop on poor marginal lands. It is a hardy drought-resistant plant and is grown under a wided range of climatic conditions. Two types are recognized:

1. The red-stemmed grass is the true lemon-grass and a selection 'OD-19' made at the Lemon Grass Research Station, Oodakkali (Kerala) is recommended for high yield,
2. The white-stemmed (var.albscens) yields oil or low citral content. The crop is best propagated through seed raised in nurseries; 10kg of the old seedlings are planted in rows, 40 to 15x 10 cm apart, during rains and the first harvest is ready after 90 days. In Kerala, 3 harvests are obtained in the first year and 4 to 5 harvests during each of the 3 to 5 succeeding years; the crop is cut after every 60 to 65 days, except during the dry season. The fields are manured librally with ash and spent grass (obtained after the distillation of the oil); farmers seldom apply inorganic fertilizers. The herbage contains 0.35 percent oil on

fresh-weight basis. The grass yield ranges from 18 to 25 tonnes per hectare, giving 60 - 72 kg of oil.

Citronella Grass (Cymobopogon Winteriaruns Jowitt)

It is a stemless perennial grass. The oil is mainly used in soaps, Cosmetics, deodorants and mosquito-repellent creams. It is a recent introduction into India and its cultivation. mainly in the lower hills of Assam, in Karnataka and southern Gujrat, covers about 2,000 hectares. A part of out requirement is still met by imports

Java citronella is grown up to 1,000 m above sea level on well-drained sandy-loanto clayey-loamy soils with pH varying from 5 to 7.5 As a rainfed crop, it is propagated by using rooted slips, and is planted during the rainy season in rows, 60 to 45 cm x 45 to 30 cm apart, depending on the rate of growth and the soil fetility. Usually, the leafy portion is removed at planting during the monsoon season and the plants begin to tiller in 30 days after planting. A healthy one-year -old clump yields 60 to 80 slips. The crop needs a large quantity of nitrogenous fertilizers, When grown on medium soils, it is given 60 kg of P, 40 kg of K and 20 kg of N per ha at planting, supplemented with 80 to 100 kg of N per hectare annually as top-dressing in 3 to 4 split doses. The crop is irrigated after every 10-15 days during the dry season and the first harvest is count 20 cm above the ground after 90 days of planting; usually

3 cuttings are obtained annually (4 under Assam conditions) for 3 to 5 year after planting.

Celery (Apium Graveolens Linn)

Celery is a native of the Mediterranean region, introduced into India during late ninteenth century. India is now the principal grower (of the annual type) and exports large quantities of celery seeds (worth 17.5 millions to the American and European markets. About 8000 ha is put under this crop, mainly in the Amritsar, Gurdaspur and Jallundhar districts of the Punjab State and to a smaller extent in the Saharanpur district of Uttar Pradesh. The clery seed is used in ground form as a dry seasoning powder and for the extraction of an oleoresin used to flavour a large variety of canned food products. The celery seed oil commands a larger market mainly in the confectionery industry.

Whereas the bulk of celery seed is exported, a few local firms also produce its essential oil and olioresin on a small scale.

Celery is an erect, branchin herb, about 100 cm tall. it is a rabi crop which remains for 2 months in the nursery and for another 4 to 4 1/2 months in the field. Nursery is raised during early November. The seed - rate used is 2 kg. per hectare. The nursery - beds are kept moist and free from weeds through periodic irrigation followed by interculture. The seedlings grow up to 10 cm tall by the end of December and are ready for transplanting. The seedlings are usually planted 45 cm x 20 cm apart in early January in well - prepared fields, to which 30-50 tonnes of farmyard manure per ha is added during the preperatory tillage. On medium soils, about 80 Kg N, 40 Kg of P and 20 Kg of K per ha is applied to the crop; half of N along with the entire quantity of P and K is given to the rows at the time of planting and the remaining N is given as a top - dressing after one month. The crop requires 10-12 irrigations, each about 5 cm deep. Once estalished the crop requires 3 to 4 hoeings to keep down weeds. The plants bear flowers in umbels during early March and the fruits mature in late April. The Crop is harvested when about 80 per cent of the umbels begin to turn light brown. The harvested crop as stacked in the field for few days and is then threshed to obtain the seeds. The average grain yield ranges from 10 to 12 quintals per ha.

The celery (seed) on distillation yields to 2.1 to 2.3 percent of an essential oil containing selinene,d-limonene and sesquiterpenes. Oleoresin is prepared by using the method of the solvent extraction of the seeds. The seeds yields glycoside opiin. The crop remains remarkably free from pests and diseases.

Patchouli (Pogostemon Cablin Benth)

Patchouli is a native of humid Indo-Malayan tropics. The plant is small bushy herb which yields fragrant leaves containing a very sweet smelling oil. It is grown in small pockets mainly in Karnataka and Tamil Nadu. The oil of Patchouli is used to manufacture soap, cosmetics and incense and for imparting lasting oriental perfumery notes to many fancy products.

Two plants types of Patchouli are mainly recognized, viz. Jahore type which yields a poor leafy growth but produces a superior quality of oil; the other is Singapore type that gives more foliage and, therefore, more oil. It is a perennial crop, remaining in the field for about 3 years and gives 2 to 3 crops of leaves annually. It is a good catch crop for young orchards and can be raised as an intercrop in plantations where the over head shade is not heavy.

Patchouli requires deep, well-drained, fertile, slightly acidic soils, rich in humus; its growth is luxuriant in regions experiencing mild summer (24-280C), and a good rainfall ranging from 150 to 300 cm. Its sursery is raised rainy season and the beds are kept continuously moist. Under favourable conditions, about 85-90 per cent cutting per forth roots in a fortnight and they are ready for planting in the field in six to eight weeks at 90 x 90 cm spacing. The crop requires a liberal amount of organic matter and fertilizers; usually 10-12 tonnes of farmyard manure with 100 kg of P per ha is incorporated into the soil at the planting time, followed by 80 to 100 kg of N per hectare to the crop annually as top dressing in two split appications. The first crop is ready for harvesting in the next 4 to 6 months as indicated by the browning of the lower leaves, and the herbage is cut 10-25 cm below the apex in the morning hours. Usually, one or two growing branches are left unplucked to ensure a better growth of the succeeding harvest. The harvested leaves are dried in thin layers in sgade for 3-4 days and they develip their characteristic odour. Mature stalks are removed before distillation. Ageing improves the odour and the dry HA-77 leaves are therefore stored for a few months before distillation. A good crop stand yields about 2 tonnes of dry leaves (with 3 to 3.5 percent oil) per annum, yielding about 50-60 kg of oil per hectare.

Golden nematode (Meloidogyne incognito) seriously damages this crop. No effective meaasure to control the nematode are known.

Vetiver or Khus (Vetiveria Zizanioides (Linn Nash)

Khus is a tall perennial grass found wild in the drier tracts of western India. Its spongy, much-branched fine root lets contain a fragrant oil, whcih is a perfume by itself. The dry aromatic roots are made into curtains, mats, fans, etc. to emit scented cool aroma when moistened. The oil is used as a vlauable fixative for blending perfumes and socmetics. A large bulk of the oil is produced by distilling the wild-growing plants found in Bharatpur (Rajasthan), Musanagar, Biswan and Nawabganj etc. in western Uttar Pradesh. The cultivation of khus is scattered over small areas in the Trichur, Palghat, Kozikode, Wynad and Trivandrum district of Kerala, in the Tirunelvelly, Madhrai and Coimbatore districts of Tamil Nadu and in the kurnool and East Godavari districts of Andhara Pradesh

In southern states, khus is grown as a rainfed crop in well-drained sandy-loam soils in moderately humid localities which received 100-200 cm of rainfall annually. However, a luxuriant growth of healthier roots is obtained from plants growing under warm and damp conditions on rich, partially inundated, masrshy land (Bharatpur). The field are laid out into beds of convenient size and 15-20 cm-long rooted slips are planted. With the onset of the monsoon rains on both the sides of the ridges, made 45 cm apart. The planting of 2 to 3 slips is done in spring in pits when the crop is raised under irrigation. The crop is given 10-12 tonnes of farmyard manure or compost at planting, supplemented with ash and groundnutcake or ammonium sulphate, one month after planting to stimulate growth.

Khus is a 12 to 18 month crop and the roots are dug out during dry months before autumn. The aerial parts are first cut at a height of 15 to 20 cm and are removed, the clumps are then dug out and beaten. The soil is further dug out up to a depth of one metre to remove the remaining rootlets. The roots are light to yellowish brown containing usually 0.6 to 0.8 per cent of dark brown viscous, persistently fragrant oil. The yield is 3 to 5 tonnes of fresh root, yielding about 20 kg of oil per hectare.

Jasmine

Among the perfume yielding jasmines, juhi (Jasminum curiculatum Vahl) and chameli (J officinale Linn) are commonly used for producing attars which sell at fancy prices. Jasmine ' concrete' and absolutes' are used to impart a gentle pleasing aroma to innumerable high-grade perparations. In the Western countries, Spanish (alsocalled French) jasmine (J. officinale Linn var grandiflorum Bailey) is largely cultivated; it has 7 to 11 leaflets and the flower bud has a dull creamy to punish spot on the posterior most petal. A high yelding clone of the Spanish jasmine has been recently developed at the Tamil Nadu Agricultural University, Coimbatore. It blooms from March to December and is reported to yield about 12 tonnes of fresh flowers per hectare annually against 1.6 to 3 tonnes of flowers obtained from the Spanish jasmine in India. The crop remains in the field for 10 to 15 years.

The jasmines prefer well drained, rich sandy-loam to clayey-loam soils and remain in loom longer in a mild climate; the var. grandiflorum is more sensitive to fros. It is raised from 20 cm long stem cutting prepared from near mature wood and planted in deep pits at 1.5 x 1 m spacing during the rainy season. The growing plants are pruned during January February and July to induce lateral branching and flowering, and are given farmyard manure liberally. The plantation needs fortnightly irrigation during dry months. Picking is done during the early morning hours and the precentage recovery of the concrete ranges from 0.24 to 0.38 by using the solvent extraction method. Fresh flowers lose their fragrance soon, and it is essential that the solvent extraction apparatus as available at the site where the jasmine plantation is raised for perfumery aromatics.

Kewara (Pandanus Odoratissimus Linn)

Kewara is a large indigenous shrub, 3 to 6 m tall, bearing white or creemy dioecious flowers including its enclosing spathe contains a fragrant oil. The kewara attar and kewara water are commonly used at ceremonial functions in perfuming aerated waters, other drinks and confectionery products. Most of the cultivation is confined to the Ganjam district (400 ha) in Orissa where it is drains and ponds. The plant thrives in clayey loam soil in the tropical climate, usually receiving heavy rainfall.

Kewara is propagated from shoots, branches and leaves which readily from roots during the rainy season. It bears flowers in the fourth or fifth year and has an economic life of 20 years. The crops needs no special care, except periodic pruning. The flowers are borne from June to September. A plant may produce 15 to 40 flowers in a season. A flower takes 15 days to mature and grows grammes. The blossom contains 0.1 to 0.3 per cent oil. The attar is mosly produced over sandalwood oil or paraffin base.

Davana (Artemisia Pallens Wall)

It is a small (50 cm tall) annual indigenous herb with divided pluish green fragrant leaves. The oil of the herb is prized in perfumery for its sweet, persistent fruity fragrance. It is cultivated on a limited scale in karnataka for making bouquets and producing oil. It is a 4 month rabi crop raised in fertile well drained red loamy soils under equable climate receiving mild winter rains and with clear sunny weather ar maturity. Seeds are small (about 6000 g) and are kept in a moist piece of cloth for 1-2 lays for germination. The sprouted seed are thinly broadcast in the nursery in early November abd the seedlings establish themselves in 7-10 days. Five week old seedlings are planted in the field. The crop is given mainly their usual height in 10 weeeks afterplanting. The crop is harvested on bright sunny days and the harvested herb is air dried. The air dried herb is chopped into 3 to 4 pieces and distilled at prssure of 2 kg per sq. cm for 8 to 12 hours. The yield of fresh herbage is about 30 tonnes per ha. The harbage loses about four fifths of its moisture on drying; the averageoil content of the dry herb is 0.2 per cent. Thus 10 to 12 kg of brownish viscous oil is attained from one hectare. Its quantity improves with age.

Henna or Mehandi (Lawsonia Inermis Linn)

It is a persnnial hedge plant, native to North Africa. It is cultivated in the Pali, Sojat abd Nagor districts of Rajasthan and the adjoining districts of Gurgaon and Faridabad in Haryana. The crop is grown in sandy loam to loamy soils in the hot and dry climate on marginal land. Two varities are known, viz. Hinna (odorous) and Rajni (more colouring). A part of the produce is exported.

Mehndi is raised through seeds as well as through cuttings; the former method is preferred. The seeds have a hard coat and are kept under a moist piece of cloth for 8-15 days till they sprout (the average germination being 20 per cent). The sprouted seeds are mixed with fine sand and sown broadcast in a well prepared nursery during March. The seedbeds are kept moist and free from weeeds. The seedlings grow 20-30 cm tall in the next 3 months and are transplanted in wet field during the monsoon season at 15 x 30 cm or 30 x 30 cm spacing. The land is given 40 tonnes of farmyard manure and 40 kg of N per ha at planting and a similar quantity thereafter in 2 split doses annually to boost vegetative growth.

The field are bunded during the rainy season to conserve moisture. Usually the plants in third year begin to yield the leaf crop which continues to start economic yields for the nest 25 years or so. Normally, 2 harvests are taken branches are cut near the ground level and dried, preferable in shade. The dry branches are beaten on yield under rain fed conditions is 1 tonne per ha; higher yields up t 2.5 tonnes per ha are obtained when raised as an irrigated crop. Termites, ants and mites damage the crop; the dusting of the crop with BHC (10 percent) is recommended as a preventive measure.

Sweet Flag or Bach (Acorus Calamus L)

It is a perennial indigenous undershrub which inhabits stagnant pools and shallow creaks all over the country. Its long aromatic rhizomes contain an aromatic oil (Ascerone 82 percent) used for lending oriental notes in perfumery; the oil has germicidal properties and is used in insecticidal formulations. It is a 10 month crop cultivated in clayey to clayey loam soils on about 500 ha confined to the koratgere Taluk of the Tumkar district in Karnataka. Field are puddled with 40 tonnes if farmyard manure or with sullage and bunded like rice field for impounding water. The growing tops of the plants obtained from the previous crop are usually planted in March-April in soft mud at 30 x 30 cm spacing and the field are flooded with 5 cm deep water. As the crop grows, the depth of water in the field is raised to 10 cm till about a month before harvest. The crop is given weeding almost every month for the first 4 to 5 months when the plants close the rows and produce a thick cover. Fertilizers are seldomused; some farmers apply 40 kg of N in 2 splits 30 and 60 days after planting. The leaf tips begin to turn yellow as the crop matures. The rhizomes are then dug out. The rhizomes lie mostly near the surface and grow 30 to 50 cm long. They are washed, cut into 6 to 10 cm long pieces and rubbed with hessain to remove the leafy scales and fibrous roots before drying them in the sun. The crop yield ranges from 2.5 to 4 tonnes of dry rhizomes per ha. The produce can be stored for a long period.

Linaloe (Bursera Delpechianum Boiss Ex. Engl)

It is a small Mexican tree whose wood (7-9 percent) and berries (3 percent) yield a sweet smelling essential oil on steam distillation. The characteristic odour of the oil due to the presence of 35-44 percent of easter (linalyll acetate) and 32-48 per cent of free alcohols (linalool) resembling the odour of lavender. The oil is used in the manufacture of high quality soaps and cosmetic products.

Linaloe is a dioecious plant which grows about 6 meters tall abd 1 meter in girth at 20 years of age. It sheds its leaves at the commencement of winter and gives out new leaves and flowers in April. The berries ripen in Aughst September and are collected before dehiscence. In its natural habitat, the plant grows in tropical serub forests on dry eroded land and is sensitive to frost and water logging. Its growth is better on fertile forest land. Spring rains benefit the crop. Cutting, about 0.5 m in length and 1 cm in diameter, are made from the female mother plants during February March and planted in pots, baskets or polythene bags in a nursery in shade. It sprouts in 3-4 weeks and, as such, is planted in pits during the rainy season.

About 300 plants are planted per ha. and they need irrigation in the succeeding summer season. The plants bear flowering twigs at 3 or 4 years of age. The flowering twigs are clipped. In the sixth year, the plants develops a crown spread of about 2m and commences giving the commercial crop. ipe beries are collected during automn and dried in shade. The dry fruits split in two, exposing the kernels. The essential oil is confined to the husk of the fruit. The dry berries can be stored for long and distilled at convenience. They yield 2.5 to 3 per cent oil on fresh weight basis. The yield of oil is around 20 kg/ha from the sixth year onards for a growing life span of about 50 years

Lemon Gum (Eucalyptus Citriodora Hook)

It is an Australian tree, about 25 m tall, with a clean silvery green trunk and strongly-scented narrow leaves. The plant is coppiced at a height of 90 cm to get a larger yield of foliage which contains an aromatic oil. On an average, the foliage has up to 0.8 percent of oil, containing 60-80 per cent of citronellal that imparts to it the lemon like odour. Commercial plantations exist in the Nilgiri Hills. A plantation is raised on well drained gravelly soils both in tropical plains and in the sub-temperate hills up to about 2000 meters above sea level. Seeds may be sown during early spring either in polythene bags in the nursery or direct in the field. About 10-20 cm tall seedlings are translanted in the field (without exposin their roots) during the rainy season at 45 x 30 cm spacing. The land is usually given 50 kg each of P and K per hectare at planting, supplemented with about 100 kg of N per hectare in 2 to 4 split doses anually as top dressing. The terminal branches are cut to induce the plants to produce more lateral branches. During harvesting, the plants are cropped in April and November and a small harvest is also gathered during the rainy season. Fresh leaves and tender branches are distilled. The average yield from the third year onwards is about 20 tonnes per hectare per annum. This field, in turn, gives about 100 kg. of oil. The price of oil depends upon the content of citronellal in the oil. The Tamil Nadu Cinchona Department has located trees whose foliage is found to possess 85-90 per cent of citronellal and this oil fetches better price.

Muskdana or Ambrette (Abelmoschus Moschatus)

Abelmoschus moscha tus (L.) Medic, Ma lva cea e (Syn. Hibiscus abelmoschus L.) is a tropical weedy shrub native to India valued for its scented seed. Ambrette is a close relative to Okra, a popular horticultural crop. The genus Abelmoschus has six species distributed in the South and South East Asia and in North Australia. Abelmoschus moschatus Medic., A. manihot (L.) Medic., and A. esculentus (L.) Moench, contain wild and cultivated forms, and A. ficulneus, A. crinitus, and A. angulosus, are only wild. Abelmoschus manihot. In Hindi, it is popularly known as mushkdana, kasturi bhendi (kasturi= musk; bhendi= lady's finger). In other Indian languages it is known as gukhia korai (Assamese), kasturi bhenda (Telgu), kattukasturi (Malylam), varttilai kasturi (Tamil), lalkasturika (Sanskrit). The area under ambrette is presently low in India but is increasing rapidly with seed exports to France, Germany, Japan, Singapore, Spain for its use as an aromatic oil. Indian drug manufacturers are introducing new herbal drugs containing ambrette for medicinal use

Botany

Erect hispid herbs or undershrubs, 0.5-2.5 meters high, with a long slender tap root. Leave extremely variable, lower suborbicular in outline, cordate, lower or palmately 3-7 lobed, upper narrower, hastate or sagittate at the base with linear-oblong or triangular lobes. Flowers regular, bisexual, involucral bracts 8-12, hairy yellow with purple centre. Fruits capsule fulvous hairy, oblong lanceolate, acute. Seeds subreniform and blackish.

Uses

Ambrette oil obtained from seeds possess an odor similar to that of musk and its aromatic constitents have long been used in perfumery industry. Different grades of essential, or aromatic absolute, are marked in Europe as high-grade perfumes (Singh et al. 1996) The seeds are valued for the volatile oil present in the seed coat. Seed analysis report 11.1 percent moisture, 31.5 percent crude fiber; 14.5 percent lipids, 13.4 percent starch, 2.3 percent protein, volatile oil (0.2-0.6 percent) and ca/ 5 percent resin.

Analysis of volatiles report myricetin-3-glucoside and a glycoside of cyanidin in flowers, an aromatic constituent in seeds, beta-sitosteral and its beta-D-glucoside, myricetin and its glucoside in leaves and petals and beta-sitosterol from dry fruit husk. In India, roots, leaves (rarely), and seeds of ambrette are considered valuable traditional medicines. The bitter, sweet, acrid, aromatic seeds are used as a tonic and are considered "cooling, aphrodisiac, opthalmic, cardiotonic, digestive, stomachic, constipating, carminative, pectoral, diuretic, stimulant, antispasmodic, deodorant, and effective against "kapha" and "vata," intestinal complaints, stomatitis; and diseases of the heart, allays thirst and checks vomiting. According to Unani system of medicine seeds allay thirst, cure stomatitis, dyspepsia, urinary discharge, gonorrhea, leucoderma and itch. Roots and leaves are cures for gonorrhea . Even use against venomous reptiles has been reported.

Cultivation

Ambrette is cultivated as pre-kharif crop in India. It is usually sown in March–April but as late as the first week of July in Central India. Seed rates of 41g/kg are optimum. Application of dried Neem leaves (500Kg/ha) at last ploughing increased oil content and quality. April sown crop start flowering in September; fruits ripen from November to January and are harvested when fully mature. Applications of fertilizers improves growth of plant and seed yields but studies conducted by SOPAM indicate the use of chemical inputs resulted in negative impact on oil content and quality. Harvested capsules are sun dried and seeds dehisce when the capsules burst. The oil for perfumery is extracted by steam distillation of crushed seeds.

❐

Economic Medicinal Plants

Electronics, space travel and genetic-manipulation have, no doubt, opened new vistas for betterment of mankind but at the same time we have been ignorant, to some degree, about our diverse biological resources which constitute the apogee of the evolutionary process. We have been ignoring the importance of such resources, particularly plants resources in day to day welfare of mankind. Admittedly, plants have given us food, shelter and protection from diseases. Out of these three distinct roles played by plants, the role to protect us from diseases needs special mention in the present context. Little we may realize, each time we purchase medicines from the chemists, that one chance out of two is that it owes its origin, in some way or other, from medicinal plants. This is about the modern allopathic medicines. Age old traditional system of medicines such as Ayurveda system is based upon medicinal properties of the plants owes its origin in India since the dawn of civilization.

HISTORY OF MEDICINAL PLANTS & TRADITIONAL SYSTEMS OF MEDICINE

God has created the nature in which he has embedded a well programmed controlling and sustaining mechanism to protect His creation. This has led to interdependence between animal kingdom and plant kingdom in natural way. Many plants contain elements or active-principles-obviously natural chemical molecules, which fight out pathogenic agents/factors both in animals and plants. Interestingly, the truth was known to mankind since the primitive age which he utilized to protect himself in a rudimentary way. It was then concretized and put to medicinal practices by the Indian scholars of our ancient era like Charaka, Dhanwantary, Sushruta etc. Their dedicated efforts gave birth to so called ayurvedic system of medicines.

Thereafter in later stages, scholars from Egypt like Harun Rashid gave birth to another herbal system of medicine called Unani. Similarly, Homeopathy system of medicine invented by Samuel Hahneman also depends mostly on

Herbal plants. Chinese and Tibetan traditional practitioners also found out various medicinal properties of plant. However, Ayurvedic system occupies an unique position among all the traditional systems of medicine. Therefore, India unquestionably occupies a premier position in the use of herbal drugs utilizing about 540 plant species in different formulations. In the 19th century, Major Kirtikar and Brigr. Basu wrote a great book named "Indian Medicine Plants" which contributed enormously to the whole world. In the early forties of this century, Lt. Col. Ramanath Chopra, the then Director of Regional Research Laboratory of Jammu expressed the scientific value of the plant in his book " INDIGENOUS DRUG&OF INDIA".

EFFICACY AND ADVANTAGE OF HERBAL MEDICINE

1. Unlike modern allopathic medicines, traditional herbal medicines do not have adverse or side effects and are completely safe. Reason being that they originate from the NATURE and then act on animal body which is again from the nature. Hence, herbal medicines are well accepted and work with synergism in human body to fight out the diseases causing factors or elements.
2. Herbal medicines have shown excellent results without any ambiguity in ailments like Jaundice, Dyspepsia, Rheumatism etc. where there is no substitute, till now, in allopathic medicine.
3. The medicinal plants are available easily even in our court-yard.
4. After 1940's, there was a boost is modern allopathic medicine with advancement in science and technology. Many new and more potent antibiotics have been discovered. Many wonder drugs have come up. But unfortunately these drugs are not free from adverse reactions and very often they are not safe for prolonged use. Sometimes the efficacy of certain drugs either falls to zero or becomes doubtful due to some undesirable reactions which are often irreversible. On the other hand, the efficacy of herbal medicine goes without any doubt and their healing effects are sustainable.

Some Important Medicinal Plants Used in Traditional System of Treatment

In India the popularity of the herbal medicine formulated by various Indian scholars went unabated up to 1940s that is till the beginning of modern allopathic system of medicine. It is worthwhile to mention briefly the medicinal properties of some common plants used in ayurvedic system of medicine.

1. TULASI: (Occimum sanctum) Tulasi is not only most popular holy plant in Indian household but also proved to be a 'Wonder Drug' against all sorts of cough and cold problems. Tulasi symbolises sanctity and purity
2. YASTIMADHU: (Glycirrhiza glabra) Yastimadhu or Licorice is a very popular name in Ayurvedic system of medicine. It is used as restorative, urinary tract sedative and against cough and cold.

3. VASAK: (Justicia-Adhatoda Vasika) It is a household remedy for cough and cold and its leaf extract is used in anti-cold preparation.
4. NEEM: (Azadiracta indica) Like Tulasi Neem is also a holy plant and its fruit kernels, leaves and barks used in traditional Ayurvedic medicine as potent antimicrobial agents. The chewing of neem twig is very popular practice in India to fight tooth decay and gum troubles.
5. GUGUL:(Commiphora mukul) & RASNA (Vanda roxbergii) Gugul is a resinous substance exuded from Gugul plant which has potent anti- rheumatic and anti-cholesterol activity. Rasna extract is very effective against Gout and all kinds of Rheumatism. Both Gugul and Rasna are widely use in all anti-rheumatic preparations and found to be very effective.
6. TRIFALA: (Amla, Haritaki, Bahera) This trio are super megastar in Ayurvedic system of medicine and are used as all disease fighter and prophylactic against a host of diseases like constipation, dyspepsia, liver troubles etc.
7. ASHWAGANDHA: (Withania somnifera) Ashwagandha is a single super star in the field of health restorative like Panax ginseng of Korea. It finds application in many Ayurvedic formulation.
8. ARJUN: (Terminalia arjuna) -The extract of Afjun bark is a well proven anti-hepertensive drug and well established as a Cardiac Tonic.
9. SHANKHAPUSHPI: Evolvulus occinoides) -Shankhapushpi is found all over the country in rainy season in open grass land or on stony wasteland. Its sharbat is beneficial in mental fatigue and memory revitalising. It has also anti-pyretic property. It has the reputation in curing mental disorder. A team of scientists of BHU proved that shankhapushpi is very good against haemotemesis and hypertension.
10. ARNI :(Sans. Agnimantha, bot. -Clerodendrum phlomidis) In south India its leave juice is used to treat gonorrhea and syphilis. Adivasis, particularly, Santals rub the plant over their body in dropsy.
11. BRAHMI: (Bacopa monnieri-Linn) The plant is well known for its potency to increase one's memory and said to improve intellect, used against epilepsy I insanity and other nervous disorders. The leaves are used as diuretic and aperients and contain alkaloids like brahmine and herpestine and saponin-hersaponin which showed cardiotonic action in frog.
12. PUNARNAVA: *(Boerhavia diffusa):* Punarnava is one of the major constituents of many ayurvedic medicines. It is well known in Indian house-hold for its medicinal properties. Roots of B. diffusa considered to be a potent expectorant, diuretic and laxative. It is also used in asthma. Fairly good diuretic in dropsy associated with

bright's disease. The drug exerts more powerful action as compared to other diuretics on certain types of ascites such as those of liver and chronic peritonitis. Active constituent of B diffusa is punarnavine.

13. PIPPALI: (Piper longum) : Fruits are used as spice and also used as preservative in pickles. Roots and fruits are used against diseases of respiratory tract. It is also used as analgesic and anti-inflammatory in muscular pain. It also posseses the properties like sedative, carminative, cologogue in obstruction of bile duct and gall bladder. In Indian house- hold powder of dried fruit is taken with honey for relief from common cold and cough.
14. GOKSHURA OR IKSHUGANDHA :(Tribulus terrestris) : Leaves and tender shoots are used as pot herb. Fruits are source of flour used in times of scarcity. Leaves are rich in calcium, but poor in iron supplying cheap supplement to rice diets. Fruits are used in ayurvedic as tonic and diuretic. It is used in painful micturition and urinary calculus. It is also prescribed in bright's disease. Herb contains saponins such as diosgenin, gotogenin, chlorogenin, ruscogenin, and 25 D-spirosta-3, 5- diene.
15. NIRGUNDI:(Vitex negundo) : Leaves are used as tonic and vermifuge; smoked for relief from cold and catarrh and headache. Leaves and root possess tranquilizing effects and form a constituent of famous ayurvedic preparation Vishagarbha taila. Extract of leaves show anti-cancer activity against Ehrlich ascites tomour cell. Root is used as tonic, febrifuge and in rheumatism. It is also used as demulcent in dysentry and piles. Flowers are used in liver complaints, fever and diarrhoea.
16. MANDUKAPARNI: (Centella asiatica) : It is a diuretic and tonic. It is also use in treatment of leprosy. A glycoside-asiaticoside proven to be the active principle in treatment of leprosy has been isolated scientists.
17. SHATABARI: (Asperagus recemosus) : A very common name in ayurveda and widely used as tonic in ayurvedic medicines. It is also used as diuretic and galactogogue. Fresh root juice is mixed with honey and given for dyspepsia. Roots form a constituent of medicinal oils for nervous and rheumatic complaints.
18. VIDARI:(Oriya-BhuinKakharu.bot.-Ipomoeamauritiana):Tuberous roots contain a resin similar to Jalap resin and are considered tonic, aphrodisiac, demulcent, lactagogue and cholagogue. Powdered root is given in diseases of spleen and liver, debility, fatty deposition and menorrhagia.
19. MADHUNASHINI: (Gymnema sylvestra) : Leaves, when chewed paralyse for few hours the sense of taste for sweet and bitter substances. In ayurveda, G. sylvestra is being used as anti-diabetic drug with doubtful integrity. Leave powder is cardiac stimulant and diuretic..

20. ASHOKA: (Saraca asoka syn-S. indica) : Ashoka is a well known medicine in ayurveda for treatment of uterine disorders. Due to its stimulating effect on endometrium and ovarian tissue and hence it is useful in menorrhagia due to uterine fibroids. Flower is used as uterine tonic. It is also used in biliousness, heamarrhagic dysentry.
21. MANDUPARNI OR COMMON YEW: (Taxus baccata) :'Leaves and various parts of the tree possess anti-cancer property. Taxus leaves and its parts are being exported from Northern states to USA and France for preparation of anti-cancer and anti-malarial drugs. Many of the ayurvedic preparation contain manduparni which is becoming rare due to its export demand..
22. GULUCHI: (Tinospora cardifolia) : Stem is a constituent of several ayurvedic preparations used in general debility, dyspepsia, fever and urinary diseases. Dry twigs with bark intact constitute the drug. The bitter principle present in the drug show anti-spasmodic, anti-pyretic and anti-inflammatory properties. The decoction of guluchi plant is given in gout. The drug possesses one fifth of the analgesic effect of aspirin.
23. CHITRAKA: (Plumbago indica or zeylanica) Root is abortifacient, vesicant, and diuretic and used in dyspepsia, piles, diarrhoea and skin diseases. The paste of root is applied in opening of abscesses. Infusion of roots used in influenza and black-water fever.
24. GHRITA KUMARI: (Aloe barbadensis; syn A. vera) : A well known medicine plant in India. Fresh juice of leaves is cathartic and refrigerant and used in liver and spleen diseases and in eye troubles. It is believed to cool the brain-therefore it is used as a hair tonic. Leaf extract inhibits the growth of mycobacterium tuberculosis. It is found to be useful in X-ray burns, dermatitis and cutaneous leishmaniasis and other skin disorders. The jelly of Aloe vera is being used by many Multi National companies in their sun ray protecting creams. Its jelly is now found to be a good culture medium for tissue culture. It will cut down the cost of culture medium which is being exported from foreign countries.
25. GAMBHARI: (Gmelina arborea) : It is found in the forests of Orissa plentily. Its wood is used for furniture making. Its root is one of the Dashamularishta.
26. MITHIPATTI (Scoparia dulcis) : In Bastar region it is called Mithipatti or Ghodatulsi Infusion of the leaves used in fever, cough and bronchitis. Its juice is used as gargle in toothache. Anti-diabetic compound, amellin, occurs in the leaves and stems of green plants. It is helpful in anaemia, albuminaria, ketonuria, retinitis associated with diabetes.
27. PASHANABHEDAKA (Homonoia riparia; Oriya Jamla, Tam. -Kattalari) : Root laxative, diuretic, used in piles, stone in bladder

and vesicle calculi, strangury, and !Jsed in urinary discharges. Tender leaf is used as vegetables.

Recent Research on Medicinal Plants & Revival of Herbal Medicine

Being convinced that modern allopathic medicines, though potent, are not safe and also being convinced that these drugs are not sustainable in the context of its incompatibility in the natural system the gamut of modern allopathic drugs is being reviewed differently in recent past.

The revival of herbal medicines and its productive blending with modern medical science have been given serious thoughts.

The recent findings on the properties of medicinal plants are very amazing. Here we may mention a few of such findings.

A: ON HUMAN

1. SADABAHAR :.The most common Indian plant Sadabahar whose botanical name is Catharanthus rosea syn-Vinca rosea found to contain an important cytotoxic alkaloids vincrystin in smaller quantity and vinblastin in larger quantity. Vincrystin found to be clinically effective against leukemia and vinblastin against Hodkin diseases. The credit goes to USA and Canadian scientist who initiated resJ3arch in 1950s on isolation of alkaloids from common Rosy Periwinckle or Catharanthus rosea or vinca rosea. After the discovery of vincrystin the survival rate of children suffering from leukemia has jumped over to about 80 %. The clinical effectiveness of vincrystin in leukemia among children created a huge demand for Vinca rosea in USA.
2. ASHWAGANDHA: A team of Doctor from Kasturba Medical College, Manipal have reported that an alcoholic root extract of Ashwagandha has shown anti-tumour activity. They have also reported that Ashwagandha Injection can also augment the effect of radiation on tumor regression and delayed its growth.
3. RAKTA CHITRAKA: The same team led by Prof. P. Umadevi also reported that the extract of Rakta Chitraka (Plumbago Indica) a well known herbs in traditional Indian medicine found to have effective anti-tumor property and augmenting the effect of radiation given concurrently in arresting the growth of Tumour. Rakta Chitraka is being prescribed for cancer treatment in Siddha system.
4. MUSTARD : Mustard a popular condiment and oil-seed in India may have potential anti-cancer property according to a preliminary study at the National Institute of Nutrition, Hyderabad. Such anti-cancer property may be attributed to chemical compound phenyl-iso- thiocyanate present in mustard seed.
5. NEEM: Extensive researches in India well as abroad on Neem (Azadiracta Indica) has opened new vistas in Herbal medicines due to its versatile- properties.

Neem extract has shown activity against Rodent-Malaria caused by Plasmodium berghei prevalent in West Africa according to Scientist of University of Nizeria and African Bio-Science Net Work. Researches are being continued to investigate the activities of Neem and other plants against deadly parasite, Plasmodium falcifarum, found in African countries.

Indian researches on versatile applications of Neem are very promising. It is an established fact the chewing of Neem twig fights mouth Bacteria/ protozoa causing tooth decay, Gingivitis and Pyorrhea. India is the first country to manufacture Neem-based tooth paste and soap.

It has been found by the scientist of Defense Institute of Physiology and Science (DIPAS) and National Institute of Immunology (NII), New Delhi that Neem oil acts as an effective spermicidal contraceptive without any hazardous side effects. The contraceptive formulation called Nm-76 prepared from Neem oil extract which is undergoing trials and expected to be a safe and effective vaginal-spermicide. NIL scientist have clinically tried two Neem based products-PRANEEM OIL & PRANEEM POLYHERBAL CREAM which are effective as vaginal contraceptive and vaginal anti-microbial.

A team of Indo-American scientist from NII, New Delhi and Harvard Medical School, USA have shown that a sugar like extract from Neem bark can stop infectivity of AIDS-VIRUS in human blood cells, cultured in laboratories. No doubt, this findings may bring a new hope in the treatment of AIDS.

A group of researchers have shown Neem leaves extract acts as a sedative and anxiolytic in low dose of 10 to 200 mg/kg of body wt. in experimental rate.

Scientists of Malaria Research Institute New Delhi have reported that Neem oil is an excellent and low cost mosquito repellent. 5% Neem oil mixed with kerosene burnt in lamp. repels mosquitoes effectively without causing any harm to human body, unlike mosquito repellent mats and coils. A cream developed from Neem oil when applied to human body nullify the bites of sand fly that spreads Kalazar prevalent in Bihar.

B: ON PLANTS

Recently it has become a serious concern that the chemical pesticide leave high percentage of residual poison in the edible agro-horticultural product leading to serious health hazards. This is one of the bad effects of so called green revolution. Now it is high time that we should seriously think about alternative pesticides and. fungicide which are safe both to human and environment.

It is a matter of pleasure that such alternative pesticides are heading their way by the dedicated efforts of scientist and in near future these will come in a big way and may totally replace the hazardous chemical pesticide. These may be called as bio-pesticide which are of two types: 1) Microbe-based and 2) Plant Extract-based. As we are presently concern about the medicinal plant, we may cite a few examples where plant extracts are processed as pesticides.

1. Extract of marigold leaves (Electra of Ecomax Agrotech) is effective against soil nematodes and it is used as soil spray.
2. Aqueous extract of neem seed powder when sprayed on plants can effectively control a number of plant insects and fungal infections.
3. REPLIN-a spray insecticide formulation enriched with neem extract prepared by ITC agro-Industry, Hyderabad successfully tested in the field and found to be effective against steam borer and leaf folders.

C: ON ANIMAL

Even the veterinary surgeon depends upon plant for the treatment of the animal. Scientist from Calcutta have discovered anti-filarial activity in a drug isolated from the plant Acacia auriculoformis. The drug contains two active compounds acaciaside A and acaciaside B. These two saponins at a concentration of 4 mg. per ml. killed 97 percent of micro-filaria-the slender pre-larval forms of the filarial nematode in 100 minutes. The compound could also kill all the adults in 35 minutes. This report is published by the scientists ion the Indian journal of experimental biology.

NATIONAL RESEARCH INSTITUTES ON MEDICINAL PLANTS

Following R & D labs. and institution are engaged specifically on identification, isolation of chemicals and improving agro technique for cultivation of medicinal plants.

1. Central Institute for Medicinal-Lucknow & Aromatic Plants (CIMAP).
2. National Botanical Research Institute. -Lucknow
3. Regional Research Laboratory-Jorhat, Tiruvantpuram, Bhubaneswar, Jammu.
4. Central Drug Research Inst. -Lucknow
5. Council for Scientific and Industrial Research (CSIR) -New Delhi

DATABASES FOR ASSESSMENT OF LOCAL HEALTH TRADITIONS

The web-based Referral Browser basically aims to provide support for assessment of folk health traditions. This will help to promote best health-related practices in a specific area for human, plant and animal health care. The browser will procure references from Ayurveda, Siddha, Unani and modern pharmacology for a resource used in folk health practice and is subjected to evaluation/assessment.

SPECIALISED REPORTS & CHECKLISTS

FRLHT has come out with state wise checklists and specialised reports on medicinal plants in conservation sites. While specialised reports have been prepared and published on the medicinal plants of Karnataka, Kerala and Tamil Nadu, checklists have been prepared for Andhra Pradesh, Maharashtra, Madhya Pradesh, Arunachal Pradesh, Himachal Pradesh, Meghalaya and Uttranchal. The specialised reports list the species recorded in the state and the species found in the MPCAs, their habit and the system of medicine in which they are used. Specialised reports also has the distribution and the forest type maps of the respective state, the botanical profile of the state and the MPCA and the habit wise analysis of the medicinal plants.

INFORMATION PRODUCTS

CDs on Medicinal plants of southern India

Three CDs on medicinal plants of Karnataka, Kerala and Tamil Nadu have been designed for the use of researchers working in the field of conservation. The CDs incorporate data on checklist of medicinal plants in each of these States. It also provides information on threat status of the species, synonyms, different systems of medicine they are used in and forest type where the plants occur. There are around 900 images. Information is also available on primary health care uses for 128 species and propagation techniques for 200 species. More than 65, 000 regional names have been included, in different languages like Sanskrit, Hindi, Marathi, Telugu, Kannada, Malayalam and Tamil, along with maps to show the occurrence of individual species in various forest types. The search of a species can be done either from botanical or regional name. It can filter the species depending on the forest type, threat status, system of medicine and by the language.

Clinically Important plants of Ayurveda (CIPA)

Clinically Important Plants of Ayurveda is now available as a CD-ROM, which contains detailed information of 3500 pharmaceutical preparations for 200 indications. It has plant pictures, botanical and regional names, Sanskrit synonyms and its complete reference, plant properties and English meaning of all technical Sanskrit terms. This would be useful for pharmaceutical industries, Ayurveda practitioners and researchers.

Plants of Caraka Samhita

This bilingual database incorporates 12, 873 plant references from Caraka Samhita which are grouped into 620 species. This was carried out based on a guideline prepared for grouping plant names as anonyms, synonyms and variant names. In the database, each plant reference is provided with its English translation and all the technical terms are supported with a dictionary of its English meaning. Classification of medicinal plants, 1,700 formulation information, plant picture, various botanical correlations and its identity status, habit and trade information of selected species, commentator 's opinion of plant identity, etc. are the important features of this database.

A multimedia CD was designed with necessary visual effects highlighting the importance of Caraka Samhita. A brochure on this CD is also available to support dissemination activities.

Database on plants of Ayurveda for BAMS course

All classical information pertaining to detailed and non-detailed list of plants mentioned in the BAMS (Bachelor of Ayurvedic Medicine and Surgery) syllabus were compiled from 20 classical texts. There are 370 plants in the syllabus which are incorporated in the database. Botanical names, regional names, classical references like Sanskrit slokas, interpretation of the slokas into English, and usage of these plants as single drugs are incorporated into this database.

Modern botanical information such as morphology, distribution, propagation methods and pharmacognosy information inclusive of its plant biochemistry and pharmacology are provided. This database is aimed to provide all required information for graduates and postgraduate students of Ayurveda.

Database on Ayurveda formularies

The database of the Ayurveda formularies incorporated in the Ver. 1 of CIPA (Clinically important plants of Ayurveda) CD. The second version of the CIPA will have 4, 000 more Ayurvedic formulation compiled from 7 classical texts covering about 150 plants.

MEDICINAL PLANTS AS A SOURCE OF RAW MATERIALS FOR ALLOPATHIC MEDICINE

Besides the direct applications of extract, powder, seed powder etc. of medicinal plants on the diseases, as mentioned in traditional system of medicines, many medicinal plants are used in pharmaceutical or drug industries to extract intermediary raw materials in manufacturing of various allopathic medicines.

1. There are sorrye plants which contain 4 to 8 % of diosgenins, the steroidal saponins and examples being Diascorea floribunda, Dioscorea deltoidea the common yam or khamb-alu in Oriya. Diosgenins when subjected to appropriate chemical reactions converted to cortisone a steroidal hormones for therapeutic purposes..
2. Reserpine an alkaloid extracted from Rouwlfia serpentina root (Sarpagandha) is used for manufacturing anti-hypertensive and sedative drugs.

TO CONSERVE AND CULTIVATE MEDICINAL PLANT-A GLOBAL NEED

It is now a need to preserve the medicinal plant which are in this spasm of extinction and to cultivate medicinal plants on commercial basis due to the following reasons.

1. It is being observed that many useful 111edicinal plants have become either endangered or becoming extinct particularly in the tropical eco- system of developing countries. It is apprehended that the modern allopathic system of medicine will suffer a serious set

back if certain medicinal plant species go totally extinct. Therefore, it is high time that our policy makers should seriously think about the preservation of such species in the form of herbarium and Gene Bank.

2. Increased demand for medicinal plants Iike Sadabahar, Rouwlfia, Occimum sanctum, Neem, Ashwagandha, Panax ginseng etc. warrants a development of improved agro-techniques for large scale commercial cultivation in tropical countries. It is interesting to know that there is a substantial demand from Ayurvedic. Allopathic and Homeopathic medicine manufacturers for medicinal plants. The estimated demand of various medicinal plants from leading Ayurvedic medicine manufacturer alone in India like Charak, Zandu. Dabur, Baidyanath etc. amounts to about Rs. 1000 crores per year. The export demand in India for Vinca rosea for preparation of vincrystin in USA is about Rs. 5 million.

3. The justification for commercial cultivation for medicinal plants may also be attributed to rampant deforestation.

CULTIVATION OF MEDICINAL PLANTS- A NEW ENTREPRENEURIAL OPPORTUNITY IN RURAL AREAS

Commercial cultivation of most demanded medicinal plant will lead to sustainable employment generation in the rural and tribal areas of India vis-a-vis enormous ur. 1employment problem and secondly it will boost up our forex earning through export ultimately both leading to over all economic development. Therefore, it may be concluded without any doubt and ambiguity that cultivation of medicinal plants offers an opportunity for entrepreneurial venture in a big way, particularly for S & T entrepreneurs.

AN OVERVIEW OF INDIAN NOVEL TRADITIONAL MEDICINAL PLANTS WITH ANTI-DIABETIC POTENTIALS

Diabetes mellitus is the most severe metabolic pandemic of the 21st century, affecting essential biochemical activities in almost every cell in the body and increasing the risk of cardiac problems. It is estimated that in the year 2000, 171 million people had diabetes, and this is expected to double by year 2030. Conventionally, insulin-dependant diabetes mellitus is treated with exogenous insulin and non insulin-dependant diabetes mellitus with synthetic oral hypoglycemic agents like sulphonylureas and biguanides. However the hormone fails as a curative agent for complications of diabetes and synthetic oral drugs produce adverse health effects. Different medicinal systems are using the active plant constituents, which discovered as natural hypoglycemic medicine, came from the virtue of traditional knowledge. Herbal drugs are considered free from side effects than synthetic one. They are less toxic, relatively cheap and popular. In India, medicinal plants have been used as natural medicine since the days of Vedic glory. Many of these medicinal plants and herbs are part of our diet as spices, vegetables and fruits. Historically, in 'Atharva-Veda' (about 200 B. C.) description of medicinal plants was made under a separate chapter 'Ayurveda'. Sushruta (about 400 B. C.) compiled classification of 700 herbal drugs under 37 classes in 'Sushruta Samhita' (A compendium of ancient Indian surgery). Charak (about 600 B. C.) made the scientific classification of herbal drugs based on remedial properties in his renowned treatise 'Charaka Samhita' (A compendium of general medicine). In which he described 50 classes of herbal remedies comprising 500 crude drugs. The medicinal values of plants have been tested by trial and error method for a long time by different workers. Even today great opportunities are still open for scientific investigations of herbal medicines for cure of diabetes and its complications.

TRIALS FOR ANTI-DIABETIC POTENTIALS OF MEDICINAL PLANTS

Recently the plants and herbs are being used as decoctions or in other extracted forms for their blood sugar lowering potential. There are some useful reviews on Indian medicinal plants having blood sugar lowering potentials. Many useful herbs introduced in pharmacological and clinical trials have confirmed their blood sugar lowering effect, repair of â-cells of islets of Langerhans. Details of some potent Indian herbs, their recently reported pharmacological and clinical hypoglycemic efficacy, active chemical constituents, their mechanism of action and available toxicity status are described chronologically as follows:

AEGLE MARMELOS LINN. COOREA (FAMILY: RUTACEAE)

Hindi name: Bel; Common name: Holy Fruit Tree

The trees grow throughout deciduous forest of India and ripen fruits are commonly use for delicacy. Aegle marmelos is widely used in Indian Ayurvedic medicine for the treatment of diabetes mellitus. Hypoglycemic effect of root bark decoction (1ml/100mg) has been observed in normal fasted rats. Leaf extract produced anti-hyperglycemic activity in alloxan diabetic rats along with decreased cholesterol and blood urea. In diabetic rats leaf extract exhibited insulin like activity. Aqueous leaf extract has been shown to improve the functional state of pancreatic cells in streptozotocin induced diabetic rats. Aqueous leaf extract (250 & 500mg/kg, orally) produced hypoglycemic effect and increased plasma insulin level of STZ-diabetic rats. LD50 (lethal dose) observed greater than 10. 0g/kg at oral administration to rats. Anti-hyperglycemic activity caused by leaf extract (250mg/kg, orally) in glucose fed hyperglycemic rats (Sachdewa et al., 2001). Aqueous fruit extract (250mg/kg, twice daily for one month) produces anti-hyperglycemic effect along with decreasing glycosylated haemoglobin level in STZ induced diabetic albino wistar rats. Hypoglycemic and antioxidant activity of leaves have been observed in diabetic male albino rats. Fruit extract (125 and 250mg/kg, orally twice daily for 30 days) produced anti-diabetic, anti-hyperlipidaemic and antioxidant activity in STZ diabetic rats along with partial repair of damaged pancreatic islets (Kamalakkanan et al., 2005). Treatment of severely (fasting blood glucose level >250 mg/ml) diabetic rats for 14 days with aqueous extract (250mg/kg, orally) of Aegle marmelos seeds reduced the fasting blood glucose by 60. 84% and urine sugar by 75% than their pretreatment levels.

ALLIUM CEPA LINN. (FAMILY: LILIACEAE)

Hindi name: Pyaj; Common name: Onion

The plant is cultivated throughout India. Onion bulb and leaves are the important part of diet. Ether soluble fraction of onion (0. 25mg/kg, orally) has been observed to lower blood sugar level in normal rabbits and exhibited potent antioxidant activity (Auguati, 1973). In a clinical study treatment of diabetic patients by juice of Allium cepa bulb, controlled the blood sugar level. Dipropyl disulphide oxide and onion oil produced significant hypoglycemic effect. Significant blood sugar lowering produced by petroleum ether extract (2g/kg) from onion bulb in glucose, induced hyper-glycemic rabbits. A sulphur containing amino acid, S-methyl cystein sulphoxide (at a dose of 200mg/kg for 45 days) from onion showed potent hypoglycemic activity in alloxan induced diabetic rats. S-allyl cystein sulphoxide from onion significantly reduced blood glucose level of alloxan induced diabetic rats. Prolonged administration of freeze dried onion powder (3%) with a diet produced anti- hyperglycemic, hypolipidemic and antioxidant activity in STZ-diabetic rats. Onion callus cultures showed greater hypoglycemic potential over natural onion bulb. Prolonged administration of a diet containing onion produced hypoglycemic and antioxidant effect in diabetic rats. Allium cepa juice (0. 4g/100g b. w. for 4 weeks) exhibited anti-hyperglycemic and antioxidant effect in alloxan induced diabetic rats, it also repaired hepatic and renal damage caused by alloxan.

ALLIUM SATIVUM LINN. (FAMILY: LILIACEAE)

Hindi name: Lahsun; Common name: Garlic

The plant is cultivated all over India. It is an important part of dietary ingredients. Allicin (0. 25mg/kg, orally) from garlic exhibited pronounce hypoglycemia in mild diabetic rabbits. In alloxan induced diabetic rabbits ethanol, ethyl acetate and petroleum ether extract (0. 25mg/kg, orally) produced antihyperglycemic activity. Treatment of alloxan diabetic rats with the antioxidant s-allyl cysteine sulfoxide isolated from garlic ameliorates the diabetic condition almost to the same extent as did glibenclamide and insulin. It also significantly stimulates in vitro insulin secretion from â-cells isolated from pancreas of normal rats. Extract (500mg/kg/day) of Allium sativum bulb proved to be effective for treatment of l-thyroxine (l-T4) induced hyperglycemia in rats. Alloxan induced diabetic rats fed a diet containing Allium sativum (12. 5%) for 15 days were able to reduce blood glucose as compare to control group. Oral administration of a laboratory diet containing 0. 05% of ajoene (derived from garlic) for 8 weeks has been observed to produce anti-diabetic effect in genetically diabetic KK-A(y) mice. The levels of plasma glucose significantly suppressed about 73. 8%. Two garlic compounds garlic oil (100mg/kg body weight) and diallyl trisulfide (40mg/kg body weight) given every other day for 3 weeks to STZ-diabetic rats significantly raised the basal insulin concentration and increased the insulin sensitivity. Herbal extract of garlic (20mg 100 g-1 body weight, orally, daily for 5 weeks) produced hypoglycemia, probably by interfering with food intake of both normal and STZ-diabetic rats. S-allyl cysteine, a key component of aged garlic, found potent antioxidant and inhibited AGEP (accumulation of advanced glycation end products) formation. Bis (allixinato) oxovanadium (IV) from garlic found to be the most potent anti-diabetic agent in type 1 diabetic mice on both intraperitoneal injections and oral administrations (Adachi et al., 2006).

ALOE VERA (LINN.) BURM. F. (FAMILY: LILIACEAE)

Hindi and Common name: Aloe

The herbs are cultivated throughout India for its variety of medicinal properties. Dry sap of plant produced prominent anti-hyperglycemic response in type 2 diabetic patients (½ teaspoonful, orally for 4–14 weeks), and in alloxan induced diabetic Swiss albino mice (500mg/kg, twice daily for 5 days). In a clinical study, it was reported that oral administration of aloe might be a useful adjuvant for lowering of blood glucose in diabetic patients. Aloe vera leaf pulp extract showed hypoglycemic activity on type 1 and type 2 diabetic rats, the effect being enhanced in type 2 diabetes as compared with glibenclamide. Plant extract (200 and 300mg/kg, orally) produced hypoglycemic activity along with controlled carbohydrate metabolizing enzymes in normal fasted, oral glucose fed and STZ-diabetic rats. Oral administration of ethanolic extract (300mg/kg b. w.) to STZ-diabetic rats for 21 days resulted in a prominent reduction of fasting blood glucose along with improved plasma insulin level of diabetic rats. Administration of the five phytosterols from Aloe vera namely, lophenol, 24-methyl-lophenol, 24-ethyl-lophenol, cycloartanol and 24-the fasting blood glucose levels 64%, 28%, 47%, 51%, and 55% respectively. Oral administration of Aloe vera gel extract (300mg/kg b. w. per day for 21 days) to STZ-diabetic rats resulted in a significant reduction of fasting blood glucose and improved the plasma insulin level.

ANDROGRAPHIS PANICULATA (BURM. F.) NEES (FAMILY: ACANTHACEAE)

Hindi name: Kalmegha; Common name: King of Bitter

This is an annual herb that grows throughout India. Plant extract effectively produced hypoglycemic and anti-hyperglycemic activity in normal rats. Different doses (0. 1, 0. 2, and 0. 4g/kg b. w.) of plant extract effectively reduced the fasting serum glucose level of STZ-diabetic rats. Antihyperglycemic and antioxidant activity of plant extract (400mg/kg b. w, twice a day for 14 days), has also been reported in diabetic rats.

The andrographolide from plant increases the glucose utilization and lowers plasma glucose in diabetic rats lacking insulin. Significant reduction in blood glucose level (52. 90%) observed when hyperglycemic rats treated with 50mg/kg body weight aqueous extract of Andrographis paniculata. This effect enhanced when freeze-dried material used at a dose of 6. 25 mg/ kg body weight, it reduced 61. 81% blood glucose level. The anti-diabetic potentials of plant restored the impaired estrous cycle in alloxan-induced diabetic rats.

ANNONA SQUAMOSA LINN. (ANNONACEAE)

Hindi name: Sharifa; Common name: Sugar apple tree

The plants grow throughout India and commonly use by tribal communities of Northern India for the treatment of diabetes. Aqueous leaf extract produces hypoglycemic activity in streptozotocin-nicotinamide induced dia betic rats. Ethanolic leaf-extract (350mg/kg b. w., orally 10-day) administration to STZ-diabetic rats has been shown to lower fasting blood glucose level to (73. 3%), and treatment of severely diabetic rabbits with leaf- extract (350mg/kg, for 15 days) reduced fasting blood glucose by 52. 7% and urine sugar by 75%. Annona squamosa fruit pulp extract (2. 5 and 5. 0g/kg b. w.) has been observed to improve the glucose tolerance of alloxan diabetic rats. Further more, fruit pulp (5g/kg b. w.) brought down urine sugar, urine protein and glycol-hemoglobin in diabetic rabbits. Oral administration of aqueous leaf-extract to diabetic rats for 30 days significantly reduced the levels of blood glucose and increased the activity of plasma insulin and antioxidant enzymes.

AZADIRACHTA INDICA A. JUSS. (FAMILY: MELIACEAE)

Hindi name: Neem; Common name: Indian lilac tree

This is an evergreen tree grows throughout India. Aqueous extract is known to produce antihyperglycemic and hypoglycemic activity in diabetic dogs. Fresh leaves decoction induced antihyperglycemic activity and increased the peripheral glucose utilization in normal rats. Leaf extract of Azadirachta indica has been reported to produce the hypoglycemic activity in normal rats without altered serum cortisol level (Chattopadhyay et al., 1999). Crude ethanol extract (250mg/kg, for 2 weeks) potentially lowered the blood sugar level of alloxan diabetic rats. Leaf extract has been observed to produce anti-hyperglycemic activity in streptozotocin diabetic rats without altered serum cortisol level. Petroleum ether extract of seed kernel (2gm/kg b. w.) & seed husk (0. 9gm/kg b. w.) restricted oxidative stress in heart and erythrocytes caused by streptozotocin in diabetic rats. Dianex, a polyherbal formulation consists of the aqueous extract of Azadirachta indica has been well tolerated in laboratory animals at higher doses (up to 10 g/kg in mice, acute toxicity; up to 2. 5 g/kg in rats, sub-acute toxicity studies for 30 days) without any toxic manifestation. Beta-sitosterol, a steroid obtained from Azadirachta indica, may be responsible for its hypoglycemic property. In a clinical study of type 2 diabetes powdered part, aqueous extract and alcoholic extract of Azadirachta indica at high dose for 14 days exhibited hypoglycemic activity.

CINNAMOMUM TAMALA (HAMM.) NEES. & EBERM. (FAMILY: LAURACEAE)

Hindi name: Tejpat; Common name: Bayberry

The plant is cultivated in different parts of India and use as spice. Aqueous leaf extract induced potential blood sugar lowering effect in 18 hours fasted and glucose induced hyperglycemic rabbits at a dose of 500mg/kg. Oral administration of powdered leaves (20gm for 15 days) exhibited hypoglycemic effect in patients of type 2 diabetes mellitus along with insulin released from pancreatic â-cells. In a clinical study, leave powder produced hypoglycemic response in type 2 diabetic patients. Ethanolic extract (210mg/kg) of leaves induced potential hypoglycemic effect in 18 hours fasted albino rats. Alcoholic extract of leaves produced hypoglycemic activity in alloxan induced diabetic rats when administered orally for two weeks at a dose of 250mg/kg.

COCCINIA GRANDIS (LINN.) VOIGT (FAMILY: CUCURBITACEAE)

Syn. Coccina indica (White & Arn); Hindi name: Kunderi; Common name: Ivy Guard lowering effect has been observed in patients treated with homogenized freeze dried leaves. Ethanol extract (250mg/kg) of whole plant produced hypoglycemic activity in fasted, glucose fed and diabetic albino rats. Hypoglycemic effect of alcoholic extract (250mg/kg, orally) of Coccinia indica was observed in fasted and glucose fed hyperglycemic male albino rats. Alcoholic leaf extract produced hypoglycemic effect in normal fed and 48 hours fasted rats, response mediated by suppression of gluconeogenic enzyme glucose-6-phosphatase. Pectin (200mg/100gm/day) isolated from fruits, exhibited blood sugar lowering effect and an increase in the glycogen content of liver in normal rats. Ethanol (60%) leaf extract (200mg/kg, orally) lowered the blood sugar level of diabetic rats due to suppressed glucose synthesis, through depression of glucose-6-phosphatase, fructose-1-6-biphosphatase and enhanced glucose oxidation by shunt pathway through activation of glucose-

6-phosphate dehydrogenase. Leaf extract was produced hypoglycemic, and insulin secretogouge activity in diabetic patients. Dried extract (500mg/kg, p. o. for 6 weeks), of plant exhibited anti-hyperglycemic activity in diabetic patients. Extract mimic insulin like activity and improved the functional status of enzymes in glycolytic pathway and lypolytic pathway. Potent antioxidant and hypolipidemic activity exhibited by ethanolic leaf extract administered at a dose of 200mg/kg for 45 days to streptozotocin induced diabetic rats.

FICUS BENGALENSIS LINN. (FAMILY: MORACEAE)

Hindi name: Bargad; Common name: Indian Banyan Tree

Plants grow throughout India and in the Indian tradition it is considered as a holy tree. In a chronic toxicity test extract (25 & 250mg/kg), produced reversible hepatic damage while the acute LD50 (lethal dose) found to be 9. 47g/kg body weight when given intraperitoneally. Leucocyanidin (3-O-â-D-galactosylcellobioside) a dimethoxy derivative isolated from bark, lowered blood sugar level and increased serum insulin in normal and moderate diabetic rats. It also inhibits the degradation processes of insulin. Alcoholic extract of stem bark at a dose of 25, 50 & 75mg/day/100g, b. w. lowered the blood sugar level 47 to 70%, and also restored the normal levels of serum urea, cholesterol and total protein of alloxan diabetic albino rats. Glucoside of leucopelargonidin isolated from bark has been reported to induce hypoglycemic, hypolipidemic and serum insulin raising effect in moderately diabetic rats. 3-O-alfa-L- rhamnoside (250mg/kg, single dose study & 100mg/kg/day, long term study), a dimethoxy derivative isolated from bark, lowered blood sugar in fasted and glucose induced hyperglycemic rats, along with enhanced insulin secretion from â-cells. Leucodelphinidine derivative isolated from bark exhibited hypoglycemic activity in normal and alloxan diabetic rats. 3-O-á-L-rhamnoside isolated from the bark has been showed its median effective dose (ED50) as 100mg/kg with 12% hypoglycemic action in normal rats. Hypoglycemic and hypercholesterolemic effect of aqueous bark extract was observed in alloxan induced mild and severe diabetic rabbits. Lethal dose (LD50) of this was found to be 1gm/kg, when administered orally for 3 months in rats. Leucopelrgonin (100mg/kg/day for one month) isolated from bark lowered the fasting blood sugar (34%) and glycosylated haemoglobin (28%) of alloxan diabetic dogs.

GYMNEMA SYLVESTRE (WILLD) R. BR. (FAMILY: ASCELPIADACEAE)

Hindi name: Gudmar; Common name: Periploca of the wood

Plants are grown in tropical regions of India and used as household remedy for diabetes. Oral administration of a water soluble fraction G-54 isolated from Gymnema sylvestre administered to 27 type 2 diabetic patients reduced their insulin requirement, lowered the fasting blood sugar and glycosylated haemoglobin content. Two water soluble fractions (GS-3 and GS- 4) obtained from leaves were found to double the pancreatic islets and â-cell numbers in diabetic rats. Alcoholic leaf extract (500mg/kg, orally) lowered maximum blood sugar in fasted, glucose fed and diabetic rats along with insulin released from pancreatic â-cells. In rats the insulin secretion from islets of Langerhans and several pancreatic â-cell lines induced by alcoholic extract in absence of other stimulus. Gymnemic acid IV, isolated from leaves produced potent hypoglycemic effect in STZ-diabetic mice. Leaf extract has been observed to produce anti-hyperglycemic and hypoglycemic effects of in corticosteroid-induced diabetes mellitus, without altered serum cortisol concentration. A polyherbal formulation containing aqueous extracts of Gymnema sylvestre produced prominent hypoglycemic activity in normal and diabetic rats at a dose of 100–500mg/kg/day, orally for acute, 6 hours and for long-term, 6 weeks studies. Gymnemic acid IV isolated from the leaves has been observed to produce hypoglycemic, anti-hyperglycemic, glucose uptake inhibitory and gut glycosidase inhibitory effects.

MOMORDICA CHARANTIA LINN. (FAMILY: CUCURBITACEAE)

Hindi name: Karela; Common name: Bitter gourd

The plant is an annual climber grown mostly in tropical India and commonly use as vegetable. Charantin (50mg/kg, orally) isolated from Momordica charantia has been resembled insulin lower blood sugar level (maximum 42% at 4th hour) of rabbits. In a clinical study of type 1 and type 2 diabetic patients the polypeptide-p isolated from fruit, seeds and tissue exhibited hypoglycemic activity without any side effect. The subcutaneous injection of (0. 5unit/kg) lowered the blood sugar in gerbils and langurs. Charantin obtained from Momordica charantia induced hypoglycemic effect and also stimulated the insulin release and blocked the formation of glucose in blood stream. Hypoglycemic effect and delayed cataract development was reported in alloxan diabetic rats treated with fruit extract (4g/kg/Day orally for 2 months). Ethanolic extract (200mg/kg) of Momordica charantia was produced hypoglycemic activity in normal and streptozotocin diabetic rats; this was occurred possibly due to inhibiting glucose-6-phosphatase and fructose-1, 6-biphosphatase in liver, and stimulating hepatic glucose-6-phosphate dehydrogenase activities. Oleanolic acid and momordin from plant, produced antihyperglycemic effect by inhibiting glucose transport in intestine of rat. Fruit aqueous extract (200mg/kg, orally for 6 weeks), and exercise potentially lowered blood sugar of type 2 diabetic and hyperinsulinemic (insulin resistance) rats. Seed aqueous extract produced prominent reduction in blood glucose, glycosylated hemoglobin, lactate dehydrogenase, glucose-6-phosphatase, fructose-1, 6-bisphosphatase and glycogen phosphorylase along with increased hemoglobin, glycogen content and hexokinase, glycogen synthase activity. Anti-diabetic properties of plant such as charantin, vicine and polypeptide-p have the potential to be a part of dietary supplement for patients of diabetes. From Momordica charantia the major compounds, 5b, 19- e po xy -3 b, 2 5 d ih yd ro xy cu cu rb it a - 6 , 2 3 (E) - di en e(4) and 3 b- 7 b ,25dihydroxycucurbita-5, 23(E) -dien-19-al(5) administered at a dose of 400mg/kg produced hypoglycemic effect in ddY mice strain.

OCIMUM SANCTUM LINN. (FAMILY: LAMIACEAE)

Hindi name: Tulasi; Common name: Holy Basil

It is a tropical annual herb grown all over India and use for household remediation. Oral administration of alcoholic extract of leaves of Ocimum sanctum lowered blood sugar level in normal; glucose fed hyperglycemic and STZ-diabetic rats, along with increased insulin release. Ocimum sanctum leaf powder was produced potent hypoglycemic and hypolipidemic effect in normal and diabetic rats. Alcoholic extract of leaves significantly lowered the blood glucose in normal and alloxan diabetic rats. Administration of plant extract 200mg/kg in STZ-diabetic rats for 30 days led to decreased in plasma glucose level by 26. 4%. Plant extract lowered blood glucose level along with inhibited cortisol level. From leaf extract the aqueous butanol and ethylacetate fractions stimulated insulin secretion from perfuse rat pancreas, isolated rat islets and a clonal rat â-cell line in a concentration-dependent manner.

PTEROCARPUS MARSUPIUM ROXB. (FAMILY: FABACEAE)

Hindi name: Vijayasar; Common name: Indian Malabar

Plants grow throughout India and are use as hypoglycemic plant in folklore medicine. Aqueous bark extract lowered blood sugar and improved glucose tolerance of diabetics with no side effects observed. From alcoholic extract of bark the ethyl acetate soluble fraction caused blood sugar lowering and repaired the alloxan induced pancreatic â-cells damage in albino rats. From plant the (-) -epicatechin (30mg/kg, i. p.) produced anti-hyperglycemic effect in alloxan induced diabetic rats. The (-) epicatechin, from bark increased the cAMP content of the pancreatic islets associated with increased insulin release, conversion of proinsulin to insulin and cathepsin B activity in rats. Marsupin and pterostilbene, two phenolic constituents of plant potentially lowered blood glucose at same level as compared to metformin in STZ- diabetic rats. Aqueous extract (1g/kg, orally) of bark has been observed to produce anti-cataract activity in alloxan diabetic rats. Plant extract was prevented the hyper-triglyceridaemia and hyper-insulinaemia (insulin resistance) in type 2 diabetic patients. Aqueous extract (250mg/kg, orally) of dried wood has been reported to produce hypoglycemic effect in acute and sub-acute study.

SWERTIA CHIRAYITA (ROXB. EX FLAM) KARST. (FAMILY: GENTIANACEAE)

Hindi name: Kirayat Chirata; Common name: Bitter Stick

The herbs grow abundantly in Himalayan regions of India and are used for treatment of various ailments by the tribes. 95% ethanol extract (250mg/kg) of plant potentially lowered the blood sugar level in fasted, glucose fed and tolbutamide pretreated animals. Hexane fraction (250mg/kg, b. w. orally for 28 days) of plant, lowered blood sugar of albino rats with increased glycogen content of liver and insulin released from pancreatic â-cells. Swerchirin (50mg/

kg, orally) isolated from hexane fraction of plant exerted potent hypoglycemic activity in normal and STZ-diabetic albino rats. A xanthone isolated from the hexane fraction of Swertia chirayita identified as swerchirin (1, 8-dihydroxy-3, 5-dimethoxyxanthone) exhibited blood sugar lowering effect in fasted, fed, glucose fed hyperglycemic and tolbutamide pretreated albino rats. Effective dose (ED50) of Swertia chirayita has been reported to be 23. 1mg/kg/oral, lower maximum 40% blood sugar level of male albino rats of body weight 140–165g. Swerchirin (50mg/kg, b. w. orally) isolated from crude extract lowered maximum 60% blood glucose at 7 hour post-treatment, along with depleted aldehyde-fuchsin stained b-granules and immunostained insulin of islets of Langerhans. Swerchirin isolated from plant was found to be superior blood sugar lowering agent over tolbutamide. Alcoholic extract (250mg/kg, once daily for two weeks) exhibited hypoglycemic effect in alloxan induced diabetic rats.

SYZYGIUM CUMINI LINN. (FAMILY: MYRTACEAE)

Syn. Eugenia jambolana (Linn.); Hindi name: Jamun; Common name: Black Berry

Plants grow in different parts of India. The ripe fruits are used as part of dietary component. Oral administration of fruit pulp induced hypoglycemic activity in normal and STZ-diabetic rats along with insulin released from â-cells. Seed powder provided good symptomatic relief to 30 patients of diabetes (type 2) and regulated blood sugar level. Increased activity of hexokinase and decreased activity of glucose-6-phosphate in liver produced blood sugar lowering effect at oral administration of aqueous seed extract (2. 5g/kg, b. w. for one month) to alloxan diabetic rats.

Aqueous seed extract (2. 5 & 5g/kg, b. w. for 6 weeks) has been observed to produce hypoglycemic and antioxidant activity, and increase in haemoglobin content in rats. Alcoholic seed extract injection (20mg, intraperitoneally) reduced the blood sugar level to 37. 17% at 3 hour and 46. 68% at 6 hour of administration in alloxan diabetic mice along with enhanced insulin secretion. Decreased plasma glucose concentrations in STZ-induced diabetic mice was observed at oral administration of fruit extract (200mg/kg, for 50 days).

Blood sugar lowering, hypolipidemic activity, increased serum insulin, increased glycogen content of liver and muscles and a fall in glycosylated haemoglobin level produced by ethanolic extract (100mg/kg b. w. orally) of seed.

Ethanolic seed kernels extract (100gm/kg b. w.) has been observed to improve glucose tolerance, and produce hypoglycemic and hypolipidemic effect in STZ-diabetic rats. Syzygium cumini was produced prominent fall of blood sugar in mice. Aqueous and ethanolic extracts of the fruit-pulp has been reported to produce antihyperglycemic effect in alloxan diabetic rats, and 24. 4% raise in plasma insulin level in mild diabetic and 26. 3% in severely diabetic rabbits.

TRIGONELLA FOENUM-GRAECUM LINN. (FAMILY: FABACEAE)

Hindi name: Methi; Common name: Fenugreek

Plants are commonly cultivated throughout India. The leaves are used as vegetable and seeds as spice. Major alkaloid trigonellin from fenugreek seeds produced hypoglycemic activity. Ethanol extract (0. 8g/kg, i. p.) of leaves has been observed to reduce blood glucose concentration in alloxan induced diabetic rats. Lethal doses (LD50) of aqueous leaf extract were 1.9g/ kg at intra-peritoneal and 10g/kg at oral administration. 4-Hydroxyisoleucine, an insulinotropic compound isolated from seeds increased the insulin release in glucose fed hyperglycemic rats and humans.

Seeds powder treatment normalized the enhanced lipid peroxidation and reduced the susceptibility to oxidative stress associated with depletion of antioxidants in liver of rats. Maximum 46. 64% decrease in blood sugar level of diabetic rats was observed at oral administration of seed extract (1g/kg, for one month).

From fenugreek seeds, the soluble dietary fibre (SDF) fraction at (0. 5g/ kg, orally administered twice daily, for 28 days) inhibited platelets aggregation in type 2 diabetic rats and produced beneficial effect in dyslipidemia.

Restored activity of glutamate dehydrogenase, NAD linked isocitrate dehydrogenase and D-b-hydroxybutyrate dehydrogenase reported at oral administration of seed powder (5%, for 3 weeks) in alloxan diabetic rats. It a ls o re pa ire d th e li ver a nd k idney da m a ge c a use d by a llo xa n. 4 - hydroxyisoleucine:5, an amino acid, isolated from seeds, produced anti-hyperglycemic effect and decreased the 33% plasma triglyceride, 22% total cholesterol (22%) and 14% free fatty acids.

ACTIVE HYPOGLYCEMIC CONSTITUENTS FROM PLANTS

Many active compounds have been isolated from the plant and herb species of India. These active principles are dietary fibres, alkaloids, flavonoids, saponins, amino acids, steroids, peptides and others. These have produced potent hypoglycemic, anti-hyperglycemic and glucose suppressive activities.

The above effects achieved by either insulin release from pancreatic â-cells, inhibited glucose absorption in gut, stimulated glycogenesis in liver or increased glucose utilization by the body. These compounds also exhibited their antioxidant, hypolipidemic, anticataract activities, restored enzymatic functions, repair and regeneration of pancreatic islets and the alleviation of liver and renal damage. Some active constituents have been obtained from plants possess insulin like activity and could be provide alternate for insulin therapy. Chemical structures of few active compounds having anti-diabetic potentials from above mentioned plants are provided.

Metabolic imbalance causing diabetes mellitus is a characteristic of materialistic world. Differences in social structure, psychic stress, obesity, hormonal imbalance and heredity are optimizing the growth of pandemic. Increasing population with diabetes has a huge requirement of effective remediation.

The Indian flora has a vast variety of medicinal plants, which are used traditionally for their anti-diabetic property. However, careful assessment including sustainability of such herbs, ecological and seasonal variation in activity of phyto-constituents, metal contents of crude herbal anti-diabetic drugs, thorough toxicity study and cost effectiveness is required for their popularity.

These efforts may provide treatment for all and justify the role of novel traditional medicinal plants having anti-diabetic potentials.

BIO-INFORMATICS ON MEDICINAL PLANTS AND TRADITIONAL KNOWLEDGE

Medicinal Plants Master Database

A comprehensive master database on medicinal plants of India has been systematically built up at FRLHT over the last 8 years. Currently, this database incorporates more than 7, 500 botanical names which are linked to more than 1, 40, 500 *Vernacular names* in 13 different languages like Tamil, Kannada, Malayalam, Hindi, Sanskrit, etc. Each such correlation can be traced back to a published reference.

This database also incorporates more than 10, 000 authentic digital images of plants duly linked to their botanical names. An important feature of this database is a fully-referenced distribution database which provides information on geographical distribution of nearly 6, 000 plant species. Through a system of assigning a unique ID number to each botanical name and linking various aspects of information, for each species, to this unique ID, data relating to several different aspects like propagation, trade, pharmacognosy etc can be quickly accessed for a specific plant entity with search being initiated with the help of a botanical or vernacular name.

This multi-faceted database forms the backbone for undertaking and promoting sustainable use and informed conservation action for native medicinal plant species and also acts as a platform for designing various research projects relating to the management of this valuable natural resource.

This database is also linked to referenced information on the plant materia-medica of traditional systems of medicine as well as to pharmacognosy and pharmacology of the plant entities.

PHARMACOGNOSY DATABASE ON INDIAN MEDICINAL PLANTS

A computerised database called Labguru has been created for storing and retrieving referenced literature on pharmacognosy and pharmacology of medicinal plants. Labguru is a stand-alone database with an easy-to-use interface, linked to the master database.

This database is a valuable literature source for researchers and industry alike. Data compilation is from published sources such as texts and on-line databases. This is an ongoing evolving activity in the laboratory at FRLHT.

Database on metals and minerals used in Indian medicines

Mineral and metal medicine is used by traditional practitioners all over India. These are potent medicinal materials which need accurate identification of materials and careful processing for their proper use. Therefore it was decided to develop a user-friendly and easily retrievable database on mineral and metal medicine by compilation of relevant references from authentic traditional texts of Ayurveda that are difficult to procure at one place for most users. Correlating the traditional names of metals minerals to modern geological entities helps to understand the identity of the minerals used.

AYUSH Databases

FRLHT in the last 10 years has been documenting and developing traditional knowledge databases on the materia medica of Indian systems of medicine.

Medicinal plant databases have been already initiated on Ayurveda, Siddha, Unani system and Homoeopathy. The current FRLHT databases have screened a limited number of the known medical texts written across the period 1500 BC to 1900 AD and therefore much work yet remains to be done.

In the next 5 years we would also like to initiate new database work on diagnostics and other speciality areas like panchakarma and rasayana, as these fields are critical for effective application of Ayurveda and Siddha.

The main goal of the databases is to serve the needs of students and teachers of Indian systems of medicine, medical practitioners, researchers, community enterprises, community health NGOs and pharmaceutical companies.

Database of plants of Susruta Samhita

The database of plants of Susruta Samhita has 9, 650 references. This data has been converted from the previous data environment to the present one to support access to various database tools. A checklist of the plant names was prepared and a report is made available in Sanskrit and English scripts.

Database on plants of Siddha medicine

The bilingual database has an extensive collection of information pertaining to a therapeutic information of plants mentioned in 5 texts of 2, 350 records, simple remedies mentioned in 6 texts of 1, 800 records, formulation data of 3,013 records and 36, 000 records of dictionary file which has Tamil names of plants.

A separate nighantu file in Tamil script and a glossary of the technical terms are also incorporated in this database.

Database on plants of Homoeo medicine

This database could complete compilation of plants and products information of 80 plants mentioned in Homoeo medicine from 15-20 sources as text document.

Database on plants of Unani medicine

A hard copy of the Arabic and Urdu names appearing in the classical texts of Unani medicine was prepared from the FRLHT's nomenclature database. Verification on botanical names and spellings of Arabic names and Unani names were carried out.

❒

Our Medicinal Plants

KNOWLEDGE RELATING TO MEDICINAL PLANTS

Mere knowledge is difficult to protect legally, as it is intangible. One kind of protection is by means of asserting an intellectual property right, such as a patent, copyright, or trade secret. In the case of medicinal plants, traditional knowledge relating to these plants does not fall within any of these established categories. On the other hand, the use of technology, including biotechnology, to develop a useful product using this traditional knowledge is generally protected. The issue of bio-piracy in relation to such useful and financially productive knowledge has come into Knowledge relating to medicinal plants prominence as a result of the cases challenging the patent granted on neem and on turmeric.

In the turmeric case, the US Patent and Trademark Office granted a patent on the "use of turmeric in wound healing". India successfully challenged this patent by showing that this use of turmeric was well known and that nothing new had been invented. The documents relating to this traditional knowledge of India were unknown to the US Patent and Trademark Office. When they were brought to the attention of the Office they were considered to be "prior art" and the patent was revoked.

In the case of neem, the patent challenged referred to improving the storage stability of an insecticide containing neem seed extracts. This patent could not be revoked as the patent holder (W. R. Grace & Co.) had improved on existing knowledge. While neem-based insecticides were well known, they did not have the storage-stability claimed in the patent. The patented composition could thus be distinguished from the traditional knowledge.

The cases of turmeric and neem are illustrative of the dilemma facing India in relation to the traditional knowledge of medicinal plants. On the one hand, traditional knowledge is not documented in an easily accessible form so as to be considered "prior art". On the other hand, where traditional knowledge is available as to the property of a particular plant, it can be modified so as to be distinguishable from the original traditional knowledge for legal purposes. The end result is that a particular company may get the sole right to manufacture and sell the active chemical compound derived from a plant, although communities may have used the plant for the same or similar purpose over a long period of time.

To prevent this, the preparation of databases of traditional knowledge is being actively pursued. This would solve the problem of showing traditional knowledge to be "prior art" (the turmeric case). But this does not solve the problem faced in the neem case that of the modification of traditional knowledge. Information as provided by traditional knowledge is often all that is needed to provide the necessary input for research and development by a pharmaceutical company, which may use it to make a product that is legally "new", but is considered to be bio-piracy by the community concerned.

One solution to this would be to have pre-conditions in place for access to the databases. This would take the form of a legal contract between the researcher and the database owner. This contract may necessarily vary from region to region or community to community, but it would nevertheless be based on certain common provisions. For example, the contract would require the researcher to give an undertaking to give credit to the community as the source of the information, to share any future benefits arising out of the use of such knowledge, etc. The contract would be have to be signed by every person accessing the database, irrespective of country or community or reason for access, before he or she is permitted to look at the database.

Apart from the above non-statutory methods of protecting knowledge, the Biological Diversity Bill, 2000 requires prior approval of the National Biodiversity Authority for any foreigner or non-resident Indian who wishes to obtain knowledge associated with any biological resource occurring in India. Its prior approval is also necessary for any person who wishes to apply for any intellectual property right anywhere in the world for an invention based on information on a biological resource obtained from India (except in the case of a patent application, where the approval may be obtained anytime before the sealing of the patent). The Parliamentary Standing Committee that considered this Bill has recommended that a ceiling of 90 days be provided to the Authority for granting its approval.

The Patents (Second Amendment) Bill, 1999 has a limited form of protection for traditional knowledge. It states that an Indian patent may be opposed or revoked if the invention was anticipated having regard to the knowledge, oral or otherwise, available within any local or indigenous community in any country. This would need to be reciprocated by other countries for Indian traditional knowledge to be adequately protected.

India has adopted a combination of methods for the protection of medicinal plants. Wherever a pluralistic legislative framework is adopted, the efficacy of the system depends to a large extent on the amount of friction between the parts. As each legislative proposal has been promoted by a different

Governmental Department, it could be difficult for the national interest to be promoted without close co-operation between the different Authorities involved.

CONSIDERING THE ROLE FOR INDIA

The global context briefly sketched above suggests several tremendous opportunities for India, a country unrivaled in terms of diversity of medical systems and practices, in addition to being a major storehouse of biological diversity, with 2 of the 14 megabiodiversity areas of the world located within its borders. The global market would appear to be more receptive than ever to the mounting of a concentrated Indian effort at supplying it with medical materials and know-how. Such an effort would also appear to be increasingly remunerative for the country. India is of course already an active participant in the global medicinal plants market having been for some time the world's largest supplier of raw materials (though an insignificant supplier of finished products) (Patnaik 1994). Of the 74 species accounted for in one of the studies mentioned above, India was known to be exporting 22 and importing 8 (Handa 1992), while the German study quoted earlier, which is now underway, has found India to be Germany's largest trading partner by far (Lange 1996). Moreover, medicinal plants are one of the most important components of the non-wood forest products sector which supplies over 80% of India's net forest annual export earnings.

Despite these promising indications, however, it is unclear whether India is truly exploiting her comparative advantage in the medicinal plants sector and tapping the full potential of an expanding consumer base. In addition, several concerns arise in relation to the current consequences of participation in the market, with regard to the sustainability and equitability of prevailing practices in the sector.

Although only micro-studies are currently available in this regard, most of these indicate that current practices are both unsustainable, as they rapidly deplete the natural supplies of the country's plant base, and inequitable, perpetuating impoverishment for those charged with stewarding and harvesting the resource, while a few profit in dramatic disproportion to their inputs. Negative impacts on local primary health care, as plants become diverted to national and international markets, have also been cited in some cases. To add to all of these negative aspects, the market in India has been shown to be highly inefficient and imperfect.

The need of the hour, then, is to replan India's participation in the expanding global market, in light of the interests of all the stakeholders who are affected and who play a role in this sector. There is a need to collate all the available information regarding medicinal plants development in the country in order to obtain a comprehensive overview which will provide the necessary insight for coordinated and effective action.

Such an overview could form the basis of a renewed development of India's medicinal plants sector, and a strategic exploitation of her comparative advantage in the global market on a sustainable and equitable basis.

ORIGINS AND OBJECTIVES OF THE REVIEW

It was with the intention of providing such a comprehensive overview that the International Development Research Centre and the World Bank's Department of Agriculture and Natural Resources commissioned the authors to conduct a state-of-the-art review of the medicinal plants sector in India.

Medicinal plants, of course, do not presently constitute a sector as typically defined in international development discourse; generally they have been defined as a forestry sub-sector, or less often, as a sub-sector in health care. However, this review takes up medicinal plants as an independent sector for two reasons: 1) to emphasize that none of the various 'homes' to which medicinal plants have been assigned provide a sufficient base of expertise for their sustainable and equitable development; and 2) to provide an organizational framework for the community of researchers and stakeholders, to whom this paper will be circulated, to think through this area of common interest and move forward together.

This review then is a mapping exercise, which tries to identify the who, what, how, where, why and when of medicinal plants development in India, in order to supply a comprehensive understanding and overall picture to researchers, NGOs, health care workers, private companies, conservation and development agencies, policy makers and other interested stakeholders. It is intended to provide a framework and knowledge base, and an initial way forward, for those interested in seeing India exploit her comparative advantage in the global market, both sustainably and equitably.

LIMITS AND CONSTRAINTS FACED

There is no dearth of interest in medicinal plants amongst the Indian research community. As a single example, the IDRC Medicinal Plants Network, a South-Asia focused initiative operating from New Delhi, already maintains an active database of over 900 Indian researchers and development specialists working on medicinal plants projects after only one year of active compilation.

When a call for proposals in the field was issued, over 250 responses were received within the subscribed period, a tremendous number considering that the grants were of the magnitude of only USD 15, 000.

Unfortunately, however, this interest has not resulted in the development of a strong and high-quality knowledge base for the sector. Instead, one finds in a review such as this one several instances where information is either unobtainable or unreliable. Several factors contribute to this situation.

The most important among these is the highly secretive and complex nature of the trade in raw materials. Most experts consulted agreed that the largest part of the trade occurs in the informal sector, and is absent from official statistics and trade catalogues. As previous authors have also found, nearly everyone involved in the medicinal plants trade is very hesitant to divulge information which is essential to a complete understanding —such as prices, supply sources, points of transformation, and transport routes. As a result, despite assiduous efforts, we still cannot claim to have a complete picture of the trade scenario, and have most likely erred in the direction of conservatively estimating the volumes of materials under trade.

Information available regarding the formal sector is also limited. Most data is available only in aggregate form, such as numbers of species being exported or overall value of the trade to India. These statistics unfortunately supply little information about how the market actually works, and may even obscure such vital information to policy makers such as seasonal fluctuations and the like. In addition, in most cases, no explanations are given for how the aggregations were calculated or verified (i.e. dry weights or fresh weights; exchange values in effect; self-reporting by companies or based on registration with governments, etc.). The lack of methodological explanation makes it virtually impossible to compare and synthesize related sets of information; or to understand why two sets of statistics, purporting to cover the same phenomena over the same time period, give differing results.

Moreover, these statistics rely exclusively on market price as an indicator of value, a narrow approach which neglects environmental, cultural, personal, and long-term methods of assigning value. The social context of the market which is extremely important in the medicinal plants sector, involving as it does, a complex market spread across time and space, is there by lost. This constraint is related to a general lack of strategic focus in the bulk of current socio-economic research on medicinal plants in India. The largest group of scientists currently working with medicinal plants appears to be those in the natural sciences—including botanists, taxonomists, and chemists; and the applied sciences such as biotechnology and health care. In most instances where economic or social analysis has been undertaken, it has been by these same scientists, the majority of whom are untrained and unqualified to conduct such research.

While laudable as an attempt to bridge the disciplinary barrier, this has unfortunatelyalso resulted in a generally lower quality of socio-economic analysis related to medicinal plants as against other resources, with analysis tending to oversimplify complex market and policy realities such as the frequently suggested solution: cut out the middleman. In addition, there is a regrettable absence of any 'research community' or peer group working on socio-economic and policy aspects of medicinal plants, such as that which exists with regard to agro-technology, biotechnology, and the like, which would assist in defining higher standards of quality.

ABRUS PRECATORIUS L. (FABACEAE)

Syn : Abrus minor and A. pauciflorus Desv. *English names:* Indian liquorice, Crab's eye. Sanskrit name: Krishna gunja.

Vernacular names: Asm : Latuwani; Ben: Rati, Kunch; Guj: Gumchi; Hin and Pun: Rati; Kan : Gurgunn, Gulaganji; Ori : Kaincha, Gunja; Mal: Kunnikkura; Tam: Kunthamani; Tel: Gumginja.

Trade names: Rati, Kunch.

Traditional use: SANTAL:

(i) grind the roots, make small pills, encase the pills in molasses and eat the same to treat night-blindedness;

(ii) make a plaster by grinding the roots of white-fruited variety and apply the plaster on the painful part of inflammated sections of the gum;

(iii) to treat white-coloured urine they drink a mixture made by grinding roots of the following:

a. white-fruited A. precatorius, b. Indigofera pulchella,

c. Panicum repens and

d. Spatholobus roxburghii;

e. to treat gravel they drink a mixture made of the following:

- roots of A. precatorius,
- the refuse of molasses,
- exudation from a sapling of Diospyros tomentosa,
- exudation from Acacia catechu,
- little saltpeter, and
- pinch of sulphur;
- to treat the variety of childbed complaints (usually caused by anaemia) characterized by profuse diarrhoea, roots of A. precatorius are used in preparing two different varieties of mixtures; the ingredients of the mixtures are given below:

First variety: roots of A. precatorius, Elaeodendron roxburghii, Coix lachryma- jobi, Piper longum, Ruellia suffruticosa, white onion, rhizome of Zingiber officinale; Second variety: roots of A. precatorius, Coix lachryma-jobi, Embelia robusta, Piper longum, bark of Casearea tomentosa, Elaeodendron roxburghii, Gmelina arborea, Emblica officinalis, white onion, leaves of Ocimum sanctum, rhizome of Curcuma angustifolia and Zingiber officinale- all these are ground together, boiled and mixed with the refuse of molasses;

- roots as abortifacient and in paralysis;
- apply leaf-paste with lime-water (2:1) on swelling of glands;
- grind the leaves of white-flowered A. precatorius, warm slightly and plaster on the loins to kill pain there;
- grind leaves of A. precatorius along with leaves of Lawsonia alba and Tamarindus indica (1:1:1), add a little salt, boil a little and apply the plaster on the whole body to get relief from muscular pain caused by over-exhaustion;

- make a paste of leaves of A. precatorius along with roots of Carissa carandas and Gossypium arboreum, warm the paste slightly and plaster the same over the whole body of the patient suffering from stealth convulsions;
- leaf-paste in leucoderma;
- seed-paste in skin diseases;
- seeds after some processing as contraceptive. MUNDA: Root-paste in gonorrhoea. ORAON: dried root-powder as mild purgative.

AGNI PURANA:

(i) husks of A. precatorius along with the same of Vitis vinifera and the decoction of Polyalthia longifolia, Moringa pterigosperma, payomuca and tripha/a (fruits of Terminalia belerica, Terminalia chebula and Emblica officinalis) destroys all intestinal worms;

(ii) the mixture of powder of A. precatorius, marine salt and pathya in warm water removes all fevers;

(iii) consumption of the seeds of A. precatorius along with the fruits of Melia azadiracta, Holarrhena antidysenterica (leaves). Acorus calamus (young leaves) and Glycyrrhiza glabra (powder of stem) causes vomiting;

(iv) regular drinking of A. precatorius along with Acorus calamus, G/oriosa superba, vasa, nisagada, Zingiber officinalis, Glycyrrhiza glabra and marine salt daily in the morning enhances memory of young boys;

(v) A. precatorius can enhance the span of a man's life, if it is eaten with marine salt and some other plants (Tinospora cordifolia, pathya, citraka, dried rhizome of Zingiber officinalis).

Modern use: Roots: emetic and alexiteric; Decoction of roots and leaves: for cough, cold and colic; Seeds: purgative, emetic, tonic, aphrodisiac, used in nervous disorder and cattle poisoning; Poultice of seeds: as suppository to bring about abortion; Paste of seeds: applied locally in sciatica, stiffness of shoulder joints and in paralysis.

Phytography : Copiously branched climber with slender branches; leaves alternate, pinnately compound with numerous deciduous leaflets; flowers small, in dense racemes on axillary peduncles or short branches; pods 2. 5-3. 7 by 1. 0-1. 25 cm; seeds bright scarlet and black or whitish or black or mixed black and white, large like pea.

Phenology: Flowering: August and September; Fruiting : January to March (even up to May).

Distribution: Occurring throughout greater parts of India, ascending the outer Himalaya up to 1200 m, occasionally planted in gardens.

Ecology and cultivation: Naturalised in tropical countries.

Chemical contents: Root and Leaf: glycyrrhizin, isoflavanquinones, abrusquinone A, B & C; leaves taste sweet and roots less so; roots also contain precol, abrol, abrasine and precasine. Seed: poisonous, principal constituents being 'abrin'; a fat-splitting enzyme, haemaagglutinin, urease; alkaloid (abrin), a glucoside (abralin) and a small quantity of fatty oil have also been isolated from seed.

Pharmacologically, abrin is considered to be intensely poisonous. Besides abrin, a seed contains hypaphorine, two steroids-one oily and the other crystalline-â-sitosterol, stigmasterol, 5 B-cholanic acid, abricin, abridin, cholesterol, lectins and toxic proteins.

Remark: Root is used as an adulterant of the root of Glycyrrhiza glabra (Fam. Fabaceae).

AEGLE MARMELOS CORR. (RUTACEAE)

Syn: Feronia pellucida Roth, Crataeva religiosa Ainslie

English names: Wood apple, Bael tree.

Sanskrit names: Bilwa, Shriphal.

Vernacular names: Asm and Ben: Bel; Guj: Biliva phal, BiI; Hin : Shriphal, Bel; Kan: Bilwa patre, Bil patre; Kon : Belfoll; Mal: Vilvam, Koovalam; Mar: Bel; Ori : Bela; Pun: Bil; Tam: Vilvam, Vilvamaram; Tel: Bilambu, Maredu; Urd: Bel.

Trade names: Bel, Shriphal.

Traditional use: SANTAL: (a) leaves of this plant along with {i} many other plant materials for the treatment of continuous fever; (ii) the molasses and fruits of Gryllus monostrosus for the treatment of diseases without premonitory symptoms; {iii} the fruits of Nigella indica and black pepper to treat a patient of convulsions; (iv) the leaves of Melia azadirac hta and the seeds of Semecarpus ana cardium to treat nausea; (v) the fruits of Randia dumetorum and Nigella indica, oilcake of Bassia latifolia, salt and Carum ajowan for treatment of constipation with meteorismus; (vi) the bark of the following plants -Pterocarpus marsupium, Bauhinia vahlii, Spatholobus roxburghii, Terminalia tomentosa, Dalbergia latifolia and fried rice for treatment of chronic stomachache and (vii) the bark of Odina wodier, salt and Carum ajowan to treat watery diarrhoea; (b) various parts of fruit for making the following medicines: (i) for curing the patient of cholera, a medicine prepared with the following, is administered: the old fruit of A. marmelos, bark of Melia azadirachta, the resin of Shorea robusta and pulverized kernel of a mango stone; (ii) a sherbet prepared with the ripe fruit of A. marmelos and sugar candy is administered to the patient of dysentery; (iii) to treat the complaints of a mother after child-birth, a plaster made of the following is applied: top of the fresh unripe fruit of A. mermelos, leaves of Ocimum sanctum, little ginger and 84 blac_ peppers; (iv) a patient of puerperal fever is given a liquid drink made with the entire contents scraped out of a ripe fruit of A. marmelos, juice of old dried fruits of Mangifera indica, two ounces of a kind of red ants and a little salt; (v) a thick mixture, made with twin fruits of A. marmelos, melted hail and earth excavated by rats, is smeared on the breasts of a young mother to check the flow of milk when the breasts pain or suppurate; and (c) the bark of old trees of A. marmelos and Melia azadirachta are used to prepare an antidote for the poison of all kinds of snake bite; ATHARVAVEDA : the unripe fruit medicinal, but ripe fruit harmful; CHARAKA SAMHITA: the unripe fruit increases the digestive power, but the ripe fruit is difficult to digest; KURMA PURANA: (i) regular drinking of fruit juice ensures long span of life and golden colour of the skin; (ii) brushing the teeth with young branch of this plant is beneficial;

MATSYA PURANA : the paste of this plant is a good steriliser for clothings, beds, furniture, coat of armour, ornaments, canopy and fans made of wools and furs; BRAHMAVAIVARTA PURANA : consumption of ripe fruits of this plant helps to eliminate the ailment caused by excessive bile, but drinking water immediately after eating the fruit aggravates the bile-disorder; AGNI PURANA : (i) this plant is of great medicinal value; (ii) inhaling the oil, obtained from this plant, increases the poetic acumen of the inhaler and enables him to live a long life; (iii) for treatment of gastroenteritis, the patient should drink (a) the water containing the decoction of A. marmelos, Aconitum heterophyllum and Holerrhena antidysenterica, (b) the fruit juice of A. marmelos, Mangifera indica, Dolicos lablab, Woodfordia fruticosa, shunthi along with buttermilk and molasses; and (iv) it can cure a patient suffering from fever and its associate pains and cough.

UNANI: Ingredient for 'Belgiri'.

HOMOEOPATHY: Destroys phlegm and a good remedy in fevers associated with catarrhal symptoms, also good for dropsy, bleeding piles, dysentery, diarrhoea, bowel complaints and is a good laxative.

Modern use: Fruits: chiefly used in (i) chronic diarrhoea and dysentery; (ii) as a good laxative, and the sherbet prepared from the pulp is good for bacillary dysentery; Half-ripe fruit: astringent, digestive and used in diarrhoea. It is also antidiuretic, anthelmintic, antipyretic, carminative, tonic.

Phytography: Deciduous glabrous tree, up to 8 min height and 1 m in girth, bark shallowly furrowed and corky; leaves alternate, with straight sharp axillary thorns (buds), trifoliate, aromatic; flowers in axillary panicles, greenish white, fragrant; fruit hard-shelled, up to 5 cm in diameter, greyish or yellowish, scented, pulp orange, sweet and gummy; seeds numerous, oblong, compressed, testa mucous.

Phenology: Flowering: April-May; Fruiting: persistent, ripening by February.

Distribution: Found in the plains and submontane regions of India, wild in the sub-Himalayan tract, often planted.

Ecology and cultivation: Wild; often planted.

Chemical contents: Bark of root and stem: umbelliferone, other coumarins, â-sitosterol, aurapten, marmin, lupeol, two unidentified alkaloids and two unknown compounds-their proportion varies with the age of the bark; Stem: yields a good gum; Heartwood: a ferro-quinoline alkaloid, /dictamine, marmasin and â-sitosterol; Leaves: ã-sitosterol, aegeline, aegelenine, lupeol; sitosterol, rutin, marmesinin, â-sitosterol, glucoside and essential oil; Fruits: psoralen, aegelinol, furanocoumarin, marmelide, â-sitosterol and essential oil; Ripe fruits: xanthotoxol, scoparone, scopoletin, umbelliforone, marmesin, skimmin and â-sitosterol glucoside.

Adulterants: Umonia acidissima Correa, Garcinia mangostina L. and Puilica granatum L. are used as substitute of Aegle marmelos Correa.

ALLIUM SATIVUM L. (ALLIACEAE)

English name: Garlic.

Sanskrit names: Arishta, Lashuna, Mahausada, Rason.

Vernacular names Asm : Naharu; Ben: Rasun; Guj : Lasan, Shunam; Hin : Lashun; Kan : Belluli; Kon : Lossun; Mar: Velluli, Velluthulli; Mar: Lasun;

Ori : Rasun; Tam: Vellaipundu; Tel: Tellagadda.

Trade names: Rasun, Lashun.

Traditional use : UPAVARHANA SAMHITA : good for health; AGNI PURANA: a mixture of this plant, ginger and Moringa oleifera is helpful for eye and also as eardrop.

MATSYA PURANA : of great medicinal value, should be stored in forts.

UNANI: an ingredient of 'Seer (Lahsan) '.

HOMOEOPATHY: Mother tincture, a good remedy for cough and cold, pain in the chest, swelling of glands, psoas, iliacus and erosion of old diseases at the adimanic stage.

Modern use: Bulb: antidiabetic, antiinflammatory, anticancer, effective in rheumatism, catarrhal conditions; Raw garlic: decreases glucose, cholesterol, phospholipids, triglycerides, useful in dyspepsia, cryptococcal meningitis, rickettsia; applied externally as resolvent to indolent tumours, internally given with common salt in nervous diseases, headache; Liniment: beneficial in infantile convulsion and other spasmodic affections; Juice: applied to bruises and sprain, relieves earache, allays pain in otorrhoea; preparation have been given to pulmonary phthisis, bronchitis, gangrene of the lung and whooping cough; Garlic juice: good for treatment of laryngeal tuberculosis, lupus and duodenal ulcer; Inhalation of fresh garlic juice: useful in pulmonary tuberculosis, dyspep-sia, flatulence and colic; in external application, the juice is used as a rubifacient; in skin diseases, as an eyedrop and in earache.

Phytography : Hardy perennial bulbous scapigerous herb; stem flat, dry, lower portion of the plant forms bulb which consists of several smaller bulbs called cloves, surrounded by a thin white or pinkish sheath; leaves flat, narrow green; heads bear small white flowers and bulbils.

Phenology: Flowering and Fruiting: Winter.

Distribution: Cultivated throughout India since ancient days; also cultivated in Pakistan, Bangladesh and almost in all tropical countries.

Ecology and cultivation: It favours a richer soil and higher elevation (1000-1300 m), well-drained, moderately clayey loam is best suited for cultivation;

requires a cool, moist period during growth and a relatively dry period during maturing of the crop; takes 4-5 months to mature, harvested during February to April. Yields good results, if treated with farmyard manure and top-dressing of ammonium sulphate mixed with superphosphate. It grows as a late irrigated crop; in South India, it is rotated with ragi.

Chemical contents: Garlic: protein 6. 3%, fat 0. 1 %, carbohydrate 29%, Ca 0. 03%, Fe 1. 3 mg/100 g, vitamin C 13 mg/100 g, and also Cu-peptides, 2 mercapto-L-cysteins, anthocyanins, glycosides of kaempferol and quercetin, polysaccharides, allinase, sterols, hydrocarbons, alliin (nonvolatile sulpher amino acid), sativin I & II, scordinines A & B; Essential oil: the bulbs, on distillation, yield 0. 06-0. 1 % of an essential oil containing allyl-propyl-disulphide, diallyl disulphide and two sulphur containing compounds.

ALOE BARBADENSIS MILL. (LILIACEAE)

Syn : Aloe indica Royle, A. littoralis Koening., A. vera Tourn. ex Linn. *English names:* Barbados aloe, Curacas aloe, Indian aloe, Jafarabad aloe. Sanskrit name: Ghritakumari.

Vernacular names: Asm : Chalkunwari; Ben: Ghritakumari; Guj : Kumarpathu, Kunvar; Hin : Ghee kunvar; Kan : Lolesara; Kon : Kantikkor, Katkunvor; Mal: Kattarvazha kumari; Mar: Korphad; Ori : Gheokunri; Pun: Ghikur, Kawargandal; Tam: Alagai, Chirukuttali, Kuttilai; Tel: Chinnakata banda, Kala banda, Kittanara.

Trade names: Ghritakumari, Ghee kunvar.

Traditional use: TRIBAL: Leaf-pulp: in liver troubles, jaundice, fever, gonorrhoea, spleen disorder, rheumatism, piles, dysmenorrhoea, sterility in women; Leaf-mucilage: mild laxative, to cure hardening of breast tissues, in insect stings.

AYURVEDA: alternative, bitter, cooling, purgative, sweet, tonic, anthelmintic, useful in eye diseases, tumours, enlargement of spleen, liver troubles, vomiting, skin diseases, bilious-ness, asthma, leprosy, jaundice, strangury, ulcer; Flowers: anthelmintic.

UNANI: Gheekawar is useful in inflammation of spleen, lumbago, muscular pain, ophthal-mia, digestive, purgative; Leaves good for piles and biliousness.

Modern use: Aloe: in menstrual diseases, stomach pain, tonic after pregnancy, uterine disorders, high fever; Pulp: menstrual suppressions, nervous imbalance; Aloe com-pound: in treatment of women sterility; Mucilage: painful inflammation; Root: colic pain; Aloe mixture with other plant extracts: for treating obstruction of lymphatic system.

Phytography : A coarse-looking plant with a short (30-60 cm high) stem; leaves succulent, green, large (37 cm long, 10 cm broad, 2 cm thick), densely crowded; flowers in racemes, bright yellow, tubular, stamens frequently projected beyond the perianth tube.

Phenology: Flowering: September-December; Fruiting: scarce.

Distribution: A native of North Africa, Canary Islands and Spain; naturalised in India; many varieties are found in a semi-wild state in all parts of India; also cultivated in pots and gardens.

Ecology and cultivation: Xerophyte; propagated by suckers.

Chemical contents: Plant: aloin, aloe-emodin and resins.

Adulterant: Aloe candelabrum Berger is used as substitute for Aloe barbadensis Miller.

ALSTONIA SCHOLARIS R. BR. (APOCYNACEAE)

Syn : Echites scholaris L., E. pala Ham.

English names: Devil's tree, Dita bark.

Sanskrit names: Saptapa rni, Sa pta pa rna , Sa ra da, Vishala lva ka , Vishamachhda, Ayugmaparna, Gandhiparna, Payasya, Jivani, Kshalrya, Madagandha, Grahashi, Grahanashana.

Vernacular names: Asm : Chatiar; Ben: Chhatim; Hin : Chatian, Salni chatian; Kan : Saptaparna, Maddale, Kodale, Elele kale, Janthalla, Hale; Ken: SantnarUkh; Mal: Ezhilampala, Mukkampala, Pala; Mar: Salvin; Ori : Chhatiana, Chhanchania; Silgandha; Pun: Satona; Sin: Rukattana; Tam: Elilaipillai, Mukumpalei, Pala, Wedrase; Tel: Eda kula, Pala garuda.

Trade names: Chatiyan, Shaitan wood, Saptaparni.

Traditional use: MUNDAS OF CHOTANAGPUR : Bark: in colic pain; SOME PARTS OF INDIA: Plant: used in the treatment of leprosy; Twig: hung in the room of the newly confined woman to lessen the activities of evil spirit on the new born.

ATHARVA VEDA: preventive and curative of diseases caused by change of season. CHARAKA SAMHITA and SUSHRUTA SAMHITA: good for headache, sores, and some other diseases; A YURVEDA : the following uses are recommended: (i) Bark: dermal sores, ragging fever, discharge of sperm with urine, hiccup, insufficiency in breast milk, gout, cold congestion, dyspepsia; (ii) Latex: caries, pimple, pyorrhoea; (iii) Flower: asthma, respiratory troubles.

UNANI: Ingredient of 'Kashim'.

HOMOEOPATHY: Malarial fever, anaemia, indigestion, general debility and other stomach ailments.

Modern use: Bark: known in commerce as Dita bark and is used in medicine as bitter, febrifuge and astringent, in treatment of malarial fever, chronic dysentery, diarrhoea and in snake bite; Milky juice: applied to ulcers.

Phytography: Large (20 m high, 3 m girth), evergreen tree with straight, often fluted and buttressed base, branches whorled, bark yellow inside and exudes milky bitter latex; leaves simple, whorled-usually 7 in a whorl, coriaceous, whitish beneath, obovate or elliptic or oblong, obtuse rounded or obtusely acuminate, 30-60 pairs of horizontal veins joining an intramarginal one; cymes peduncled or sessile, umbellately branched; flowers aromatic, 0.8-1. 25 cm in diameter, greenish white, pubescent; follicles 30-60 cm long and 0. 3 cm in diameter, pendulous, in clusters.

Phenology: Flowering: Autumn; Fruiting: Winter.

Distribution: Throughout moist regions of India, especially in West Coast forests, in the Himalaya it ascends up to 1000 m; also found in Bangladesh and Pakistan. Planted in the gardens.

Ecology and cultivation: Also grown as an ornamental.

Adulterants: Alstonia macrophylla Wall. and A. venenata R. Br. are used as substitute for A. scholaris.

ANACARDIUM OCCIDENTALE L. (ANACARDIACEAE)

English name: Cashew nut.

Vernacular names: Asm : Kaju badam; Ben: Hijli badam, Kaju badam; Guj, Hin, Mar and Pun: Kaju; Kan : Gerupappu; Godambi; Kon: Kaz; Mat: Kashumaru, Parankimara, Andiparuppau; Ori : Lanka badam; Tam: Mundiri, Munthirikai; Tel: Jidimamidi, Muntha mamidi.

Trade names: Cashew nut, Kaju.

Traditional use: Cashew nut shell-oil: mild purgative, used in folk medicine for treatment of hookworm, cracks on soles of feet, warts, corns, leporus sores.

Modern use: Cashew nut: used in mental derangement, sexual debility, nervous prostration following seminal emission, morning sickness in pregnancy, palpitation of heart, rheumatic percarditis, loss of memory as a sequel to small pox; Kernel: good for week

patients suffering from I incessant and chronic vomiting;Kernel-oil: antidote for irritant poisons; Liquor made from fruit: diuretic.

HOMOEOPATHY : for boils, warts, wounds and different types of cracks in legs; used sometimes in case of leprosy.

Phytography : Small tree with short, thick, crooked trunk; leaves simple, alternate, petiolate, entire, hard, 10-20 cm by 7. 5-12. 5 cm; panicles terminal, bracteate, pubescent; branches long, naked to the tips; flowers yellow with pink stripes, 0. 8 cm in diameter; cashew apple red or yellow-is the swollen, enlarged pedicel which bears the nut.

Phenology: Flowering: March-April; Fruiting: April-May.

Distribution: Native to tropical America, naturalised in the hotter sea-shores of India; Pakistan, Bangladesh and Malaysia.

Ecology and cultivation: Introduced; grows in plains, especially towards the coast, very occasionally ascending up to 1200 m; being extensively planted by clearing scrub jungles in the plains.

Chemical contents: Bark: exudes gum; Flower: polyphenols; Cashew shell: yields gum, oil and liquid (CNSL); Liquid-free nutshell: syringic and gallic acids, galocatechin; Defatted nutshell: naringenin, prunin-6″-O-p-coumarate; acid, caffeic acid, quinic acid, polyphenols, bioflavone.

ANDROGRAPHIS PANICULATA (BURM. F.) WALL. EX NEES (ACANTHACEAE)

Syn : Justicia paniculata Burm. f.

English names: The great king of bitters, the creat. *Sanskrit names:* Bhunimba, Kirata.

Vernacular names: Ben: Kalmegh; Guj : Kariyatu; Hin: Kirayat; Kan: Nelabaru; Mar: Olikiryata; Tam and Tel: Nelavemu.

Trade names: Kalmegh, Kirayat.

Traditional use: Plant:. febrifuge, alterative, anthelmintic, anodyne, useful in debility, diabetes, consumption, influenza, bronchitis, itches and piles; in Bengal, household medicine known as 'Kalmegh', made from leaves, is given to the children suffering from stomach complaints.

HOEMOEPATHY: used for treatment of different ailments of head, mind, eyes, nose, mouth, tongue, throat, abdomen, stool, urine, fever and other modalities.

Modern use: Drug constitute stem, leaf and inflorescence: as a tonic and in the treatment of fevers, worms, dysentery and also beneficial to liver and digestive ailments; it is reported that it has some antityphoid and antibiotic activity; Decoction: used for sluggishness of liver and in jaundice.

Phytography : An erect herb with square stem, glabrous below, glandular hairy above; leaves linear, lanceolate, glabrous and distinctly pedicelled; flowers white or pale purple; capsules compressed transversely; seeds bony.

Phenology: Flowering and Fruiting: September-May.

Distribution: Throughout India in the plains and hills; Bangladesh, Pakistan, all South- East Asian and SAARC countries.

Ecology and cultivation: Common in stony lines in forests and in wastelands. Culti-vated as an ornamental.

Chemical contents: Plant: kalmeghin, bitter principle andrographolide; bitterness is due to nonbasic principle.

Adulterants: It is used as adulterants for Chirata, and is a substitute for quinine.

Remark: Whole plant is bitter.

ABROMA AUGUSTA (L) LT. (STERCULIACEAE)

(now known as Ambroma L. f.)

Syn : Abroma augulata Lam., A. wheeleri Retz., A. fastuosum Gaertn., Theobroma augusta L.

English name: Devil's cotton.

Vernacular names: Asm : Bon kopashi; Hin and Ben: Ulat kambal; Tam: Sivapputtutti.

Trade name: Ulat kambal.

Traditional use: Seed: yields fatty oil, rich in linoleic acid and lowers cholesterol level in blood.

HOMOEOPATHY: used to control mind, different ailments of head, heart, eyes, ears, nose, face, mouth, throat, stomach, abdomen, urinary organs, male and female sexual organs, respiratory organs, neck, back and limbs, skin diseases, fever; to regulate appetite and sleep.

Modern use: Fresh and dried root-bark: used as uterine tonic and emmenagogue; regulates menstrual flow; Fresh juice from root-bark: useful in congestive and neuralgic forms of dysmenorrhoea, amenorrhoea, urinary trouble, bronchitis, broncho-pneumonia, carbuncles and poisonous boils; Leaf: used in diabetes, rheumatic pain and sinusitis.

Phytography : Shrub, branches downy; leaf simple, cordate, 10-15 cm by 10-12. 5 cm, base 3-7 costate, repand-denticulate while the upper narrower leaves are entire, glabrescent above and tomentose below, petiolate, petioles 1. 25-2. 5 cm long, stipules linear, as long as the petiole, deciduous; flowers axillary, pedunculate, peduncle 3. 5 cm long; capsules 5-angled, 5-winged, obpyramidal, thrice as long as the persistent calyx; seeds albuminous, numerous.

Distribution: Widely distributed in hotter parts of India up to 1500 m; Bangladesh, Pakistan and the adjacent countries.

Ecology and cultivation: Plant prefers hot and moist climate; sometimes planted, occasionally found as an escape.

Chemical contents: Plant: fixed oil, a little resinous matter, alkaloid (minute quantity) and water-soluble bases.

ACANTHUS ILICIFOLIUS L. (ACANTHACEAE)

Syn : Acanthus doloarius Blanco, Dilivaria ilicifolia Nees

Sanskrit name: Harikasa.

Vernacular names: Ben: Hargoza, Harkachkanta; Kan : Holeculli; Mal: Payinaculli; Mar: Maranda, Maraneli; Ori : Harkamcli; Tam: Kalutai mulli; Tel: Alei.

Trade name: Harkasa.

Traditional use: TRIBES OF SUNDARBANS: Root (boiled in mustard oil) : in paralysis of limbs; FOLKS OF GOA: Leaf: as fomentation in rheumatism and neuralgia. tender shoot: in snake bite; Root: in asthma, paralysis, leucorrhoea and debility;

Leaf: as fomentation in rheumatism, neuralgia and in snake bite.

Phytography : Erect herb; stems up to 1. 5 m, in clumps, little divided, glabrous; leaves shortly petioled, oblong or elliptic, base usually spinous, toothed or, pinnatifid, rigid, glabrous; spikes 10-40 cm, terminal, commonly solitary; flowers mostly opposite, bract and bracteoles present, sepals 4, outer 2 elliptic rounded, inner 2 broadly lanceolate, subacute, petals 5, blue, united, 2-lipped, corolla tube short, pubescent within, stamens 4, didynamous, shorter than coroll_ lip, filaments stout, anthers 1-lobed, bearded, carpels 2, united, ovary 2-chambered having 2 ovules in chamber, style short, bifid; capsules shining chestnut-brown, ellipsoid, compressed, 0. 6-0. 8 cm long; testa white, very lax.

Phenology: Flowering and Fruiting: almost throughout the year.

Distribution: Mangroves of Indian peninsula; Sri Lanka, Bangladesh, Pakistan and the adjoining areas.

Ecology and cultivation: Commonly grown on the river banks, tidal canal sides, low swampy areas in the mangrove forests and its vicinity; wild.

Chemical contents: Plant: acanthicifoline, oleanolic acid, â-sitosterol, lupeol, quercetin and its glucopyranoside, trigonellin; Root: saponin, glycoside of 3á-OH-lup-20(29) -ene.

ACONITUM FEROX WALL. (RANUNCULACEAE)

Syn: Aconitum virosum Don., A. napellus var. rigidum Hook, f & T.

English names: Wolf's bane, Indian aconite.

Sanskrit names: Vatsanabha, Visa.

Vernacular names: Hin: Bish, Mahoor; Guj and Mar: Vachang; Kas: Mohra; Tam: Vasnumbi; Tel: Vasnabhi.

Trade name: Bish.

Traditional use: AYURVEDA : Root: used in the mrityunjaya rasa (used to treat the fever supposed to be caused by deranged vayu, i.e., wind, sannipatika jvara, i.e., remittent fever, hingulesware-rasa, anandabhairav agnitundi vati, etc.

Vatsanabha has been used in medicine from a very remote period. It is regarded as healing and stimulant. It is used in a great variety of affections, but is specially recommended in fever, cephalagia, affections of throat, dyspepsia and rheumatism. HOMOEOPATHY: remedy for clotting of blood in heart or in lungs, pneumonia, Iymptisis, pleurisy, eye trouble, earache, toothache and urinary trouble.

Modern use: Extremely poisonous; used in leprosy, fever, cholera, nasal catarrah, tonsillitis, sore throat, gastric disorders, debility, etc., also used as a sedative and diaphoretic; applied in the form of paste in cases of neuralgia and rheumatism.

Phytography : Perennial erect herb growing up to 2 m in height; roots look like the navel of children; leaves alternate, simple, rounded or oval, may be palmately 5-lobed; flowers borne on branched racemes, bracts and bracteoles present, large helmet-type, helmet vaulted with short sharp beak, pale dirty blue in colour, zygomorphic, floral parts arranged spirally on an elongated receptacle; follicles erect, usually densely villose-sometimes glabrous.

Phenology: Flowering and Fruiting: July-November.

Distribution : Alpine Himalaya including Nepal; endemic.

Ecology and cultivation: Temperate to alpine regions of the Himalaya in the altitude of 3300-5000 m.

Chemical contents: Root: pseudoaconitine (a toxic alkaloid), indactonitine, chasmaconitine, bikhaconitine.

Adultcrants: Indian aconite root is known as 'bikh' or 'bish', the name which is applied to aconite from more than one species, and different authors have ascribed it to different species.

Remarks: Vulnerable due to excessive collection for medicinal uses. Collection in wild state should be banned and measures for cultivation should be initiated.

ACORUS CALAMUS L. (ARACEAE)

Syn : Acorus griffithii Schott., A. belangeii Schott, A. casia Bertol.

English name: The sweet flag.

Sanskrit name: Vacha.

Vernacular names: Asm, Ben and Hin : Boch; Gui : Godavaj, Vekhand; Kan : Baje, Baje gida; Kon: Waikhand; Mal: Vayambu; Mar: Vekhand; Ori : Bacha; Pun: Bari, Boj, Warch; Tam: Vasamboo; Tel: Vasa.

Trade name: Boch.

Traditional Use

Santal : Use the plant in the following ways: (i) they mix and grind black pepper, cloves, root of Carissa carandus lo along with little of the rootstock of A. calamus lo, then stir the same in pure mustard oil-the emulsion, thus prepared is anointed daily over the whole body of the patient suffering form epilepsy with foaming and groaning, as soon as the fit comes on; a few drops of this emulsion should be poured into the nose of the patient; (ii) for the treatment of indigestion, they take pills made by grinding 100 black peppers, little amount of ginger and the root of A. calamus together; (iii) also use in the treatment of asthma, bronchitis, cold and cough, dry cough, epilepsy, haemopty-sis, indigestion, phthisis; BIRHOR : Rhizome in alopecia, Root as massage, in fever, hysteria, pain in neck, teething trouble of children, malaria and cancer.

Agni Purana : This plant is of great medicinal value; it recommends the following uses: (i) for treatment of epilepsy, this plant should be boiled with Costus speciosus, shankhapushpi, along with the juice of Bacopa monnieri; the substance thus obtained should be administered to the patient; (ii) drinking the decoction of this plant, Piper peepuloides, Staphyles emodi Wall., and Cyperus parviflorus Heyne and pippalimula is good for the patient of rheumatic arthritis; (iii) the powder or decoction of this plant helps curing chronic enlargement of spleen; (iv) decoction of the plant is beneficial for the patient of dropsy; A YURVEDA: Rhizome: bitter, healing, emetic, laxative, diuretic, carminative; improves voice and appetite; good for oral diseases, abdominal pain, epilepsy, bronchitis, hysteria, loss of memory, rat bite and worms in ear.

Siddha System: Fresh root for bronchial asthma.

Unani: An ingredient of the medicine called 'Waje-Turki'; useful in flatulent colic, chronic dyspepsia, catarrhal, in burn wounds, carminative, anthelmintic and as bitter tonic.

Modern use: Rhizome: aromatic, bitter, carminative, emetic, stimulant, stomachic, useful in dyspepsia, colic, remittent fevers, nerve tonic, in bronchitis, dysentery, epilepsy and other mental ailments, glandular and abdominal tumours and in snake bite.

Phytography: Perennial, erect, aromatic herb, common on river banks and marshes, ascending to 3000 m; rhizome cylindrical or slightly compressed, about 2. 5 cm in diameter, much-branched, externally light brown or pinkish brown but white and spongy within; leaves distichous, large, 1-2 m in length, base equitant, margin waved; spadix sessile, cylindric, densely flowered, not completely enclosed by spathe, spathe 15-75 cm in length, narrow, leaf-like; flowers small, bisexual; berries few-seeded; seeds oblong, albuminous.

Phenology: Flowering and Fruiting: July-August; fruiting very rare.

Distribution: Throughout India; ascending the Himalaya up to 2000 m; Sri Lanka, Pakistan and Bangladesh.

Ecology and cultivation: Probably introduced; found from the coast to

1200 m; often near village wells and along watercourses; confined to marshy areas; gregarious herb from a stout horizontal rhizome; wild and cultivated.

Chemical contents: Dry rhizome :1. 5-3. 5% of a yellow aromatic volatile oil-calamus oil; the oil contains â-asarone, small quantities of sesquiterpenes and sesquiterpenes alcohols; Rhizome: also contains choline (0. 26%), flavone, acoradin, 2, 4, 5-tri-MeO-benzaldehyde, 2, 5-di-MeO-benzoquinone, galangin, calameone, acolamone, isoacolamone, epoxyisoacoragermacrone; Aerial parts: lutcolin-6, 8-c-diglucoside; chemical constituents vary in ecotypes and polyploides.

Adulterants: The powdered drug has been adulterated with siliceous earth, ground marsh mallow root and cereal flowers.

Remark: Rhizomes are valued for indigenous medicine.

ARECA CATECHU L. (ARECACEAE)

English names: Areca palm, Areca nut, Betel nut, Pinang palm.

Sanskrit names: Gubak, Phalam, Poag, Pooga, Poogi.

Vernacular names: Asm : Tambul; Ben: Supari, Gua; Guj : Supaari; Hin : Kasaili,

Supari; Kan : Adike, Bette; Kon : Maddi; Mal: Adakka, Pugam, Pakka;

Mar: Supari Ori : Gua; Tam: Kamubu, Pakku; Tel: Poke, Vakka.

Trade names: Areca nut, Betel nut, Supari. There are over 150 trade types.

Traditional use: SANTAL: (i) a patient of small pox is given to eat the areca nut when the pustules subside; (ii) a mixture for biliary colic is prepared with areca nut as a constituent; (iii) an ointment for chancre and syphilis is made by pestling areca nut with the root of Gymnema hirsutus, leaf of Piper betel and then cooking the same in mustard oil or butter; TRIBALS also use this plant in rhagadas, venereal sores, syphilis, dysentery, cholera, small pox and for fractured bones.

References to this plant are found in the BHAGVA TA along with the plants of Musa paradisica and Borassus flabellifer. CHARAKA SAMHITA :

Fruit: useful in the diseases caused by bile; SUSHRUTA SAMHITA : Fruit: beneficial in the diseases caused by phlegm; but overuse of this may distort voice of a man; CHACRADATTA : Paste of unripe fruit: may be used as liniment; Extract of unripe fruit: useful in small pox; HARITA SAMHITA : sesame oil in which extract of unripe fruit has been boiled should be used; A YURVEDA : various preparations of unripe and ripe nuts are useful in toothache, pyorrhea, gum diseases, in treatment of worms, while extract of young leaf mixed with mustard oil is useful as liniment in rheumatism; BRAHMAVAIVARTA PURANA : brushing the teeth with twig of this plant is beneficial; AGNI PURANA : (i) immortality can be attained by consuming decoction of this plant along with the powder of root, bark, leaf and fruit of margosa and juice of Wedelia calendulacea; (ii) alkaloids of this plant are beneficial medicine.

UNANI: Ingradient of 'Futal (Chalia)'.

Modern use: Nut: chewing facilitates salivation, it being a good source of fluoride prevents tooth decay, but constant use might cause oral carcinoma; shows antimicrobial activities; Aqueous extract of nut: exhibits vascoconstriction and adrenalin p. Qtentiation in rats; Extract of leaf and fruit: spasmogenic.

Phytography : Tall, slender, unbranched palm with a crown of leaves; stem annulate; leaves pinnate with a conspicuous sheet; flowers in spadix, male many at the upper portion, female much longer and a few at the base; fruits are single-seeded berries with flesh and fibrous pericarp and a stony seed, 3. 8-5 em long, smooth, orange or scarlet when ripe.

Phenology: Flowering: August-January; Fruiting: about a year later.

Distribution: Cultivated in the coastal regions of India, Bangladesh, Pakistan, Sri Lanka, Myanmar and other tropical and subtropical countries.

Ecology and cultivation: This palm requires a moist tropical climate with heavy (500 cm/year) rainfall provided with good drainage. It can be grown in drier areas (rainfall 50 cm/year), if properly irrigated. It is a shade-loving plant, especially in the earlier stages and is very sensitive to drought. It grows on a variety of soils, but saline or alkaline soil, light and sandy soil are not suitable for it, but slightly saline sandy soil is good.

It is generally cultivated as a mixed crop with coconut and plantain or along with Erythrina indica. The betel nuts are sown in October/November with a distance of 10-15 em between two nuts. Transplanting is normally done after two years, occasionally after 3 or 4 years. Transplantation is done in July in the highlands and from February to April in lowlands. The second transplantation takes place when the first have come into bearing. In a fully planted grove, a distance of about 2 m each way is kept between the betel nut tree.

Chemical contents: Nut: alkaloids-arecoline, arecaidine, guvacine and isoguvacine.

Adulterants: Fruits of Areca triandra Roxb. and Areca nagensis Griff. are substitutes for Areca catechu L.

Remark: Stem and leaves are used in various ways. vascoconstriction and adrenalin p. Qtentiation in rats; Extract of leaf and fruit: spasmogenic.

ARISTOLOCHIA INDICA L. (ARISTOLOCHIACEAE)

English name: Indian birthwort. Sanskrit name: Ishvari. *Vernacular names*: Ben and Hin : Isharmul; Mal: Isvaramuli; Mar: Sapasan;

Tel: Eswaramuli.

Trade name: Iswarmul.

Traditional use: Root: tonic, stimulant, emetic, emmenagogue, in fever, in powder form is given with honey for leucoderma; Root-decoction: in impotency; Crushed root: applied on itching; Juice of leaf: in snake bite, used for cough; Seed: inflammations, biliousness and dry cough.

UNANI: a constituent of 'Majnoon-e-Flasfa'.

Modern use: Plant: used as abortifacient; EtOH (50%) extract: diuretic and anti-inflammatory; Dried stem and root: used as drug, which should be used in minimal doses; the drug promotes digestion and controls menstruation; in higher doses, it may prove lethal, it is used as a stimulant, tonic and for fevers; in moderate doses, it is used as a gastric stimulant and in dyspepsia; Root: considered as a stimulant, tonic and emmenagogue and also used in intermittentfever and in bowl troubles of children; shows antifertility activity in experimental animals.

Phytography : Twining herb, semiwoody, having more or less swollen nodes; leaves cordate or ovate, exstipulate; flowers irregular, often offensively smelling, perianth globose with a purple dilated and trumpet-shaped mouth with a strap-shaped brown purple appendage or lip behind; fruit a subglobose capsule.

Phenology: Flowering: June to October; Fruiting: November to March.

Distribution: Found throughout the subcontinent, mainly in the plains and lower hilly regions from Nepal to Bangladesh.

Ecology and cultivation: Found in open scrub jungles; wild.

Chemical contents: Root: a crystalline substance-probably a glucoside, a micro-crys-talline principle glucosidic in nature named isoaristolochic acid, allantoin, 0. 05% carbonyl compounds and a small amount of an oil, with the odour of isovanillin, ishwarone, ishwarane, aristolochene.

ASPARAGUS RACEMOSUS WILLD. VAR. JAVANICUS BAKER (LILIACEAE)

Syn : Asperagus tetragonus.

English name: Asparagus.

Sanskrit names: Shatavari, Shatamuli.

Vernacular names: Asm : Shatamul; Ben: Shatamuli; Guj : Satawari; Hin : Shakakul, Sada bori, Shatamuli, Satwar; Mal: Shatavali; Mar: Shatavari, Shatavarimul; Ori : Shatamuli; Tam: Chattavari, Cadumullam, Shimai shadavari; Tel :Challagadda.

Trade names: Shatamuli, Asparagus.

Traditional use: SOME TRIBES OF INDIA: Root: refrigerant, antiseptic, alterative and galactogogue; roots form a constituent of medicinal oils used for nervous and rheumatic complaints; powder boiled with milk and sugar has been used in different types of neurological disorders, urinary calculi; rub the root of the plant in different diseases of urinary organs; Powder of leaf: enhances breast milk, used for the treatment of colon syndrome.

AYURVEDA : useful in different types of cardiac abnormality; beneficial for intelligence as well as on memory modulatory; Powder of root (boiled with milk) : for treatment of night blindness; .

UNANI : Ingredient of 'Satawar '.

Modern use: Root: used as demulcent, aphrodisiac, diuretic, antidysenteric, in impotency, azoospermea.

Phytography : A slender, scrambling/scandent suffruticose perennial, woody, prickly shoots with reflexed spines; cladode more or less acicular and triquetrous falcate 13-26 mm long; divaricate, finely acuminate; flowers white, sweet-scented, :t 6 mm on filiform articulate pedicels, 6-12 mm long in very short racemes; berries 2. 5-6 mm in diameter, scarlet, red on ripening.

Phenology: Flowering: September-December; deciduous or dying back to the root in the hot season; Fruiting: throughout the year.

Distribution: Throughout tropical and subtropical regions of the country,

Ecology and cultivation: Common in scrub jungles and in forests;

cultivated as ornamentals.

Chemical contents: Leaf: quercetin-3-glucoronide, sitosterol, stigmasterol, sarsasapogenin, sito-sterol D-glucoside, stigmasterol-B-D-glucoside, two sirostanolic and two furostandic saponins.

Remark: Root is used in veterinary medicine.

BACOPA MONNIERI (L.) PENNEL (SCROPHULARIACEAE)

Syn: Herpestis monniera (L.) H. B. & K., Moniera cuneifolia Michx., Gratiola monniera L.

English name: Thyme leaved gratiola.

Sanskrit names: Brahmi, Nira brahmi.

Vernacular names: Ben: Adhabirni, Birmi shak, Barmi shak, Brahmi; Hin :Barambhi, Safed chammi; Mal: Nir bramhi; Mar: Barna; Ori : Urishnaparni; Tam: Nirbrami; Tel: Sambranichettu.

Trade name: Brahmi.

Traditional use: ATHARVA VEDA: strengthens body, improves quality of semen; CHARAKA SAMHITA : invigorat-ing, life sustaining; SUSHRUTA SAMHITA : increases memory and lifespan; AYURVEDA: (a) Plant: bitter, diuretic, blood-purifier, invigorates sex; (b) Plant-extract: used in purification of blood, for anaemia, dermatitis, diabetes, filaria; (c) Plant-juice (along with ginger, sugar and bark extract of Moringa oleifera) : to children in stomach disorder; (d) Leaves (fried in ghee) : as a brain tonic, in nervous weakness, hysteria, epilepsy, insanity, anxiety neurosis, and to sharpen dull memory.

AGNI PURANA: Plant: poison-killer; Plant-juice: good for epilepsy. UNANI: invigorating and good for cold and cough.

Modern use: Plant-extract: In experiments with mice, rat and dog, it has been proved to be tranquilizer, musculature relaxant, antispasmodic, anticancer;

Powdered dried leaf: satisfactory results obtained in man in cases of asthenia, nervous breakdown, and other low adynamic conditions.

Phytography : Annual creeper, rooting at each node; stem soft, succulent, soft hairs present; branches 10-25 cm long; leaves alternate, simple, 1. 25-1. 8 cm long, sessile or subsessile, oval-shaped; flowers light blue or white, 0.8-1. 5 cm long; capsules 2-grooved, valves separating from entire column, many-seeded.

Phenology: Flowering: April-June; Fruiting: June-December.

Distribution: Marshes throughout India, ascending up to 1300 m; Bangladesh, Pakistan and Sri Lanka.

Ecology and cultivation: Grows in damp or marshy areas, on the banks of ponds and canals, in the crop fields.

Chemical contents: Plant: Becoside A & B, betulic acid, betulinic acid, d- mannitol, stigmasterol, â-sitosterol, saponin, stigmastanol, hersaponin, monnierin, nicotine, luteoline and its glucosides.

BALANITES AEGYPTICA (L.) DELILE (BALANITACEAE)

Syn : Balanites roxburghii Planch, B. aegyptica var. roxburghii Duthie.

English names: Desert date, Soapberry tree, Thorn tree.

Sanskrit name: Ingudi.

Vernacular names: Ben and Hin : Hingan; Mar: Hinganbet; Tam: Nanjunda; Tel: Gari.

Trade name: Hingan.

Traditional use : TRIBES OF PANCH MAHAL (Maharashtra) and RURAL FOLK: Bark, Leaf, Fruit and Seed: as anthelmintic and purgative; Fruit: in boils, leucoderma and other skin diseases; Fruit-pulp: in whooping cough.

Modern use: Plant: cytotoxic and antitumour principle isolated; Bark: bactericide; EtOH (50%) extract of bark: spasmolytic; Seed-kernel oil: antimicrobial, useful in burns and ulcers, spermicidal.

Phytography : Spiny tree, about 6 m high; branches glabrous or puberulous and ending in very strong ascending spines; leaves alternate, bifoliate, ashy green, leaflets coriaceous; cymes axillary, 4-to 10-flowered; flowers green, velvety pubescent; fruits ovoid, about 5 cm in length, fleshy drupes, 1-seeded; seed oily but exalbuminou8

Phenology: Flowering: November, also during February to May; Fruiting: Winter.

Distribution: Bihar, Deccan, Gujarat, Uttar Pradesh (Kanpur) and Sikkim.

Ecology and cultivation: Xerophyte, found chiefly on black cotton soil; does not thrive in rocky areas.

Chemical contents: Plant: diosgenin and yamogenin; Root: steroidal sapogenin, diosgenin, yamogenin; Stem-bark: steroidal sapogenin, nitrogen glucoside, sesquiterpene, balanitol, bergapten; Leaf: 6 diosgenin glucosides; Fruit: steroidal sapogenin, yamogenin, 5 diosgenin glycerides, 6 diosgenin glucosides, diosgenin, balanitisins A, B, C, D & E; Seed: a saponin of diosgenin, non-edible fatty oil.

Remarks: Fruit-pulp is edible and used for cleansing silk and cotton. Fruit-shell is used in fire-cracker industry. Wood is chiefly used for making walking sticks and as fuel.

BUTEA MONOSPERMA (LAMK.) TAUB. (FABACEAE)

Syn : Butea frondosa Roxb., Erythrina monosperma Lamk. *English names:* Flame of the forest, Parrot tree. Sanskrit name Palasha.

Vernacular names: Asm and Ben: Palash; Guj : Khakar; Hin : Dhak; Kan : Muttugathoras, Muttugu-mara; Mal: Chamath, Khakar; Mar: Palash; Mun : Murud ba; Orn : Murka; Ori: Palasa;. Pun: Dhak; Sad: Pal as, Paras; Tam: Samithu, Pal-asam; Tel: Moduga, Palashamu.

Trade names Palasha, Dhak.

Traditional use: KHASI and GARO : Leaf: in delirium; TRIBES OF PURULIA (West Bengal) : Seed: in ascaris; TRIBES OF MA YURBHANJA (Orissa) : Seed: as contraceptive; TRIBES OF SANTAL PARGANAS (Bihar) : Root: in tuberculosis; TRIBES OF VARANASI (Uttar Pradesh) : Leaf: in boils; Seed: as vermifuge; TRIBES OF MIRZAPUR (Uttar Pradesh) : Bark: in dysentery; Gum: in diarrhoea, dysentery; TRIBES OF SIWALIK (Uttar Pradesh) : Gum: as tonic; BHAT: Seed: as abortifacient; BHOXA: Bark: in bone fracture, Gum: in piles, urinary complaints; GARHWALI: Leaf: in boil, inflammation, Flower: in diarrhoea, dysentery, pimples, Seed: as anthelmintic; THARU: Gum: as diuretic, Seed: as cooling agent; FOLKS OF DELHI: Gum: as astringent, Flower: as aphrodisiac, astringent, diuretic, Seed: as anthelmintic; FOLKS OF KURUKSHETRA (Haryana) : Flower: in stomachache; DANG: Bark: in diarrhoea; TRIBESOFRATANMAHAL HILLS (Gujarat) : Flower: in eye complaints; KORKU (of Maharashtra) : Flower, in dysentery; TRIBES OF KHANDLA (Maharashtra) : Flower: in dog bite, urinary complaints; TRIBES OF CHANDRAPURA (Maharashtra) : Leaf: in skin diseases; TRIBES OF JHABUA (Madhya Pradesh) : Root: in dog bite; TRIBES OF SAGAR (Madhya Pradesh) : Leaf: as vermifuge, Flower: in diabetes, diarrhoea, piles; TRIBES OF EAST GODAVARI (Andhra Pradesh) : Gum: in diarrhoea; TRIBES OF NILGIRI (Tamil Nadu) : Bark: as haemostatic, in wounds, Flower: in eye complaints; TRIBES OF KANNANORE (Kerala) : Flower: in antifertility.

ATHARVA VEDA: Extract of stem: beneficial for sperms and helps securing conception; CHARAKA SAMHITA : Stem-extract: useful in leprosy, piles, gastroenteritis and menorrha-gia; SUSHRUTA SAMHITA : useful in diseases caused by vayu (wind), Seed: effective against intestinal worms; A YURVEDA

: Bark: useful against snake venom, wounds, indigestion, gastroenteritis, fever, tuberculosis, Gum: astringent, beneficial to children and women,Leaf: astringent,

sex stimulant, useful in intestinal worms, dyspepsia, piles, menorrhagia, pimples, wounds in mouth/throat, Flower: diuretic, sex stimulant, helps menstruation, useful in gastroenteritis, Seed: useful against intestinal worms.

SIDDHA : Flower-juice: used in preparation of the medicine Murukkam, Seed and Kernel: in Palac

UNANI: Ingredient of the medicine called 'Dhak(tesu) ' and 'Samaghke Dhak'.

Modern use: Plant (alcoholic extract: produces persistent vasodepression in cats, shows activity against earthworms; Bark: insecticide against house flies; Alcohol extract of bark : inhibitory against E. coli and Micrococcus pyogenes var. aureus; Gum: solution applied to check conception; Root (bark) : aphrodisiac, analgesic, anthelmintic, useful in elephan-tiasis, applied in sprue, piles, ulcers, tumours and dropsy; EtOH (50%) extract of leaf: spasmogenic; FlolYer: effective in leprosy, gout; Alcoholic extract: antiestrogenic in mice; Aqueous extract: anti- implantation in rats; along with Hygrophila auriculata leaf and root taken with milk to cure leucorrhoea; Seed (freshly powdered) : effective against Ascaris; Extract (in vitro) : anthelmintic against Asacridia galli worms; finely powdered along with Acorus calamus rhizome or mixed with juice of Cyperus rotundus rhizome: cures delirium; Saline extract: agglutinates erythrocytes of animals; Hot alcoholic extract: anti-implantation and anti-ovulatory in animals.

Phytography : Erect tree, reaching a height of 13-17 m; young stem clothed with grey or brown silky hairs; leaves alternate, petioles 7. 5-15. 0 cm long, trifoliate, leaflets 10-20 cm long, leathery, lower surface covered with dense silky hairs; racemes 15 cm long; flowers bright orange-red, thickly clothed on the outside with silvery small hairs; pods 15-20 cm by 3. 7-5. 0 cm, narrowed suddenly into a stalk longer than calyx.

Phenology: Flowering: February-April; Fruiting: May-July. Distribution: Plains of India, ascending up to 1300 m; Myanmar. Ecology and cultivation: Mesophyte; wild.

Chemical contents: Plant: flavonoids, glucosides, butin, butrin, isobutrin, palastrin; Flower: butrin, coriopsin, monospermoside, sulphurein, chalcones; Seed: palasonin, Seed oil: d-Iactone of n-heneicosanoic acid, monospermine, new phytolectin.

Remarks: An important tree for lac cultivation, but the lac produced on it is of inferior quality. Bark yields fibre, wood yields timber of poor quality; stem-bark used as fish poison by tribes of South Rajasthan. Plates and bowls are made by stitching the leaves by the tribes of Purulia and Saurashtra.

Flowers yield a yellow dye of little permanency.

Flowers are eaten as vegetables by tribes of Manbhum and Hazaribagh Districts of Bihar while fruits by Garhwalis.

Tree is sacred to the Hindus and Buddhists. Flower is an essential item of Saraswati Puja.

BAUHINIA VAHLII WT. & ARN. (CAESALPINIACEAE)

Syn : Phanera vahlii Benth.

Vernacular names: Ben: Sehari; Lod : Jom-Iar; San: Sihari-chop.

Traditional use: TRIBES OF TEHRI-GARHWAL : (i) Fruit: aphrodisiac, (ii) Seed: tonic and vermifuge; TRIBES OF BASTAR : (i) Seed: tonic; SANTAL: (i) Plant: in dysentery, stomachache, (ii) Fruit: to treat antifertility of women.

Phytography : Huge climber with many tendrils; branch lets hairy; leaves alternate, petiolate, simple, 2-cleft, cleavage goes down a quarter to one-third way from the apex, 7. 5-45. 0 cm long; racemes terminal, subcorymbose; flowers bracteate, 2. 5 cm long; pods nearly 45 by 5 cm, rusty-downy, 7-to 12-seeded.

Distribution: Foot of central and eastern Himalaya, ascending up to 800 m, Bihar, Madhya Pradesh, Maharashtra and Karnataka.

CAREYA ARBOREA ROXB. (LECYTHIDACEAE)

English name: Tummy wood.

Sanskrit name: Kumbhi.

Vernacular names: Ben and Hin : Kumbhi; Guj : Kumbi; Kan : Kaval, Doddala, Asanda; Lod : Kumbi-daru, Kumbhi; Mal: Alam, Pelu; Mun : Asanda-daru, Kumbhir; Sad: Kumbi; San: Khubati; Tam: Ayma; Tel: Araya, Duddipa.

Trade names: Kumbhi, Kumbi.

Traditional use: LODHA: (i) Root-paste: in body pain, (ii) Root-bark decoction (with long pepper) : in fever, (iii) Stem-bark powder (paste with honey) : to children in cold and cough; SANTAL : Stem-bark: (paste with margosa) : in leucoderma

Phytography : Medium-sized tree with large ovate, ovate-oblong leaves clustered at the end of the branchlets, old le_ves often red/purple; flowers large, white and pink, in dense spikes, fruits large globose green, crowded with calyx tube, deciduous.

Phenology: Flowering: March-May; Fruiting: July.

Distribution : Sub-Himalayan tract occu-rring throughout India up to an elevation of 1700 m.

Chemical contents: Bark: lupeol, betulin; Leaf: ellagic acid, hexacosanol, quercetin, â-sitosterol, â-spinasterol taraxerol and its OAc, valoneic acid, careaborin, â-amyrin; Seed: á-spinasterol, á-spinasterone, baringtogenol-C, careyagenol-E.

Remarks: Only plant named by William Roxburgh in honour of William Carey. Lodhas use fresh stem bark decoction for washing septic wounds of cattle, and keep a dry fruit in a room as snake repellant. Oraons use powdered stem, root and leaf for poisoning fish.

CATHARANTHUS ROSEUS (L.) G. DON (APOCYNACEAE)

Syn: Lochnera rosea (L.) Spach, Vinca rosea L.

English names: Madagascar periwinkle, Old maid, Red periwinkle.

Vernacular names: Ben: Nayantara; Hin : Sada sawagon; Lad: Swet chandu; Mal: Ushamalari; Mar: Sadaphul; Ori : Ainskati; Pun: Rattanjot; Tam: Sudukadu Mallikai; Tel: Billaganneru. -

Trade name: Nayantara.

Traditional use: BODO: (i) Plant: in cancer, diabetes, (ii) Leaf: in menorrhagia; LODHA : (i) Root-paste: in septic wounds, (ii) Root-decoction (with paste of long peppers) : in fever, (iii) Leaf-juice: in blood dysentery, (iv) Leaf- decoction: to babies in gripping pain; SANTAL : (i) Latex: in scabies, (ii) Seed- powder (with decoction of black pepper) : in epilepsy; ETHNIC COMMUNITIES OF EAST GODAVARI DISTRICT: Root: in cancerous wounds.

Modern use: Plant-extract: antimitotic; Root (alkaloids) : in cancer, and as emetic, hypotensive, sedative and antiviral.

Phytography : A small herb or subshrub, up to 75 cm high; leaves elliptic-ovate to oblong, 4-10 by 2-4 cm, glabrous to puberulous, base acute or cuneate, apex obtusely apiculate, lateral nerves 10-12 pairs, petiole 1. 0-1. 5 cm; flowers in axillary or terminal cymes; solitary or paired, shortly pedicellate, pink or white or white with pink or yellow ring in orifice region; mericarps 3-4 by 0. 3 cm, puberulous.

Phenology: Flowering and Fruiting: throughout the year.

Distribution: A native of West Indies; commonly grown in gardens throughout India;

Bangladesh and Pakistan.

Ecology and cultivation: Plains from the coasts, in wastelands, fallow fields, less on the hills 800-1400 m, also widely cultivated. vinleukoblastine (VLB), vincristine or vinleurocristine (VCR), ursolic acid, oleanolic acid, ajmalicine, alstonine; Stem: vinca rodine, vincoline, vinamidine, leurocolombine, vinca thicine, vincubine; Leaf: leurosine, vindoline, catharanthine, lochnerine, tetrahydroalstonine, roseoside, essential oil; Seed: vincedine, vincedicine, tabersonine.

CURCUMA LONGA L. (ZINGIBERACEAE)

Syn : Curcuma domestica Val. English name: Turmeric. Sanskrit name: Haridra.

Vernacular names: Asm : Holodhi; Ben: Halud; Guj : Halada; Hin : Haldi; Kan : Arisina; Kon : Holldi, Ghor hollad; Mal: Manjella-kua; Mar: Halede; Mun : Hatu sasang, Sasang; Orn: Balka; Ori : Haladi; Sad: Haldi; San: Oerel sasan; Tam: Manjal; Tel: Pasupu.

Trade name: Haldi.

Traditional use: ETHNIC COMMUNITIES OF ARUNACHAL PRADESH AND ASSAM: Rhizome: in migrain; SANTALS : (i) Rhizome: in hazy vision, inflammation of eye, night blindness, subnormal temperature after fever, spleen consumption, Basli rog (pain similar to rheumatism), rheumatism due to draught, lock-jaw, Rosbi (stealth convulsions with indistinct speech), chronic scabies, sores and curbuncles, infantile atrophy, indigestion, prolapsus ani and fistula ani, bronchitis, cough and cold, puerperal fever; (ii) Extract of Rhizome: in rhagades; (iii) Bulb: in drying up of lactation; (iv) Flower: in cholera, sores in throat, syphilis; (v) Dried Flower: in icterus; ETHNIC COMMUNITIES OF RANCHI and HAZARIBAGH (Bihar) : (i) Leaf: in cold, fever, pneumonia; GARHWALI: Rhizome: in pimples and feckles on face, wounds, leprosy; KUMAONI : Rhizome: in cough, insect stings, wounds; ETHNIC COMMUNITIES OF KURUKSHETRA (Haryana) : Rhizome: in body pain, headache; TRIBES OF ARAKU VALLEY (Andhra Pradesh) : Rhizome: as anthelmintic..

RIGVEDA : Rhizome: improves body complexion and apetite; YAJURVEDA

: Rhizome: is a blood-purifier, improves body complexion; CHARAKA SAMHITA laxative, useful in leprosyand against contaminuos microbes; SUSHRUTA

SAMHITA : digestive; AYURVEDA : Rhizome: effective against bacterial infection, skin diseases, intestinal worms, liver complaints, stammering, filaria, asthma, sprain, boils, wounds, conjuctivitis, thirst due to phlegm, allergic reactions, against leeches, minor ingredient of a drug for malarial fever.

SIDDHA : Rhizome: ingredient of Kappu mancal, Manchal.

UNANI : ingredient of 'Majnoor-e-falsfa', useful in gastrointestinal complaints; Powder of rhizome: used as antifertility agent.

Modern use: Rhizome: ingredient of 'Geriforte'-effective in senile pruritis,

Vitafix-useful in premature ejaculation, insect repellent against houseflies, insecticide, antifungal; EtOH (50%) extract of rhizome: antiprotozoal, spasmolytic, hypotensive, Central Nervous System depressant; daily consumption of 1 gm raw rhizome helps to fight decaying metabolism and thus prevents cancer; Essential oil from rhizome: anti-arthritic, antifungal,. anti-inflammatory, antibacterial.

Phytography : Herb with large ovoid rootstock, sessile tubers thick, cylindric, bright yellow inside; petiole 60 cm long, leav. es green, 30-45 cm by 10-20 cm; peduncle 15 cm or more long, hidden by sheathing petiole, spikes 10-15 cm, about 5 cm in diameter; bracts pale green, ovate, about 3. 7 cm long, those of the coma pale pink; flowers yellow, as long as the bracts.

Phenology: Flowering: Autumn.

Distribution: Indigenous to Paresnath (Bihar); widely cultivated in West Bengal and other parts of India; Bangladesh, Sri Lanka.

Ecology and cultivation: Tropical plant; cultivated throughout the tropics. Chemical contents: Essential oil from rhizome: curcumin.

Remarks: In Hawaii, rhizome is used against growth of nostrils, for cleaning blood and as gargle; green rhizome is given for whooping and other coughs. In Sri Lanka, Rhizome paste is used in skeletal fracture. Extensive research is being carried out on the nutritional and medicinal value of this plant.

COSTUS SPECIOSUS (KOENING EX RETZ.) J.E. SMITH (ZINGIBERACEAE)

Syn : Banksea speciosa J. Koening

Sanskrit names: Canda, Kemuka.

Ve rna cula r n a me s: B e n: Ke u; Hi n : Keb u, Ke yu, K usi ; K a n : Chengaivakoshtu; Mal: Cannakilannu, Cannakkuvva, Narumeanna; Mar: Penva, Pushkarmula; Tam: Kostam, Kuiravam, Kottam; Tel: Chengaivakohtu.

Trade name: Keyu.

Traditional use: Rhizome: bitter, astringent, acrid, cooling, purgative, aphrodisiac, anthelmintic, depurative, febrifuge, expectorant and tonic, also beneficial in asthma, anaemia, bronchitis, leprosy, flatulence, constipation, fever, skin diseases and inflammation.

Modern use: in carcino-genic tumours.

Phytography : Succulent perennial herb with long leafy spirally twisted stems, 2-3 m high and horizontal rhizomes; leaves simple, spirally arranged, ob-lanceolate or oblong, glabrous above, silky pubescent beneath with broad bright red; fruits globose/ovoid capsules; seeds obovoid or semi-globose.

Phenology: Flowering: September-October; inflorescence globose of closely packed bracts.

Distribution: Throughout India; Pakistan and Bangladesh-in moist localities and in wastelands.

Ecology and cultivation: Hills above 800 m; moist places and wastelands also.

Chemical content: Root: rich in starch.

DATURA METEL L. (SOLANACEAE)

Syn : Datura alba Nees, D. fastuosa L. var alba C. B. Clarke

English name: Hindu datura.

Sanskrit name: Dhustura.

Vernacular names :Ben: Dhutra, Dhatura; Hin : Sadahdhatura; Tam:

Vellum mattai. Trade name: Dhutra.

Traditional use: FOLKS OF PURULIA (West Bengal and Rajasthan: Seed: for treatment of leprosy; FOLKS OF RAJASTHAN: Leaf: in guinea-worms; Other uses of seed, leaf and root: in insanity, fever with catarrhal and cerebral complications, diarrhoea, skin diseases and antideptic. It is narcotic, acrid, anodyne, antispasmodic, intoxicating, emetic and useful in asthma; Root: used for treatment of bites from rabbits; Poultice made of leaf: used for epilepsy, ophthalmodynia, otalgia, lumbago, sciatica, neuralgia, mumps and painful swelling.

Modern use: Seed: aphrodisiac, narcotic and antispasmodic and useful in dontalgia, otalgia, gastropathy and skin diseases and for treatment of dandruff and lice; EtOH (50%) extract of plant: anticancer, anthelmintic, spasmogenic and blood pressure depressant;Aquous extract of plant: nematicidal; Leaf extract: antiviral; EtOH extract of leaf and aquous extract of fruit: anticholinergic.

Phytography : Coarse annual herb, may be 2 m tall, stem scented; leaf alternate, petiolate, simple; flowers axillary, peduncled, white or nearly so, 17.5 cm long and may be 12. 5 cm in diameter across the mouth; capsules subglobose, 3 cm in diameter, equally spinous on all sides.

Phenology: Flowering: throughout the year; Fruiting: with blunt spines. Distribution: Throughout India; occasionally grown in gardens. Ecology and Cultivation: Hills up to 1500 m, occasionally in the plains even to the coast; wild.

Chemical contents: Root: alkaloids, tropane derivatives; Stem: hyoscine, hyoscyamine, Leaf: hyoscine, hyoscyamine, micotianamine; Fruit (pericarp) alkaloids, â-sitosterol, triterpene, daturaolone, daturadiol; Seed: hyosane, hyoscyamine, daturaolone, fastusic acid; Seed-oil: â-Me-sterols.

DIOSPYROS PEREGRINA (GAERTN.) GURKE (EBENACEAE)

Syn : Diospyros embryoteris Pers., D malabarica (Oeser.) Kost. *English names:* Gaub Persimmon, Wild Mangostein. *Sanskrit names:* Kalaskardha, Krishnasara, Tinduka.

Vernacular names: Ben and Hin : Gab, Kata Gab; Kan : Holetupari; Mal: Panachi; Mar: Tender; Ori : Dhusarokendu, Kendu; San: Makar kenda; Tam: Katlati, Tumbi; Tel : Tinduki.

Traditional use: SANTAL : (i) Root: in gravel; (ii) Bark: in cholera; (iii) Fruit: in dysentery and menorrhagia; TRIBES OF ABUJH-MARH RESERVE AREA (Madhya Pradesh) : Fruit: in dysentery and as tonic; TRIBES OF BASTAR (Madhya Pradesh) : Fruit: in blister in mouth, diarrhoea.

HARIT SAMHITA : Bark: in gastro-enteritis; BAGBHATTA : Juice of unripe fruit: in restoring normal skin colour after burn; BHABAPRAKASA : Aqueous extract of green fruit: in healing burn-wound; BANGASENA : Powder of dried fruit with honey: licking is beneficial in hiccup in children.

AYURVEDA : (i) Bark extract: in chronic dysentery; (ii) Aqueous extract of green fruit: in menorrhagia, excessive salivation.

Modern use: EtOH (50%) extract of stem and leaf: anticancer, diuretic;

EtOH (50%) extract of stem bark: antiprotozoal, antiviral, hypoglycaemic.

Phytography : Middle-sized, profusely branched tree; stem and branches black, branchlets glabrous; leaves alternate, petioles ±0. 6 to ±0. 8 cm long, lamina thick, leathery, oblong, veines slightly elevated above; male flowers in few or many-flowered short cymes, flowers tubular, 0. 8 cm long, lobed, calyx black, silky; female flowers solitary or few together, subsessile or cymose, larger than male flowers, ovary 8-celled; fruits usually solitary, subglobose, 2. 5-5. 0 cm in diameter, brick-coloured when young, yellowish when mature, persistent calyx lobed, accrescent 4-to 8 -seeded.

Phenology: Flowering and Fruiting: Summer to rainy season, fruits take 4-5 months to mature.

Distribution Throughout India; Bangladesh, Malaysia and other South-East Asian countries, also in Australia.

Ecology and cultivation: Throughout India, abundant in Bengal; cultivated near habitational sites; occasionally found as ferals; Sri Lanka.

Chemical contents: Root: glycerides; Bark: myricyle alcohol, saponin, triterpenes; Stem: â-sitosterol, á leuconanthocyanin; Leaf: triterpenes; Fruit pulp: alkenes, triterpenes; Seed: betulinic acid, â-amyrin, fatty oil, unsaponified matter. nux-vomica. Remarks: Santals use bark in treatment of rinderpest.

Rural people of North Bengal and Bangladesh consume the leaves as vegetable. Fruits are eaten by Bhoxas, Lodhas, Monpas, Santals and Bengalees. Tribes of Bastar consume the seeds.

Boatmen rub the fruit-juice on the undersurface of boats to protect the wood from rotting, and fishermen use the same in their fishing net for the same purpose.

DOLICHOS BIFLORUS L. (FABACEAE)

Syn : Dolichos uniflorus Lam., Glycine uniflora Dalz.

English name: Horsegram.

Sanskrit name: Kulattha.

Vernacular names: Ben: Kurti-kalai; Hin and Mar: Kutthi; Kan : Hurali; Mal: Muthiva; Man: Nagakrijon; Mun : Kurthi; Orn : Anrsga; Sad: Kurthi; San: Horec; Tam: Kollu; Tel: Ulavalu.

Traditional use: SANTAL : (i) plant: dysuria, sores, tumours; (ii) leaf: in burns; (iii) seed: in adenitis, fistula ani, intercostal neuralgia, pleurisy, pneumonia, prolapsus ani; MUNOA : aqueous extract of seed: to women after childbirth; IRULA, KOTA, TOOA (Nilgiri) : seed: in menstrual complaints; RURAL FOLKS: Aqueous extract of seed: in urinary troubles and kidney stone.

CHARAKA SAMHITA : seed: useful in piles, hiccup, abdominal lump, bronchial asthma, in causing and regulating perspiration; SUSHRUTA SAMHITA. seed powder: useful in stopping excessive perspiration; BAGBHATTA: seed: useful in spermatocalcali (Shukrashman); CHAKRADATTA : decoction of seed: beneficial in urticaria; RAJANIGHANTU : beneficial in piles, colic, epistasis, flatulence, ophthalmia, ulcer.

AYURVEDA : decoction of seed: useful in leucorrhoea, menstrual troubles, bleeding during pregnancy, colic caused by wind, piles, rheumatism, heamorrhagic disease, intestinal worms; seed powder: antidiaphoretic; seed (in combination with milk) : work as anthelmintic, soup prepared from seeds is beneficial in enlarged liver and spleen.

SIDDHA : seed: used in preparing a medicine named Kollu.

Modern use: Plant extract: radiolabel reagent in ABa blood grouping of human hair; EtOH (50%) extract of Seed: spasmolytic.

Phytography : Annual herb, trailing or suberect, branched; leaves alternate, stipulate, trifoliate, leaflets membranous, ovate, ±2. 5-5. 0 cm long, young ones finely pilose; flowers axillary, may be more than one together but without a common peduncle, papilionaceous, usually yellow-may be white, ±1. 25-1. 8 style; seeds 5-6 per pod, ellipsoid, flattened.

Phenology: Flowering: August-November; Fruiting: September-December.

Distribution: Widely distributed in India, ascending up to 1000 m in Sikkim; cultivated mainly in Andhra Pradesh, Tamil Nadu, Karnataka.

Ecology and cultivation: Mesophyte; wild and cultivated.

Chemical contents: Stem and Leaf: coumesterol, a lectin-like glycoproticin, psoraliding; Leaf (bacteria treated) : dolichin A and dolichin B; Seed : â- sitosterol, coumesterol, delbergiodin, genistein, 2-hydroxy-genistein, isoferreirin, keivitone, phaseollidin, pyranoside.

Adulterant: Cassia abrus L. is sometimes confused with this plant.

Remarks: Santals use the plant in treatment of rinderpest of domestic animals. Seeds are often consumed as pulse. Santals consider eating this pulse is good for patients of dysentery and leprosy, but they prohibit eating this by the patients of measles and small pox.

DILLENIA INDICA L. (DILLENIACEAE)

Syn : Dillenia speciosa Thunb.

English name: Dillenia.

Sanskrit names: Bhavya, Bharija.

Vernacular names: Asm : Chalita, Qutenga; Ben: Chalta; Guj : Karambel; Hin : Chalta; Kan :Betta kanijala; Mar: Mota karmal; Mal: Chalita, Punna; Man: Heigri; Ori : Qu, Uvu; San: Korbhatta; Tam and Tel: Uva.

Trade name: Chalta.

Traditional use: MANIPURI : Fruit decoction: for curing dandruff and checking falling of hairs; MIKIR (Assam) : Fruit: eat to combat weakness; TRIBES OFTEJPUR (Assam) : Plant: in fever; TRIBES OF TIRAP (Arunachal Pradesh) : Leaf: in dysentery; SANTAL : (i) Root: as prophylactic at the cholera season, an ingredient of a medicine for burning sensation in the chest; (ii) Stem-bark: component of medicine for sores caused by mercury poisoning, chronic progredient sores and carbuncle, and as a prophylactic at the cholera season; (iii) Mucilage: on wounds of burns; TRIBES OF ABUJH MARH RESERVE AREA (Madhya Pradesh) : Fruit: as tonic; TRIBES OF EAST GODAVARI (Andhra Pradesh) : Fleshy calyx: in stomach disorders.

YAJURVEDA : an important plant; UPAVARHANA SAMHITA : the plant is aphrodisiac and prpmotes virility; CHARAKA SAMHITA : the fruit is sweet, acidic, astringent, removes bile, phlegm, fetid and flatulence; SUSHRUTA SAMHITA : fruit cardiotonic, tasteful, astringent, acidic, removes bile, phlegm, fetid and flatulence; RAJANIGHANTU: green fruit is acidic, pungent, hot, removes wind, phlegm, but the ripe fruit is sweet, sour, appetising and beneficial in colic associated with mucous; MATSYA PURANA : decoction of this plant can be used as universal antidote for poison;

AGNI PURANA spraying water, containing stem extract, on and around the wound caused by spider bite helps in removing the poison.

AYURVEDA: (i) Root (bark extrac_: in food poisoning; (ii) Root-bark(paste) : along with leaf-paste applied externally in sprains; (iii) Young bark and Leaf: astringent; (iv) Fruit-juice : mixed with sugar and water serves as a cooling beverage in fever, fit, and as a cough syrup; (v) Ripe fruit-juice: removes flatulence, increases quantity of semen, galactogogue, combats weakness, external application helps supuration of boil, and checks loss of hair. *Modern use:* Leaf (50% EtOH extract) : shows antiamphetamine activity; Seed-extract: antimicrobial; Seed-oil: antifungal, and its unsaponifiable matter antibacterial.

Phytography : Evergreen, round-headed tree, 9-42. 5 m high; branchlets tomentose, bark cinnamomum-like; leaf alternate, simple, fascicled at the apices of branches, petiole 3. 7 cm long, lamina 20-25 cm by 5-10 cm, oblong-Ianceolate, closely set parallel veins from midrib, upper surface glabrous, hairs present on the lower surface, especially on veins; flower terminal or leaf-opposed, solitary, white, 15 cm in diameter, sepals thick; fruit globose with accrescent calyx, 12. 5-15 cm in diameter, green when young, yellowish and sweet-scented when ripe; seeds many, compressed, embedded in hairy cells.

Phenology: Flowering: May-June; Fruiting: July-August.

Ripens in November-December.

Distribution: Sub-Himalayan tract from Garhwal to Assam, Arunachal Pradesh, Manipur, Tripura, West Bengal, Orissa, Bihar, Central and South India; Nepal, Bangladesh, Sri Lanka.

Ecology and cultivation: Plant of tropical forest; occasionally grown in gardens.

Chemical contents: Stem-bark: betulin, betulinaldehyde, betulic acid, flavonoids, dillentin, dihydroisorhamnetin, lupeol, myricetin, glucosides, B-sitosterol; Wood: betulinic acid, lupeol, â-sitosterol; Leaf: betulinic acid, cycloa rtenone, fla vonoids, n-hentria conta nol, B-sitosterol; Fruit: a n arabinogalactan, betulinic acid, â-sitosterol.

Remark: Green calyx is eaten in various forms of pickles.

DIOSCOREA BULBIFERA L. (DIOSCOREACEAE)

Syn : Dioscorea crispata Roxb., D. pulchella Roxb.. D. sativa Thunb. non L, D. versicolor Buch. Ham.

English names: Air yam, Potato yam, Air potato.

Sanskrit name: Varahi.

Kan : Heggenasu; Man: Ha; Mar: Manakundu, Karukarinda; Mun : Jo aru; Tam: Kodikulangu; Tel: Chedupaddu-dumpa; San: Bongo-sanga.

Traditional use: TRIBES OF PURULIA (West Bengal) : Tuber: in boils; SANTAL : (i) Dried tuber (powdery: as shampoo and on sores; (ii) Plant:

against madness; SIKKIMESE : Tuber: in jaundice; ETHNIC COMMUNITIES OF DEHRA DUN AND SIWALIK: Tuber: in dysentery, piles; DANG (Gujarat) : Tuber: in abdominal pain, bone fracture.

Modern use: Aerial parts (50% EtOH extract) : diuretic; Rhizome: anorexiant.

Phytography : Climber, usually twining to the left; stem slender, green or purple, with 10-15 small crisped wings, tubers large, variable in form; leaves opposite and alternate, petioles 5-15 cm long, lamina cordate, very variable in size, attaining 35 cm in length, membranous, dark green, 7-9 costate; male spikes slender, almost capillary, 2. 5-10 cm long, panicled, flowers crowded or scattered, green or purplish; female spikes 10-25 cm long, pendulous; capsules 1. 6-2. 5 cm by 0. 8-1. 25 cm, membranous; seeds with broad basal wing.

Phenology: Flowering: August-September; Fruiting: November.

Distribution: Common in the outskirts of forests throughout India, ascending up to 2000 m in the hills; Bangladesh, Pakistan.

Ecology and cultivation: Plant of tropical climate, grows in the midst of scrub jungles, rare; wild and planted.

Chemical contents: Tuber: furanoid norditerpenes, norditerpene g lu co si de s, d io sb ul bi no si de D & F, di os bu lb in B & D , a ne w dihydrophenanthrene, d-sorbitol; Bulbil: diosgenin.

Remarks: Tubers are eaten as vegetable by the ethnic communities of Meghalaya, Kameng district of Arunachal Pradesh, Purulia and Medinipur districts of West Bengal, Varanasi, Mirzapur districts and Kumaon area of Uttar Pradesh, Madhya Pradesh, Goa, Maharashtra, Ratan Mahal Hills (Gujarat), Rajasthan, Cannanore district of Kerala and Mikirs (Assam), Santals (West Bengal) and Tharus (Uttar Pradesh).

Boiled bulbils are eaten by Mikirs and Santals as vegetable.

ELETTARIA CARDAMOMUM (L.) MATON (ZINGIBERACEAE)

Syn : Cardamum officinale Salisb.; (non-Ammomum cardamum L. 1753); Alpinia cardamum Roxb.

English names: Cardomum, Lesser cardamum.

Sanskrit names: Ela, Trutih.

Vernacular names: Ben: Chhoto elach; Guj : Elachi; Hin : Chhoti elaichi; Kan : Yellaki; Mal: Cittelum, Elam; Mar: Elachi veldodi; Tam: Elam; Tel: Yelakkayalu.

Trade name: Chhoti elaichi.

Traditional use: MATSYA PURANA : a constituent of an antivenom drug. AYURVEDA : seeds abortifacient, alexiteric, aromatic, acrid, sweet, cooling, carminative, cardiac tonic, digestive, diuretic, expectorant, stimulant, and tonic, beneficial in asthma, bronchitis, strangury, haemorrhoids, renal and vesical calculi, halitosis, anorexia, dyspepsia, gastropathy and burning sensation.

SIDDHA : dried fruit, seed and stem-bark are used to prepare drugs cell 'Elam', 'Elarici'.

UNANI: preparations used as antidote to poison, astringent, exhilarant and in nausea.

Modern use: Essential oil from seed: antimicrobial; oil is used in several pharmaceutical preparations.

Phytography : Perennial leafy herb, 1. 5-3. 0 m high; rootstock thick, horizontal; leaves 30-65 cm by 5-10 cm, distichous, elliptic or elliptic-lanceolate, glabrous above, softly pubescent below, acuminate at apex, narrowed or obtuse at base; flowers white, striped with violet, in elongated, flexuous, bracts, panicles arising from the rootstock; capsules oblong or subindehiscent, marked with fine vertical ribs; seeds black, arillate.

Phenology: Flowering and Fruiting: throughout the year, mainly in late autumn and winter.

Distribution: Found in rich, moist forests of the hilly tracts, up to 2000 m; commercially cultivated in Tamil Nadu, Andhra Pradesh, Karnataka, Gujarat.

Ecology and cultivation: Plant of tropical moist climate; wild and cultivated.

Chemical contents: Seed : essential oil, terpenoids.

Remark: Fruits and seeds are used as masticator.

EMBELIA RIBES BURM. F. (MYRSINACEAE)

Syn : Embelia glandulifera Wight, Samara ribes Kurz

English names: Embelia, Embelia fruit.

Sanskrit names: Jantughna, Krimighna, Krimiripu, Vella, Vidanga.

Vernacular names: Ben: Biranga; Guj : Vaivarang, Vavading; Hin : Baberang, Vayvidang; Kan : Vayuvilanga; Mar: Vaivarang, Vavadinga; Mal: Vizhal; Pun: Baburung; Tam and Tel: Vayuvilanga.

Traditional use: GARHWALI and TRIBES OF NORTH-EAST INDIA: Seed: (Assam) : Fruit: in stomach complaints.

MATSYA PURANA : important medicinal plant; AGNI PURANA : beneficial for gastroenteritis, cirrhosis of liver, oedema, skin diseases including le pr os y a n d ef fe ct ive in k il li ng w or ms i n a l im en ta ry c a n a l ; VIJACINTAMANITANTRA: consumption of powdered fruit along with fruits of Emblica officinalis, honey and sesame-oil improves quality of sperms; BHAVAPRAKASHA: it is pungent, removes morbidity, improves blood circulation, stimulates appetite, acts against phlegm, makes the body light, kills worms of all types; RAJANIGHANTU: it is pungent, hot, light, enhances balance between wind and phlegm, beneficial in anorexia and improves digestive power.

AYURVEDA : (a) Root: acrid, astringent, useful in colic, dyspepsia, flatulence, odontalgia, stomach pain and increases exothermic metabolism; (b) Leaf: astringent, demulcent, depurative, thermogenic, useful in skin diseases including leprosy; (c) Fruit: acrid, alexeteric, alterant, anodyne, anthelmintic, astringent, bitter, brain tonic, carminative, contraceptive, depurative, digestive, diuretic, febrifuge, laxative, rejuvenating, stimulant, tonic, vulnerary, and useful in amnetia, asthma, colic, constipation, cardiopathy, dental caries, dyspepsia, dyspnoea, fever, flatulence, general debility, hemicramia, odontalgia, psychopathy, respiratory troubles and ring-worms; (d) Seed: a constituent of Vidangadi Yoga, an antifertility drug.

SIDDHA : dried fruits are used to prepare the drug Vaivitankam.

Modern use : Plant: cures abdominal tumours, and aenemeas, cystic tumours, pyorrhoea, useful against tape-worms; EtOH extract of plant: slightly active against Ecoli; one of the constituents of 'Gasex', and some oral contraceptives; Fruit: cures dental, oral, throat troubles except cancer of lips and ptyslism, constituent of some quick aboriticide; Aqueous extract of fruit: pronounced antifertility activity, anthelmintic against earthworms;Fruit-powder: expels tapeworms within 6-24 hours, if taken with curd in empty stomach, effective against giardia; Seed: antibiotic, anthelmintic, antituberculosis, alterative and stimulative.

Phytography : Large scandent shrub; branches long, slender, flexible, bark with many lenticels; leaves simple, alternate, petioles ±0. 8 cm, lamina elliptic, leathery, glabrous, shining above, silvery beneath, glandular pits present on the lower surface near the midrib; racemes axillary and terminal, laxly panicled; flowers white, may be greenish, ±0. 2 cm long; berries dull red to black, globular, small, 1-or 2-seeded; seeds globose, hollowed at the base, white spotted, albuminous.

Phenology: Flowering: peak in March-April; Fruiting: August.

Distribution: Throughout India up to 1750 m in hilly regions; common in lower hills; Sri Lanka, Malaya.

Ecology and cultivation: Grows in shola border, thickets; wild.

Chemical contents: Fruit: embelin.

Remark: Ethnic communities of Cannanore (Kerala) make bowstring with the bark.

ECLIPTA ALBA (L.) ROXB. (ASTERACEAE)

Syn : Eclipta prostrata (L.) Hassk.

English name: Trailing eclipta.

Sanskrit names: Bhringa, Bhringaraja, Kesaraja, Kayyonni, Markava, Tekarajah. *Vernacular names*: Asm : Kehoraji; Ben: Bhringaraj, Keshurti, Kesuria, Keshurey; Guj : Bhengra; Hin : Babri, Bhangra, Mocakand, Safed bhannra; Kan : Garga; Mal : Kannunni, Kaiyanni, Ka yyonni; Ma n: Oochisumbal; Mar: Maka; Mun : Bhengaj, Piri kesari; Om : Bhengraj; Ori :Kesarda; Sad: Bhengrait; San: Banda-kansa; Tam: Garuga, Kaikesi, Karipan, Kayyantakara; Tel: Galagara, Guntagalyeru.

Trade name: Kesuth

Traditional use: GARO: Leaf: in gastric troubles, hepatic disorders; MANIPURI : (i) Stem-decoction: in liver enlargement; (ii) Leaf-extract: in fever and cough; TOTO: (i) Whole plant: in hepatic problems, spleen troubles; (ii) Root: in ulcers and wounds; (iii) Leaf: as antidote to scorpion sting; ETHNIC COMMUNITIES OF ORISSA: (i) Plant: in itching; (ii) Leaf: in conjunctivitis and other eye problems, in promoting hairgrowth; SANTAL : (i) Plant-decoction with paste of black pepper: in fever; (ii) Leaf-juice: on wounds; ETHNIC COMMUNITIES OF BIHAR: (i) Plant: against antifertility, (ii) Root: as antidote to snake bite; (iii) Leaf: in malaria and other fevers; ETHNIC COMMUNITIES OF ARAKU VALLEY (Madhya Pradesh) : Leaf: in conjunctivitis, eye troubles; IRULAR: Leaf: in jaundice; TRIBAL SOCIETIES OF ANAIKATTY HILLS (Tamil Nadu) : Flower bud: in fever, headache; ETHNIC COMMUNITIES OF SALSETTE ISLAND: Leaf: as cooling; TRIBAL SOCIETIES OF SAURASHTRA (Gujarat) : Whole Plant: in asthma, bronchitis, leucoderma; TRIBAL SOCIETIES OF EASTERN RAJASTHAN: Leaf: in sores, ulcers, wounds, spleen disorders; TRIBES OF KURUKSHETRA (Haryana) : Leaf: as antiseptic; GARHWALI: (i) Whole plant: in jaundice, spleen disorders; (ii) Leaf: in leucoderma, skin diseases; KOL : Leaf: in malaria; TRIBES OF BASTAR (Madhya Pradesh) : Whole plant: in liver complaints; TRIBES OF CHHINDWARA (Madhya Pradesh) : Leaf: for promoting hair growth; TRIBES OF SAGAR (Madhya Pradesh) : Plant: in toothache, headache, gland swelling, elephantiasis. disorders, prevents graying and falling of hairs.

BHAVAPRAKASHA : cures problems caused by phlegm and wind, beneficial for hair, skin, teeth and eyes, removes worms, and also effective in ja undice a nd oedema ; RAJANIGHANTU: beneficia l for ha irs, eyes, oe de ma a nd p hl eg m; KA IYAD EVAN IG HA NT U : i t re mo ve s th e problems caused by phlegm and wind and worms, beneficial for hair, teeth, skin, cures cough, jaundice and oedema; NIGHANTURATNAKARAM: in addition to the above qualities, this plant invigorates sex; VAIDYAMANORAMA : drinking juice of the plant strengthens the body and secures the foetus in womb.

AYURVEDA : cures headache, migraine; leaves are beneficial for hairs, they remove lice, blacken skin, cure pyorrhoea, chronic dysentery, oedema, nervous weakness, jaundice, anorexia, gum troubles and remove intestinal worms.

Modern use: Herb: in skin diseases; Gum resin (from herb) : anticancerous against Ehrlich ascites carcinoma; Plant(50% EtOH extract): antiviral, spasmogenic; Plant (aqueous extract) : ovicidal against Sitotroga cereale//a eggs, nematicidal, haemostatic, beneficial in body inflammation, protective against hepatotoxic action of carbon tetrachloride in female guineapigs; Plant (powder) : curative of infective hepatitis, jaundice and viral hepi1titis; Leaf(aqueous extract) : myocardial depressant, hypotensive; Leaf-juice: cures shoulder pain caused by heavy load.

Phytography : Erect or prostrate diffused annual herb with roots at each node; leaves opposite, sessile, oblong-Ianceolate, ±2. 5-1 0 cm long, very variable in form and width; heads subglobose, ±1. 25 cm broad; flowers white and compressed.

Phenology: Flowering and Fruiting: throughout the year, peak period-August--February.

Distribution: Throughout India, ascending up to 2000 m; Bangladesh and Pakistan.

Ecology and cultivation: Common on damp wastelands, low waterlogged areas, roadsides, grassy humid localities, prefers warm climate; wild.

Chemical contents: Leaf : s ti gm a s te ro l , a - te rt hi en y l me th a n ol , wedelolactone, de-Me-wedelolactone, small amount of 2-formyl-terthienyl.

Adulterants: In Sanskrit literature, three types of Bhringaraja have been mentioned-white-flowered (E. alba), yellow-flowered (Wede/ia calandulacea) and blue--flowered (not yet identified).

Remarks: Tribals use juice of leaves for tattooing purpose.

EMBLICA OFFICINALIS GAERTN. (EUPHORBIACEAE)

Read: Phyllanthus emblica L.

English name: Emblica myrobalan.

Sanskrit names: Adiphala, Amlaka, Amritaphala, Dhatri, Hatha, Nellikka.

Vernacular names: Asm : Amluki; Ben: Amla, Amlaki; Guj : Amali; Hin

: Amla, Aon, Aonala; Kan : Amalaka; Mal: Amalakam, Nelli; Man: Heikru;

Mar: Anvala; Mun : Meral daru; Orn : Amra; Ori : Amla; Pun: Ambli, Ambuli;

Sad: Aonra; San: Aohal; Tam: Nelli, Toppunelli; Tel: Amlakamu, Usirika.

Trade name: Amla, Amlaki.

Traditional use: ETHNIC COMMUNITIES OF SAGAR DISTRICT (Madhya Pradesh) : Fruit: antiemitic, used in fever, indigestion; ETHNIC COMMUNIT/ ES OF DEHRA DUN and SIWALIK DISTRICTS (Uttar Pradesh) : Fruit: in bronchitis, indigestion; Seed: in asthma; DANG (Gujarat) : Bark: on burn, wounds, stomach complaint; IRULAR (Tamil Nadu) : Leaf: against cold; BIRHoRE(West Bengal) : Fruit: in constipation, headache, liver complaint, madness; THANES (Uttar Pradesh) : Fruit: in constipation; ETHNIC COMMUNIT/ES OF GARHWAL : Fruit: laxative, cooling, in diabetes, dysentery, and as diuretic; ETHNIC COMMUNIES OF TIRAP (Arunachal Pradesh) : Fruit: in diabetes; NAGA: Fruit: in eye complaint; KHASI and JAINTIA : Fruit: in eye complaint; TRIBES OF MIRZA PUR DISTRICT (Uttar Pradesh) : Fruit: in eye complaint; TRIBES OF HAZARIBAGH DISTRICT (Bihar) : Fruit: used to revive taste; KOL (Uttar Pradesh) : Fruit: on scorpion sting; ETHNIC COMMUNITIES OF MAYURBHANJ (Orissa) : Fruit: against thirst; ORAON

: (i) Fruit: in cough; (ii) Juice of fresh fruit and (ii) Infusion of seed: in inflammation of eyes; (iv) Crushed fruit with fruit of Terminalia citrin a and Terminalia belerica macerated in a tumbler of water in the evening: a very good stomachic and tonic; MANIPURI: (i) Boiled extract of leaf: in controlling high blood sugar; (ij) Fruit: in constipation, bleeding gum, piles, blood diseases and also as brain and nerve tonic; SANTAL: (i) Leaf: in anaemia, diarrhoea, dysentery, fever, gravel, sores (agya ghao, rokoc ghao); (ii) Stem-bark: in cholera, profuse diarrhoea (haga sitka), fistula, sores (bonga khoda, nason ghao, pachiari ghao, palania ghao); (iii) Powder of male inflorescence: in nasal haemorrhage; (iv) Infusion of green fruit: in gripe; (v) Ripe fruit: in cystitis and diarrhoea.

RAJAN/GHANTU: it is acidic (amla), astringent (kashaya), pleasant(madhura), cooling and light, beneficial in burning sensation caused by deranged bile, vomiting, oedema and is rejuvenating; the fruit is appetising, antiemetic and removes fatigue, useful in constipation and flatulence.

AYURVEOA : Fruit is useful in acidity, urinary trouble, hiccup, vomiting, leucorrhoea, biliary colic, urticaria, conjunctivitis and dysentery.

SIOOHA : Root-bark, fruit-juice and dried fruit are used to prepare a medicine named Nelli.

Modern use: Fruit: pronounced expectorant, antioxidant, anticancerous; EtOH (50%) extract of fruit: antiviral, carminative, stomachic; Aqueous extract of fruit: increases cardiac glycogen level and decreases serum GOT, GPT and LDH in rats; Fruit-juice: (i) mixed with turmeric powder and honey: cures diabetes insipidus; (ii) in ghee: used for abdominal and glandular tumours; a constituent of the medicine SG-1-Switradilepa used against vitiligo, and of an antibiotic drug Septilin.

Phytography : Deciduous tree with flaky bark, greenish, grey or red; leaves distichously closely set, bipinnate, dark green, leaflets linear-oblong; flowers densely fascicled, yellowish, unisexual, males on slender pedicels while females subsessile; fruits light green when young, yellowish when mature, globose, depressed, succulent, obscurely six-lobed, one-seeded; seed trigonous.

Phenology: Flowering: February-May; Fruiting: May onwards.

Distribution: Common in the mixed deciduous forests of India, ascending up to 1500 m, often cultivated in gardens and homeyards; Bangladesh, Pakistan. Ecology and cultivation: Plant of tropical climate; predominantly wild, cultivated in Uttar Pradesh, Madhya Pradesh.

Chemical contents: Root: ellagic acid, oleanolic acid, oleanolic aldehyde, lupeol; Stem-bark: lelucodel-phinidin, procyanidin, 3-0-gallated prodelphinidin and tannin; Stem and Leaf: lupeol, â-sitosterol; Fruit: vitamin C, carotene, ri bo fl a v in e, D -g lu co se , D- fr uc to se , myoi no si to l, n ic ot in ic a ci d, D - galacturoniaacid, phyllemblic acid, mucic acid, fatty acids, D-arabinosyl, D- xylosyl, L-rhamnosyl, D-glucosyl, D-mannosyl, D-galactosyl..

Remarks: Santals use bark in rinderpest, anthrax and convulsion of cattle. Fruits are eaten raw or as pickle and used to make ink. Wood is not attacked by insects.

EUPHORBIA TIRUCALLI L. (EUPHORBIACEAE)

English name : Milk bush, Indian tree spurge.

Sanskrit names : Shatala, Trikantaka.

Vernacular names: Ben: Ganderi, Lankasij, Latadoona; Guj : Thor dandalio; Hin : Konpol, Sehund; Kan : Bantakalli; Mar: Shera; Tam: Tirukalli, Kalli; Tel: Chemudu.

Trade name: Tirukalli.

Traditional use: IRULAR: Latex: in body pain, eczema, scabies; ETHNIC COMMUNITIES OF CHAMPAKARAI and DHOOMANOOR (Tamil Nadu) : Latex: on wounds; NAYADI : Latex: in rheumatism; ETHNIC COMMUNITIES OF MADHYA PRADESH: Latex: in earache, rheumatism, warts; ETHNIC

COMMUNITIES OF CHHOTANAGPUR : Latex: in earache.

BHAVAPRAKASHA: Itis pungent, bitter, helps digestion, beneficial in oedema, deranged phlegm, epistasis, deranged bile, constipation and dyscrasia.

AYURVEDA : Root: beneficial in colic; Latex of stem and leaf: cures cough, earache, emetic, laxative and rubefacient.

Modern use: Stem-extract: antifungal; Aerial parts (50% EtOH extract) :

antiprotozoal.

Phytography : Erect tree, 3-6 m high, branches thin, cylindrical, spreading, scattered, clustered, whorled, latex extraordinarily abundant, sticky and acrid; leaves alternate, linear, caducous, petioles modified to phylloclade; involucres clustered in the forks of branches, inconspicuous, flowers shortly pedicelled, bracteoles numerous; cocci dark brown, velvety, compressed; seeds ovoid, smooth.

Phenology: Flowering: very scarce, mainly in June-July; Fruiting: July-October.

Distribution: Introduced from tropical Africa, naturalised in the drier parts of India; elsewhere largely cultivated as hedges and fuel plants.

Ecology and cultivation: Xerophytic.

Chemical contents: Root: cycloartenol, euphorbol and its hexacosanoate, ta ra xe ro ne , ti nya t ox in ; Ba rk : e up ho rb ol a nd i t s he xa co sa na te , euphorginol=taraxer-14-en-6-01, ingenol and its triacetate, taraxerone; Latex: a-amyrin, â-sitosterol, cycloartenol, cycloeuphordenol, 4-deoxyphorbol and its esters, euphol, euphorbinol, isoeuphorbol, palmitic acid, taraxerol, tinyatoxin, tirucallol, trimethyl ellagic acid; it may be noted that there are differences in chemical contents of latex of plant growing in differenet countries; Stem: campesterol, hentriacontane, hentriacontanol, kaempferol, stigmasterol, methyl ellagic acid.

Remark: The plant is worshipped as a sacred one.

FICUS RACEMOSA L. (MORACEAE)

Syn : Ficus glomerata Roxb.

English names: Cluster fig, Country fig, Gular fig.

Sa ns kr it n a m e s : A pu sh pa ph a l a s a m ba nd ha , Au du mb a r a m , Brahmavriksha, Haritaksha, Hemadugdha, Shetavalkala, Udumbara, Yajnaphala.

Vernacular names: Asm : Dimoree; Ben: Dumur, Jajna-dumur, Jaya dumur; Guj : Gudar, Umar, Umbara; Hin: Gulav, Umar; Kan: Atti; Mal: Atti, Athimaram; Man: Heibong; Mar: Umbar(a); Mun : Loa daru; Orn : Dumbari,

Ori : Dimburi; Sad: Dumbair; San: Dumbari-hesa, Loa-dare; Tam: Atti, Aththi;

Tel: Bodda, Paidi, Udumbaramu.

Trade name: Common fig.

Traditional use: MANIPURI : (i) Root-extract: in diabetes, dysentery; (ii) Latex: on boils; (iii) Fruit: in pulmonary diseases; SANTAL : (i) Bark-juice: on boils, in adenitis axillaris, epidydimitis, hydrocele, orchitis; (ii)Latex: on adenitis, muscular pain, pimps, scabies; (iii) Juice of pith: in menorrahgia, spermatorrhoea; (iv) Warts on leaves: in small pOX; (v) Leaf gall (decoction) : for washing septic wounds; BHOXA : Latex: in piles; ETHNIC COMMUNITIES OF NORTHERN INDIA: (i) Latex: in piles, pulmonary diseases; (ii) Bark and Fruit (together) : in urinary complaints; (iii) Fruit: as carminative; GARHWALI: (i) Root: in dysentery; (ii) Bark: as astringent; ETHNIC COMMUNITIES OF MOUNT ABU (R a j a s th a n): L ea f : in p ne um on ia ; E T HN IC CO MM UN I TI ES O F CHANDRAPURA (Maharashtra) : Leaf: in bronchitis; ETHNIC COMMUNITIES OF KHEDTALUKA (Maharashtra) : (i) Barkand Fruit (together) : in leprosy, urinary complaints; (ii) Fruit: in diabetes; ETHNIC COMMUNITIES OF CHHINDWARA (Madhya Pradesh) : (i) Latex: in diarrhoea; (ii) Fruit: as carminative; ETHNIC COMMUNITIES OF BANDA (Madhya Pradesh) : Latex: in dysentery, skin cracks in heels and lips.

RIGVEDA : cures piles, internal wounds, removes impurities from blood, worms from alimentary canal; YAJURVEDA : bark kills worms; ATHARVAVEDA: useful in skin diseases, including leprosy, sinus, oedema, impurities of blood and in piles; MADANADINIGHANTU : useful in antifertility, pimples and wounds; BHAVAPRAKASHA : useful in treatment of pimples and wounds; DHANVANTARINIGHANTU : removes worms, cures thrombophlebitis, syncope, burning sensation and unusual thirst; KAIYADEVANIGHANTU : astringent, sweet and heavy, cures pimples and wounds, diseases caused by deranged phlegm and deranged bile; fruits are tasteful, invigorating, astringent, cooling, cardiac tonic, useful in urinary diseases, bile disorders, menstrual disorders..

AYURVEDA: Latex: external application useful in cuts, insect bites, boils, bruises, swellings, while internal application is beneficial in haemoptysis, bleeding piles and menstrual problems.

SIDDHA : (i) Bark: used to prepare the drug atti pattai, (ii) Latex: for atti pal, and (Hi) Leaf: an ingredient of atti ilai.

Modern use: Stem-bark (50% EtOH extract) : anti-inflammatory, anti protozoal, hypoglycaemic; Leaf-powder: useful in bilious affections; Leaf-gall: beneficial in small pox.

Phytography : Spreading laticiferous tree, 9. 0-12. 2 m tall, bark reddish grey, smooth; leaves alternate, stipules ovate-Ianceolate, pubescent, 1. 25-2. 5 cm long, petioles 2. 5-5. 0 cm long, lamina simple membranous, ovate to obovate-oblong or lanceolate, 10-18 cm long, dark green, glabrous or softly pubescent above while lower surface pubescent or glabrous; fruits borne in clusters on the main trunk and leafless short branches, subglobose or pyriform, 2. 5-5. 0 cm in diameter, red when ripe.

Phenology: Flowering: Spring; Fruiting: Rainy season. Distribution: Throughout India; Pakistan, Bangladesh, Sri Lanka. Ecology and cultivation: Tropical plant; grows on the banks of streams, sides of ravines, on rocky slopes, up to 1500 m; wild.

Chemical contents: Bark: ceryl behenati gluanol-OAc, lupeol and its á-OAc, â-amyrin, â-sitosterol; Leaf: â-amyrin, â-sitosterol, gluanol-OAc; Fruit: lupeol-OAc, gluanol-OAc, glucose, hentriacontane, â-sitosterol, a sterol, ester of taraxasterol, tiglic acid.

Remarks: Some ethnic communities of Rajasthan use leaves as a galactogogue for cattle. Rural folks of Bengal, Bihar and Orissa use bark in treatment of domestic animals. Unripe fruits are eaten as a vegetable by most of the Indians, while ripe fruits are consumed by Bhoxas, Garhwalis, tribes of North-East India, hill people of Maharashtra, tribes of eastern Rajasthan, Kerala and Madhya Pradesh (Bastar).

Tribes of Chhindwara (Madhya Pradesh) use young stem as toothbrush. This tree is considered as a constituent of the sacred panchavata and as kalpataru by the Hindus. They keep a piece of stem of this plant, as a part of rite, in the labour room and also use the wood as samidh (sacrificial wood) in all yajnas. The wood is also used by the Hindus to make effigy if the corpse is lost or not available.

GMELINA ARBOREA ROXB. (VERBENACEAE)

Syn : Premna arborea Roth

English names: Cashmeri tree, Coomb teak, Malay bush beech, White teak.

Sa ns kr it n a m e s : As hvet a , B a h dr a p a r ni , Ga mb ha ri , Ga nd ha ri , Kakodumbari, Kassmari, Katphala, Nandivriksha, Sharubhadra, Shriparni, Subhadra, Vataha, Vidarini.

Vernacular names: Asm : Gomari; Ben: Gamar, Gamari, Gambar; Guj : Shewan; Hin: Gamari, Gambhari, Jugani chukur, Khambheri; Kan : Kashmirimara, Kumbalamara, Shivani; Lcd: Kashmar daru; Mal: Kambil,

Kumil, Kumilu, Kumpil; Mar: Shewan; Mun : Kasambar daru, Kasmar daru; Orn : Gambhair; Ori : Bhodroparni, Gambari; Pun: Gumhar; Sad: Gambhair; San: Kashmar daru; Tam: Gumudu-taku, Kattanam, Kumadi, Kumala maram, Perumkumbil, Umithekku; Tel: Gumar-tek, Gummadi.

Trade names: Gamar, Gamari, Gumhar.

Traditional use: MIKIR: Root: as blood purifier, Leaf: as carminative; BIRHORE : Leaf: in headache; SANTAL : in anasarca, asthma, bronchitis, cholera, colic pain, diarrhoea, dropsy, dyspepsia, epilepsy, fever, phthisis, rheumatism, small pox, sore, spleen complaints, syphilis, throat swelling, urticaria, as antidote to snake bite and some other poisons; MUNDA : Bark: to cure wounds; SORA (Orissa) : Root: in catarrh of bladder; Decoction of root: as tonic; Bark: in stomach disorder; ETHNIC COMMUNITIES OF ARAKU

VALLEY (Andhra Pradesh) : Root: in malarial fever; ETHNIC COMMUNITIES OF GODAVARI (Andhra Pradesh) : Bark-paste: on bone fracture, Leaf: in cough, gonorrhoea; ETHNIC COMMUNITIES OF DEHRA DUN (Uttar Pradesh) : Leaf-paste: on wounds.

ATHARVAVEDA : blood purifier; CHARAKA SAMHITA : useful in vomiting, dropsy and in burning sensation of the body; SUSHRUTA SAMHITA : energiser like grape, can be used as substitute of sweet date palm; BHAVAPRAKASHA : it is bitter, appetiser, brain tonic, energiser, digestive, subdues vata and kapha, removes dropsy, alleviates thirst, useful in colic pain, burning sensation of body, fever, urinary complaints, wastahge; RAJANIGHANTU : it is pungent, bitter, heavy (guru), thermogenic, removes oedema, phlegm, tridosha, burning sensation, fever, thirst, poisons; DHANVANTARINIGHANTU : bitter, thermogenic, removes bleeding tendency, tridosha, fatigue, burning sensation of body, fever, thirst; KAIYAOEVANIGHANTU : it is sweet, bitter, thermogenic, heavy, appetiser, digestive, brain tonic, removes dropsy, giddiness, colic pain, toxins, burning sensation of body, fever, alleviates thirst; flowers sweet, cooling, bitter, astringent, beneficial for the diseases caused by pitta and kapha; fruits unctuous, heavy, cooling, astringent, brain tonic, cardiotonic, removes giddiness, acidity, urinary troubles, burning sensation of body, wounds, wastage and troubles caused by vata; RAJAVALLABHAM: fruits seizing, bitter, sweet, heavy, cooling, good for hair, brain, removes burning sensation of body and diseases caused by pitta; roots are too hot; NIGHANTU RATNAKARAM: it is pungent, bitter, hot, astringent, heavy, sweet, appetiser, digestive, brain tonic, cardiotonic, removes thirst, colic pain, oedema, phlegm, toxins, burning sensation of body, fever, impurities of blood, piles, giddiness; fruits aphrodisiac, heavy, increases semen, cooling, unctuous, increases intelligence, removes urinary troubles, impurities of blood, thirst, burning sensation of body, good for urticaria, consumption, wounds, leucorrhoea.

AYURVEDA : Root: acrid, bitter, anthelmintic, galactogogue, laxative, stomachic, tonic, useful in burning sensation, dyspepsia, fever, haemorrhoids, hallucination, hyperdisia and stomachalgia; Bark: bitter, tonic, stomachic, useful in dyspepsia, fever; Leaf-paste: useful in cephalalgia, Leaf-extract: good wash for foul ulcer; Flower: acrid, astringent, bitter, refrigerant, sweet, useful in skin diseases including leprosy; Fruits: acrid, alterant, aphrodisiac, astringent, bitter, diuretic, refrigerant, sour, sweet, tonic, trichogenous, useful in anaemia, blood dysentery, constipation, leprosy, leucorrhoea, malnutrition of child and embryo, strangury and wounds.

Modern use: 50% EtOH extract of bark (and also of stem) : antiviral, hypoglycaemic. Phytography : Unarmed deciduous tree, 15-20 m in height; stem-bark whitish grey, lenticellate, young branches covered with fine white soft hairs; leaves. opposite, simple, petioles ±7. 5 cm long, lamina broadly ovate, usually 22. 5 by 15. 0 cm, more or less acuminate, glabrous above but stellately hairy beneath; panicles terminal, often 30 cm long, many-flowered;

flowers bucciniform, brownish yellow, ±3. 7 cm long, tomentose at least when young; drupes ±1. 8 cm 1000g, fleshy, ovoid, orange-yellow when ripe; seeds hard, oblong.

Phenology: Flowering: January-April; Fruiting: May-June. Distribution: Throughout India; Bangladesh (Chittagong), Sri Lanka. Ecology and cultivation: Grows in moist deciduous forests; wild.

Ch em ic a l c on te nt s: Ro ot : c er yl a lc oh o l, g me lo fu ra n , gm el in ol , hentriacontanol-I, n-octacosanol, â-sitosterol, sesquiterpene; Stem: arboreok, bromoisoarboreol, cluytyl ferulate, gmelanone, gmelinol, gummidiol, lignans, lignan hemiacetal, n-hentriacontanol-I, n-octacosanol, â-sitosterol; Leaf: apigenin, hentriacontanol, luteoHn, quercetin, quercetogenin, â-sitosterol.

Remarks: Ethnic communities of India use the plant in the treatment of rinderpest of cattle. In Sri Lanka, it is used in skeletal fracture. It is one of the best and most reliable timber-yielding trees of India. The plant is a fast grower.

GLORIOSA SUPERBA L. (LILIACEAE)

Syn : Methonica superba Lamk., Gloriosa simplex Don.

English names: Malabar glory lily, Glory lily.

Sanskrit names: Agninukhi, Agnisikha, Ailni, Garbhaghatini, Kalikari, Lanyli, Vishalya.

Vernacular names: Asm : Utatchandal; Ben: Bishalanguli, Ulatchandal; Guj : Dudhiovachnay, Varhvareli; Hin : Kalihari, Kaliari, Kulhari, Languli; Kan : Agnisikha, Akkatangaballi, Karadikanninagadde, Kolikuttuma, Sivasaktiballi, Mal: Kantal, Medoni, Mattamara, Mettonsi, Mentonni; Mar: Bachnag, Indai, Kariannag, Khadyanag, Nagharia, Nag karia; Mun : Bulung chukuru; Orn : Jhagrahi; Ori : Agnisikha, Garbhhoghhatono panjanyulia, Meherlaphulo, Panchaangula; Pun: Kariari, Mulim; Sad: Jhagar; San: Siricsamano; Tam: Akkinichilam, Kalappaikkilanku, Kalaippaikkishangu, Kannuvalikkodi, Nabhikkodi, Tel: Adabhinabhi, Agnisikha, Gangeri, Kalappagadda.

Traditional use: ETHNIC COMMUNITIES OF NORTH-EAST INDIA: Root: in gout, stomachache and as tonic; MUNDA AND ORAON: Tuber: for antifertility purpose; SANTAL : (i) Tuberous root: for abortion purpose, in intermittent fevers, wounds; (ii) Plant: in spleen complaints, syphilis, tumours; (ii) Leaf: in asthma; ETHNIC COMMUNITIES OF BIHAR: Root: in cholera, to facilitate childbirth; ETHNIC COMMUNITIES OF ORISSA: Tuber : as a b or ti fa ci en t; T RI BE S OF VAR AN AS I : Ro ot : in g ou t; TR IB ES O F PITHORAGARH: Tuber: in gonorrhoea, leprosy, piles; ETHNIC COMMUNITIES OF D EH RA D UN A ND S IWAL IK : Ro ot : a s a nt he lm in ti c; E TH NI C COMMUNITIES OF GARHWAL : Tuberous root: for abortion;

CHARAKA SAMHITA : useful in itching, skin diseases including wounds and ailments caused by vitiated kapha (phlegm) and vata (wind); SUSHRUTA SAMHITA: can be administered to a delivered mother along with spirituous drink to give relieve to her postnatal complaints, roots are poisonous; RAJANIGHANTU: it is pungent, thermogenic, eliminates deranged kapha (phlegm) and vata (wind), terminates pregnancy; DHANVANTARI NIGHANTU: in addition to the above, it is also useful in dropsy, labour pain, wounds, and as a purgative; MADANADI NIGHANTU : it is bitter, pungent, thermogenic, abortifacient, removes abdominal pain, expels the placenta, cures phlegm, skin diseases; BHAVAPRAKASHA : it is apperient, alkaline, astringent, pungent, bitter, highly potent, light, abortifacient, helps storing up energy, excites pitta (bile), it cures dropsy, piles, wounds, acute spasmodic pain, and removes worms; CHAKRADATTA : Root-paste: if smeared over ' the palms and feet of a pregnant woman, delivery of child becomes easier.

AYURVEDA : (i) roots are abortifacient, acrid, alexiteric, anthelmintic, antipyretic, bitter, depurative, digestive, emetic, expectorant, gastrointestinal irritant, highly poisonous, purgative, rejuvenating, stomachic, thermogenic, tonic, beneficial in vitiated conditions of kapha (phlegm) and vata (wind), debility, dyspepsia, flatulence, haemorrhoids, helminthiasis, inflammations, in promoting labour pain and expulsion of the placenta; (ii) root-paste is effective against paralysis, rheumatism, snake bite, insect bites; (iii) leaf-juice effective against lice.

Modern use: Root (aq. extract) : ecbolic in humans and other animals; Plant (50% EtOH extract) : spasmolytic, Central Nervous System depressant; Leaf-juice: piscicide. Phytography : Herbaceous tendril climber; rootstock tuberous, naked; stem 3-6 m long, sparingly branched; leaves sessile or nearly so, opposite or 3-nately whorled, tip tendrillar; flowers axillary, solitary, nearly 10 cm, at first greenish, becoming yellow and finally scarlet or red; capsules nearly 5 cm long.

Phenology: Flowering: October; Fruiting: throughout the year.

Distribution: Throughout tropical India ascending up to 2000 m on the hills; Indo-China, Malaysia.

Ecology and cultivation: Plains from the coast on thickets; wild.

Chemical contents: Root: colchicine, b-sitosterol and its glucoside, band t-Iumicolchicine, 2-0H-6-MeO benzoic acid; Young leaf: cholidonic acid; Flower: luterlin and its glucosides, N-formyl-de-Ac-colchicine, lumicolchicine; Seed: colchicine.

Remarks: It is getting less attention in India, though extensive researches are on abroad.

GYMNEMA SYLVESTRE R. BR. EX SCHULT (ASCLEPIADACEAE)

Syn : Periploca sylvestris Willd., Gymnema melicida Edgew.

English names: Vine, Periploca of the the woods.

Sanskrit names: Ajaballi, Ajagandini, Ajashringi, Bahalchakshu, Chakshurabahala, Grihadruma, Karnika, Kshinavartta, Madhunasini, Medhasingi, Meshashringi, Meshavishanika, Netaushadhi, Putrashringi, Sarpadanshtrika, Tiktadughdha, Vishani.

Vernacular names: Ben: Meshashringi; Guj : Dhuleti, Mardashing; Hin : Gurmar, Gumar, Merashinghi; Kan : Karhasige, Sannagera-shehumbr; Mal:

Cakkarakkolli, Madhunashini; Mar: Kavali, Kalikardor, Vakundi; Tam: Adigam,

Cheorukurinja, Kannuminayamkodi, Pasaani, Sakkaraikkolli, Shirukurinja,

Sirukurumkay; Tel: Podapatra.

Trade names: Gurmar, Merasingi.

Traditional use: KOL : Leaf: in gastric troubles; ETHNIC COMMUNITIES OF RAJASTHAN and DHASAN VALLEY: Leaf: in dia betes; ETHNIC COMMUNITIES OF KANDALA (Maharashtra) : Leaf: in urinary complaints; GOND: Leaf: in diabetes, stomachache; ETHNIC COMMUNITIES OF MADHYA PRADESH: Leaf: in cornea opacity and other eye diseases; ETHNIC COMMUNITIES OF GODAVARI DISTRICT (Andhra Pradesh) : Leaf: in diabetes, glycosuria; IRULAR : Leaf: in diabetes; CHARAKA SAMHITA: removes bad odour from breast milk, aperitive; SUSHRUTA SAMHITA : plant useful as purgative, in eye troubles; leaf extract and also the same of flower beneficial for eyes; bark useful in the diseases caused by vitiated kapha (phlegm); BAGBHAT: rootbark useful in piles; BHAVAPRAKASHA: it is bitter, appetiser, gastric stimulant, removes cough, alleviates breathing troubles, useful in curing phlegm, eyetroubles, wounds; RAJA NIGHANTU : appetiser, removes phlegm, piles, colic pain, cures dropsy, useful in eye troubles, cardiotonic, beneficial in respiratory diseases, wounds, detoxicant; fruits are bitter, sialagogue, thermogenic, cures the diseases caused by vitiated kapha (phlegm) or vata (wind); NIGHANTU RATNAKARAM : removes cough, vitiated wind, detoxicant, appetiser, useful in eye troubles. AYURVEDA : acrid, alexipharmic, anodyne, anthelmintic, antipyretic, astringent, bitter, cardiotonic, digestive, diuretic, emetic, expectorant, laxative, stimulant, stomachic, uterine tonic; useful in amennorrhoea, asthma, bronchitis, cardiopathy, conjunctivitis, con stip a tio n, c ough , dys peps ia , ha em orro ids, hepa tosp leno mega ly, inflammations, intermittant fever, jaundice and leucoderma; root emetic and removes phlegm; external application is useful in insectbite; SIDDHA : an ingredient of 'Cirukuricinver '; UNANI : an ingredient of 'Gurmarbuti'.

The fresh leaves, when chewed, paralyse the sense of sweet for sometime; for this reason it is called gur-mar, thereby meaning sugar-killer and impression has become prevalent in some parts of the country that it is useful in diabetes mellitus. Chewing fresh leaves also paralyse the taste of bitter for a while.

Modern use: Aerial parts (50% EtOH extract) : spasmolytic, hypyoglycaemic, in vitro antiviral against influenza A2 virus.

Phytography : Stout, woody, large climber; young branches slender and pubescent; leaves opposite, simple, petioles 0. 6-1. 2 cm, stout or slender, lamina 2. 5-6. 25 cm in length, elliptic or ovate, thinly coriaceous, upper surface rarely pubescent; cymes subglobose, ± 1. 25 cm in diameter; flowers yellow, ±0. 2 cm in diameter; follicles slender, ±5-7. 5 by 0. 8 cm; seeds pale brown, flat, ±1. 25 cm long.

Phenology: Flowering: August-March; Fruiting: Winter.

Distribution: Mainly in Deccan peninsula, also found in Madhya Pradesh, Maharashtra, Rajasthan; Sri Lanka.

Ecology and Cultivation: Grows in the plains from the coast, in scrub jungles and in thickets; wild.

Chemical contents: Leaf: conduritol A, gymnestrogenin, gymnamine, hentriacontane, nonacosane, penta-OH-triterpene.

Remark: In Sri Lanka, plant used in bone fractures.

GINKGO BILOBA L. (GINKGOACEAE)

English name: Maiden hair tree. Vernacular name: Hin : Balkuwari. Trade name: Ginkgo.

Traditional use: Seeds: expectorant and sedative.

Modern use: Tanakan (active principle of plant extract) : effective in induced cerebral ischemia in rats; Tebonin (a preparation containing leaf extract) : used in cardiovascular disorders, increased cerebral blood circulation, Parkinson's disease; Nut (extract) : antibacterial against Mycobacterium smegmatis. memory and boosts oxygen level in brain. It regulates neurotransmitters, increases blood flow and metabolism. It reduces migraine and vertigo. It may be useful in mental disorders, including Alzheimer 's disease. Recently a pill containing extracts from Ginkgo has been launched for eliminating excess fat (cellulite) in women.

Phytography : Tree with pyramidal form, reaching a height of 30 m; leaves petiolar, lamina fan-shaped, bilobed; dioecious; mature seeds orange-coloured and are about the size of an apricot.

Phenology: Flowering and Fruiting: Summer.

Distribution: Darjeeling (West Bengal).

Ecology and cultivation: Native of China, cultivated in Indian gardens, particularly on hills.

Chemical contents: Root-bark: Ginkgolides A, B, C & M; Plant: bilobalide, biloba none sesquiterpene; Leaf: fla vonols, bifla vonoids, diterpenes, sesquiterpene bilobalide A, â-sitosterol, ginkgolides A, B & C, shikimic acid, sequoyitol, 1, 5-MeO-bilobetin; Fruit: anacardic acids, ginnol, bilobols, cardanols.

Remarks: Chinese consume Ginkgo seeds. Endosperm of roasted seed is edible and kernel is highly nutritious. It is believed that regular consumption of Ginkgo preparation staves of ravages of age and checks senility. Ginkgo is a contemporary of dinosaurs of the Jurassic period. Because of its primitive characters, it is known as living fossil. It is a native of Chekiang in East China. It is grown by the Buddhist monasteries of China and Japan as a sacred tree. The plant was introduced into Europe in early 18th Century and later in America. Only a few trees occur in India. Perhaps it does not exist in the wild today. Because of its nutritional and medicinal properties, it is receiving increased attention. Commercial cultivation of this species should be endeavoured in

India. If appropriate measures for conservation of this important medicinal species are not taken, it is destined to be extinct in the near future.

GARCINIA XANTHOCHYMUS HOOK. F. EX T. ANDERS (CLUSIACEAE)

Syn : Xanthochymus tinctorius DC., Garcinia tinctoria Dunn.

English name: Egg tree.

Sanskrit names: Tamala, Tapinjha.

Vernacular names: Ben: Tamal, Chalta; Hin : Dampel, Tamal, Tumul; Guj : Kasamala, Ota; Kan:Deva-garige; Mal: Anavaya; Man: Heilbung; Mar: Jharambi, Dampel, Ota; Nep : Chunyel; Ori : Cheoro, Sitambu;

Tam: Kulavi, Malaippachai, Mukki, Tamalam; Tel: Sitakamraku, Evarumidi,

Tamalamu.

Trade name: Tamala.

Traditional use: Fruit: antiscorbutic, cooling, digestive, emollient, demulcent and cholagogue. Sherbet made from dried fruit is used in billiousness.

AYURVEOA : Young branch: paste as ointment on boils; Bark: astringent;

Leaf: decoction useful in diarrhoea; Young leaves (roasted in a special method) : used in dysentery; Seed: butter made from seeds useful in pulmonary affections, dysentery, goitre.

Modern use: Xanthochymol : antibacterial against Streptococcus faecallis and Klebsiella pneumoniae.

Phytography : Evergreen tree, trunk straight; branches arising in tiers, drooping, angular; leaves opposite, coriaceous, bright green, shining, 22. 5-45.0 cm by 5-10 cm; flowers polygamous, male flowers from axils of fallen leaves, fascicled with 4-8 flowers, white, thick, rough, hermaphrodites like male flowers, ovary ovoid, usually 5:chambered; fruits subglobose, pointed, dark yellow; seeds 1-4, oblong, yields a large quantity of gamboge.

Phenology: Flowering: Spring; Fruiting: Summer.

Distribution: Native to India and Myanmar; distributed widely in the lower hill forests of eastern Himalaya, Meghalaya, Sikkim, West Bengal, Maharashtra, Gujarat, Tamil Nadu, Kerala, Andhra Pradesh, the Andamans; Bangladesh, Myanmar.

Ecology and cultivation: Tropical forest; wild.

Chemical contents: Fruit: xanthochymol, isoxanthochymol, maclurin, e ux a n th on e, 1 , 5 - di hy dr ox y- a n d 1 , 3 , 5 - tr ih yd ro xy -x a n th on es , methoxyxanthones, cambogin, volkensiflavone, morello-flavone, biflavones.

Remark: In South India, fruits of this species are used in lieu of tamarind.

HOLARRHENA PUBESCENCE (BUCH. -HAM.) WALL EX DC. (APOCYNACEAE)

Syn : Holarrhena antidysenterica (L.) Wall., Echites pubescens Buch. -Ham.

English names: Bitter oleander, Conessi bark, Dysentery rosebay, Easter tree, Ivory tree, Tellichery bark.

Sanskrit names: Girimallika, Indrayava, Kalinga(ka), Kalingyava, Katuka, Katuja, Mahagandha, Mallikapushpa, Panduradruama, Pravrishya, Sangrahi, Shakrapadapa, Vatsika, Vrikshaka, Yavaphala.

Vernacular names: Asm : Dhurkhuri, Ducikhuri; Ben: Kurchi, Katuraj, Kuteswar, Indrajava; Guj : Dhowda, Kuda, Kari; Hin : Kurchi, Karchi, Karra; Kan : Beppale coodsaloo, Korchie; Lep : Fajeerip; Mal: Kodagapala; Mar: Kura, Kala-kura, Kear, Kewar, Kodago, Kuda, Dola-kuda, Pandhrakura; 'Mun :: Koraia; Pun: Kawar, Kura, Kear, Kewar; Sad: Koraia; San: Hat; Tam: Kuda-sappalai, Veppalei, Kodagapalei, Indrabam; Tel: Kodisepala, Palakodsa, Pala, Kodaga.

Trade name: Kurchi.

Traditional use: MANIPURI : Bark (boiled extract) : in diarrhoea, dysentery; GARO : Bark and Leaf: in dysentery; ETHNIC COMMUNITIES AROUND GUAHATI: Seed: as anthelmintic; BODO (of Assam) : Bark: in diarrhoea, dysentery, piles; Flower: as appetiser and in intestinal worms; Seed.. in leprosy; ASUR (of Bihar) : Bark: in snake bite; Seed: diarrhoea, fever, intestinal worms; MUNDA : Root and Leaf: in diarrhoea, bleeding from nose, haemorrhage after childbirth; SANTAL : Root: in bite of dog or jackal, blood a n d mu co us i n bo we l ex cr et io n, d ia rr ho ea , dy se nt er y, h em a t ur ia , spermatorrhoea, spleen complaints; Bark.. in bronchitis, chameleon's bite, cholera, cold, colic, fever, menorrhagia; Fruit: in anaemia, colic, constip5ltion, diarrhoea, dry cough, epilepsy, gravel, postnatal complaints, stomachache; TRIBAL SOCIETIES OF HAZARIBAGH AND RANCHI : Bark: in gastric disorder, to revive taste in tongue; ETHNIC COMMUNITIES OF ORISSA: Latex: in eczema and other skin diseases; ETHNIC COMMUNITIES OF ABUJH- MARH (Madhya Pradesh) : Bark: in menstrual complaints; TRIBAL COMMUNITIES OF SAGAR (Madhya Pradesh) : Seed: in dysentery; THARU (of Uttar Pradesh) : Bark: in fever; Bark and Seed (together) : in dysentery; KO L (o f Ut ta r P r a d es h) : S ee d: i n di ge st ive co mp la in ts ; ET H NI C COMMUNITIES OF DEHRA DUN AND SIWALIK: Seed: in diarrhoea, dysentery, fever; ETHNIC COMMUNITIES OF EAST RAJASTHAN: Bark and Seed (together) : in dysentery; ETHNIC COMMUNITIES OF MOUNT ABU: Bark: as antidote to snake bite; DANG: (of Gujarat) : Bark: in diarrhoea; VASAVA (of Gujarat) : Root: in fever; Root and Bark (together) : in gout; ETHNIC COMMUNITIES OF SAURASHTRA: Bark: in bronchitis; ETHNIC COMMUNITIES OF DAHANU FOREST DIVISION (Maharashtra) : Bark and Leaf (together) : in dysentery; Latex: as antidote to snake bite, Seed: in asthma, colic.

ATHARVAVEDA : increases semen, tightens the slackened muscles; CHARAKA SAMHITA : Bark (paste) : good for skin diseases, leprosy, ringworm, piles, fistula, adenitis; Fruit: in vomiting, beneficial in disorders caused by vitiated phlegm and bile, as galactagogue; Seed: in piles; SUSHRUTA SAMHITA: Flower: beneficial in deranged phlegm and bile, and a good remedy for leprosy; CHAKRADATTA: Bark: in diarrhoea; BHAVAPRAKASHA:

pungent, drying, refrigerant, excitant, cures piles, diarrhoea, phlegm, bile, leprosy, alleviates thirst; RAJANIGHANTU : pungent, bitter, thermogenic, astringent, c ur es d ia rr ho ea , vi ti a t ed b il e, s ki n di se a s es a nd p il es ;

DHANVANTARINIGHANTU:pungent,bitter,astringent,drying,cooling, cures skin diseases, gastroenteritis, vitiated bile; MADANANIGHANTU : excitant, digestive, astringent, beneficial in bleeding tendency, worms, skin diseases; SALIGRAMNIGHANTU : appetising, beneficial in vitiated phlegm, cures diarrhoea, skin diseases, worms; KAIYADEVANIGHANTU : astringent, cooling, drying, excitant, pungent, beneficial in vitiated phlegm, bile, skin diseases, diarrhoea, piles; Flower: refrigerant, bitter, astringent, excitant.

AYURVEDA: Bark and Seed: acrid, anthelmintic, antiperiodic, aphrodisiac, astringent, bitter, carminative, expectorant, febrifuge, stimulating, beneficial in asthma, bronchitis! blood dysentery, diarrhoea, dropsy, dysentery, fever, haemorrhages, haemorrhoides, hepatopathy, malaria, piles, rheumatism, skin diseases, urinary troubles, verminosis, vomiting; Leaf: useful in boils, bronchitis, dysentery and wounds.

SIDDHA: Root and Bark: used as constituents for the preparation of Kutacap patai.

UNANI : in the preparation of Sufuf Habis and Majnum Bawasir.

Modern use: Bark (50% EtOH extract) : hypotensive; Bark-powder: in abdominal and glandular tumours; Fruit (50% EtOH extract) : anticancer, anti protozoa, hypoglycaemic, astringent, febrifuge, useful in diarrhoea, intestinal worms, and to regulate menstruation.

Phytography : Deciduous tree or large shrub; leaves sessile or subsessile, broadly ovate to elliptic-oblong, abruptly acuminate, often unequal, rounded or obtuse at base, lateral nerves 10-15 pairs, arching near the margin; flowers white, bracts small, follicles 20-42 by 0. 8-1. 2 cm; seeds up to 1 cm long, linear-oblong, coma about twice as long as seeds, seeds brown.

Phenology: Flowering and Fruiting: May-January.

Distribution: Major parts of India up to 1500 m in the Himalaya; Bangladesh, also in Africa-mostly in drier regions.

Ecology and cultivation: Common in village surroundings; sometimes in private gardens. Chemical contents: Root-bark: holacetine; Stem-bark: L-quebrachitol, dihydroisoconessimine, kurcholessine, 3-a-aminoconan-5-ene,

7 -a-OH-conessine, holonamine; Lea f: a minoglycosteroids, aminode-oxyglycosteroids, kurchiphylline, kurchiphyllamine, kurchaline, holadysine, holadysamine, holantosines A, B, C & D, holarosine A, B, E & F.

Remarks: Tribals of East Rajasthan give root to cattle in a disease in which tongue ejects out and gets swollen. Tribals of Maharashtra eat flower and seed as vegetables. Ethnic communities of Ratan Mahal Hills use latex to curdle milk. Santal women use flowers to decorate their hairdos. Tribals of Madhya Pradesh use wood to make combs and many household articles.

❐

Cultivating Medicinal and Aromatic Plants

INTRODUCTION

Humanity has created a situation where we can truly say that our Earth is ill. There is not a single place on this planet, apart from a few very remote areas which have not been contaminated with chemical pesticides, or even with fertilisers. This condition a serious affair and has come about only in the last fifty years. Chemical supplied by the industry, and, used in agriculture, have been a result of War. Most of the fertilisers-especially the urea fertilisers-were developed during War time as explosives. Since that time, they have been used extensively in agriculture. In fact, the whole agriculture of this century has drawn upon natural reserves of humus and soil, which have been accumulated by Nature through many decades of natural vegetation growths.

Having produced those chemicals, and we know very little about their consequent effects on the environment. Chemical fertilisers are very soluble salts, which change the nature of the soil, waters, and substantially alter the ecology of the plants.

Using chemical fertilisers is similar to a non-nutritious human diet. Can plant nutrition be reduced to only a couple of minerals?

Fertiliser-based methods that reduce plant nutrition to a set of minerals imply that one can disconnect the health of a plant from its surrounding ecology, including insect pests. This approach is one that treats illnesses according to symptoms and not the cause. In this way it is similar to the modern allopathic method of treatment.

Many modern medicines are based on symptomatic treatment. The same mode of thinking has been applied in agriculture: there is a pest and the pest has to be killed, no matter what happens around it. It is not realised, that often the pest has its origin in the malnutrition of the soil. Improving the quality of the soil leads to stronger, healthier plants which in turn are more disease and pest resistant. This fact suggests that if plants were healthier, pesticides would not be necessary.

The earth is a living body. Whatever we do at this part of the planet has consequences at another. Even the people living in the Arctic have been tested positive for traces of chlorides and DDT in their bodies, although there is no farming in those remote regions of the planet. Why? Somebody in Africa is spraying DDT on his cotton crops. The rains wash the pesticidine into the river which in turn carries it into the ocean. Oceans are the circulation body of the earth; all their currents reach to every corner of the globe including the poles... and the circle continues.

We need to change the way of farming, not only of medicinal plants but also of our food, fruits and grains. Biodynamics recognises that soil itself can be alive. If we enrich the soil with life-sustaining properties the plants will carry those life forces. That, in turn, will give us life as well. Therefore, one of Biodynamics fundamental efforts is to build up stable humus in our soil through composting.

In South India, we have introduced these agricultural principles in an area of about 7000 acres. Also tea is cultivated organically. Likewise, we have taken up this method in some of the Darjeeling tea gardens.

Origin of Biodynamic Agriculture

The biodynamic system was developed in the 1920s in Europe. It draws extensively on traditional agricultural knowledge and wisdom which was present in the traditional farming communities. Rudolf Steiner (1861-1925), an Austrian philosopher, scientist, artist, educator, and the founder of antroposophy, developed this agricultural system. Biodynamic cultivation has developed into a world-wide movement since 1922.

The products from this type of agriculture are identified in the market with the Demeter symbol. On seeing this symbol affixed to a packet of carrots the consumer in Europe, the United States, Australia or New Zealand, knows this product was cultivated according to this biodynamic practice, an agricultural system which aims at quality.

Informed consumers in the industrialised countries have now realised the importance of organic and biodynamic food, and are willing to pay a premium price for food that is 100% free from any pesticides.

MEDICINAL PLANTS

India is endowed with a rich wealth of medicinal plants. These plants have made a good contribution to the development of ancient Indian materia medica. One of the earliest treatises on Indian medicine, the Charak Samhita(1000 B. C), records the use of over 340 drugs of vegetable origin. Most of these continue to be gathered from wild plants to meet the demand of the medical profession. Thus, despite the rich heritage of knowledge on the use of plant drugs, little attention had been paid to grow them as field crops in the country till the latter part of the nineteenth century.

During the past seven or eight decades, there has been a rapid extension of the allopathic system of medical treatment in India. It generated a commercial demand for pharmacopoeial drugs and products in the country, Thus efforts were made to introduce many of these drug plants into Indian agriculture, and studies on the cultivation practices were undertaken for those plant which were found suitable and remunerative for commerical cultivation. In general, agronomic practices for growing poppy, isabgol, senna, cinchona, ipecac, belladonna, ergot and a few others have been developed and there is now localized cultivation of these medicinal plants commercially. The average annual foreign trade in crude drugs and their phytochemicals is between 60 and 80 million rupees and this accounts for a little over 0. 5 per cent of the world trade in these commodities.

The curative properties of drugs are due to the presence of complex chemical substances of varied composition (present as secondary plant metabolites) in one or more parts of these plants. These plant metabolites in one, according to their composition, are grouped as alkaloids, glycosides, corticosteroids, essential oils, etc. The alkaloids form the largest group, which includes morphine and codein (poppy), strychnine and brucine (nux vomica), q ui ni ne (ci nc ho na), e rg ot a m in e(er go t) , hy po cya m in e, (be el a d on a) , scolapomine(datura), emetine(ipecac), cocaine(coco), ephedrine(ephedra), reserpine(Rauwolfia), caffeine(tea dust), aconitine(aconite), vascine(vasaca). santonin(Aremisia), lobelin(Lobelia) and a large number of others. Glycosides for man of her important group represented by dig ox in (f ox gl ove) , stropanthin(strophanthus), glycyrrhizin(liquorice), barbolin (aloe), sennocides (senna), etc. Corticosteroids have come into prominence recently and diosgenin(Dioscorea), solasodin(Solanum sp.), etc. now command a large world demand. Some essential oils such as those of valerian kutch and peppermint also possess medicating properties and are used in pharmaceutical industry. However, it should be stated in all fairness that our knowledge of the genetic and physiological make-up of most of the medicinal plants is poor and we know still less about the biosynthetic pathways leading to the formation of active constituents for which these crops are valued.

During the last two decades, the pharmaceutical industry has made massive investments on pharmacological, clinical and chemical researches all over the world in an effort to discover and still more potent plant drugs; infact, a few new drug plant have successfully passed the tests of commercial screening. However, benefits of this labour would reach the masses when the corresponding support for agricultural studies for commercial cultivation is provided. Infact, agricultural studies on medicinal plants, by its very nature, demand an equally large investment and higher priority. India, in particular, has a big scope for the development of the pharmaceutical and phytochemical industry.

The Indian Pharmacopoeia (1966) recognizes eighty five drug plants whose ingredients are used in various pharmaceutical preparations. We shall, however, confine our treatment to a few important commercially grown medicinal plants whose cultivation deserves priority in out national economy.

CINCHONA (cinchona ledgeriana Linn. and allied spp.). Sixty-five species distributed in the Andes at elevations of 800 to 2, 800 m, occur mainly in Peru, Bolivia, Columbia and Ecuador. Commercial supplies of the bank are obtained from C. ledgeriana, c. officinalis, C. calisaya, C. succirubra and their numerous hybrids. The cinchona bark yields quinine which is used as a treatment against malaria. Quinine salts are now increasingly used in soft drinks as bittters and quinidine sulphate is use in the treatment of heart troubles, such as auricular fibrillation and venticular trachycardia. Cinchona plantations cover about 1, 600 ha in the Nilgiris and the Annamalais Hills (Tamil Nadu). India, Indonesia and Zaire (the Congo) are major suppliers of quinine products to the world market; the Indian export of quinine salts earns about Rs 10 million annually.

C. ledgerianna Moens is a small tree grown at elevations between 1, 000 and 1, 900 m, mainly in West Bengal. The average total alkaloid content in the root, stem and branch (of plants 10-12 years old) is 7. 21, 6. 01 and 4. 0 per cent of which the quinine content is 5, 4 and 1. 98 per cent respectively. Under less favourable conditions, a hybrid (ledgerianna X succirubra) is preferred; the hybrid has a lower quinine content, but it produces a more robust tree, growth. C. officinalie Linn. is a weak straggling tree, about 6m high. It grows at altitudes ranging from 2, 000-2, 600 m mainly in the Nilgris. The root, stem and branch contain 1. 75-4. 16, 2. 56-4. 42 and 1. 44-2. 35 per cent of quinine respectively. A hybrid, called robusta (officinalisX succirubra) is a hardy type and, as such, is adapted to a wider range of elevations (1, 2000-3, 000 m) and temperatures; another hybrid (officinalisX ledgeriana) is grown in Mungpoo (Darjeeling District).

C. calisaya Wedd. is a large tree which is not suitable for growing under excessive cold and humid conditions, is grown at lower altitudes of 400 to 1, 000 m in the Moyar Valley (Nilgiris). The total alkaloids in the stem bark range from 3. 89 to 7. 24 per cent, of which quinine and cinchonidine are 0.78 to 5. 57 and 0. 03 to 1. 56 per cent respectively.

C. succirubra Pavon is a hardy tree which grows between elevations of 1, 200 and 2, 000 m in some parts of Annamalais and attain a heught of 18-20 meters. This species possess a remarkable ability to withstand both high humidity and drought. Its main alkaloid is cinchonidine. The total Alkolid in the root, stem and bark is 7. 6, 5. 5 and 3. 3 per cent respectively. Out of these amounts, quinine constitutes 0. 76-1. 42, 1. 1-1. 74 and 0. 8-1. 76 per cent respectively in the root, stem and bark. Cinchona prefers deep, well drained rich loamy to clayey loam, acidic soils (pH 4. 5-6) on sloping sheltered locations.

Most species prefer high humidity, a well-distributed rainfall of about 150 cms, and only minor variation in the maximum and minimum temperatures during their growing seasons. All species are susceptible to frost and succumb to water-logged conditions.

Cinchona is usually propagated through seeds. The seeds are small and light (350-400 seeds per gramme) and loose viability soon. About 50g of fresh seeds sown per square meter during February-May produce about 10, 000 seedlings in the nursery-beds, prepared with a mixture of leaf-mould and sand.

The nursery is provided with partial shade and kept moist and free from weeds. Germination takes 25 to 40 days to be completed and the seedlings grow 4 pairs of leaves in 4 to 6 months when they are transplanted in another nursery at 10 cm X 10 cm spacing. The seedling grow 30-50 cm high in the next 4 to 5 months and are planted in the field at a spacing of 2 m x 2m; the young-growing plants are provided with shade. The plantation is thinned when 4 to 6 years old and thus about 50 per cent of the stock is uprooted and debarked in two years. More bark is obtained in the 8th year by coppicing when only one strong stump is allowed to grow. The left-over trees are finally uprooted when 12-years old. The bark is moved by ringing the stem at a height of 60 cm from the ground and is dried in the open. The drying reduces its weight to 60-70 per cent.

In Indonesia, the vegetable propagation of selected clones has helped to maintain a high quinine content, thereby upgrading the average quinine content from 4 to 7. 5 per cent. Several methods of vegetative propagation, as patch and slit-budding, cincturing, layering and mould-layering, are recommended. Vegetative propagation is done during the monsoon, when root initials are produced in 40 to 60 days and the shoot is then cut off and planted.

The cinchona bark has 30 chemically related alkaloids, of which quinine (C20H24O2N2) is the most important. The alkaloids are formed during the descent of the sap and, therefore, its percentage is lowest in the twigs and it rises in the stem and is maximum in the root bark; the collar portion of about 30-45 cm in length is the richest portion. The percentage of total alkaloids increases till the age of 8 to 12 years and then begins to decline. Damping-off is reported both from nursery and fields, particularly at lower elevations.

The disease is controlled by fumigation with chloropicrin. Root-rot due to Fomeslamayensis (Murr.) Sacc. and Trott. has also been reported in nurseries; a better drainage of the nursery-beds and spraying with Bordeaux mixture help to prevent it.

ISABGOL (plantago ovata Forks.). It is an annual stemless herb, a native of Persia, now grows as a cash crop on about 16, 000 ha in the Mehsana, Palampur and Banaskantha districts of Northern Gujrat, India is the largest producer of isabgol and exports seed and huskworth Rs 25 million annually. The husk is the rosey-white membranous covering of the seed which constitutes the drug and is given as a safe laxative, particularly beneficial in habitual constipation, chronic diarrhoea and dysentery.

Isabogal is an irrigated rabi crop which remains in the field for about 4 months. The crop is grown in marginal, light, well-drained sandy-loam to loamy soils having pH between 7 to 8. It requires a cool climate and dry sunny weather or light showers cause seed shedding.

After harvesting the kharif crops, e.g. jowar (Sorghum vulgare), the land is brougt to fine tilth and laid out into beds of convenient size for irrigation. It is preferable to mix with the soil 15 cartloads of well-rotted farmyard mannure per hectare during the preparation of the land. The optimum sowing time is early November; sowing however, is extended till the end of December, but the delayed sowing decreases the yield. The seed rate is 7. 8 kg per hectare. Seeds are small and light about 6000 to a gramme and are sown by broadcast. They are covered thinly by raking the soil. A light irrigation is given immediately. Germination starts in 6 to 10 days and the crop is given the second irrigation after 3 weeks and a third one at the time of the formation of the spikes; thus the crop needs 6 to 7 irrigations.

Isabgol makes a moderate demand for nutrients. Usually, 25 kg of each N and P per hectare is given at plantation. The crop is given 1 or 2 hand- weedings during the entire growing period. The plants are about 50 cm high andeach plants gives out between 25 to 100 tillers, depending upon the fertility of soil and weather conditions. The plant bears the flowering spikes in about 60 days after sowing and matures in the next 2 months. The yellowing of the lower leaves is an indication of maturity, confirmed by pressing a spike between two figers when the mature seeds come out. The crop is harvested close to the ground in the early morning hours to avoid looses owing to seed shedding. The harvested material is stacked for 1 or 2 days, made to be trampled by bullocks, winnowed, and the separated seed crop is collected. A boldseeded crop fetches a better price. The husk, and about 30 per cent husk by weight is thus recovered. The husk contains a mucilaginous substance.

Powdery mildew sometimes attacks the crop and is brought under control by spraying the crop with wettable sulphur, e.g. 'Karathen' and 'Sulfex' two or three times at 15-day intervals after the appearance of infection. White grubs are reported to damage the roots; soil treatment with 5 per cent Aldrin or Lindane to protect the crop is given at the time of the last ploughing during the preparation of the field.

OPIUM POPPY (papaver somniferum Linn). Poppy is a native of the western Mediterranean region, introduced into India in the early sixteenth century. India produces about 70 per cent of the world's production and 90 per cent of it is exported annually. The crop can be grown under a licence issued by the Excise Department and, as such, its cultivation is restricted to about 24, 000 hectares in the districts of Neemuch, Mandsaur and Ratlam in Madhya Pradesh; in Faizabad, Bara Banki, Bareilly and Shahjahanpur in Uttar Pradesh, and in Chittoor, Jhalawar and Kota in Rajasthan.

Poppy is an annual erect plant, 60-120 cm in height, rarely branching, with ovate-oblong leaves; it bears large showy flowers and nearly globose to spherical capsules, containing small white or black kidney-shaped seeds. It is a rabi crop, and remains for about 150-160 days in the fields. It is mainly (90%)

self-pollinated, since the dehiscence of anthers takes place before the opening of the flower. A large number of the forms of variety album DC. are cultivated in India; it has ovate globose capsules devoid of apertures.

The crop is grown on well-drained, fertile, clayey loam to rich sandy- loam soils. It prefers moderately cool weather and open sunny locations; severely cold spells, frost dull cloudy weather, high winds, and heavy rainfall during the lancing period adversely affect the yield.

Land is prepared to a fine tilth up to a depth of 20-25 cm during September and the fields are laid out into beds of convenient size. Twenty-five to thirty- seven cartloads of farmyard manure is mixed with the soil during the preparation of the land, penning of sheep or goats is preferred. Seed-rate is 2.5 to 3.5 kg per hectare. The seeds are minute weighing 0. 25 to 3. 5 kg per 100. They are mixed with sand and sown thinly in rows 0.3m apart during mid-October till early November (optimum temperature 9-10 degree centigrade). The rows are covered with a thin layer of soil and are given a light irrigation, followed by another irrigation after 8-10 days when the seeds start germinating. Seed treatment with 1.0 % Agrosan protects it from seed-borne dieases. The crop is given about 15 irrigations in all, depending upon the texture of the soil and the variety sown; moisture defiency at the time of capsule formation affects the yield adversely. The crop needs a heavy nutrient supply and 50 kg N/ha is applied during the preparation of the land and another application of an equal quantity is given as top-dressing in two-split doses when the crop is one month old and at the time of the flag-leaf stage.

The seedlings are thinned out to 20-25 cm apart when they grow 5-7 cm tall. The crop is weeded and hoed weekly till the plants are about 20 cm tall and thereafter, weeding and hoeing are done once a month. The plants take 75-80 days (in Neemuch, Madhya Pradesh) and about 105 days(in Uttar Pradesh to comc into flower, depending upon the variety sown. The petals fall in 3-4 days and the growing capsule is ready for lancing in the next 6 to 10 days.

The green unripe capsules contain the maximum amount of morphine which diminishes with its ripening and yellowing; conversely, codeine and narcotine increases with age.

Lancing is done longitudinally in bright sunlight and the latex (crude opium) which oozes from the wounds dries during the following night and is scrapped with a sharp kitchen-knife in the early hours of the succeeding morning. Lancing is performed in the afternoon with a special knife, capable of making four incisions at a time, each at about 1/12 cm apart. Each capsule is lanced for 4 to 6 times. A deep incision causes the collection of the latex inside the capsule and spoils the seeds. The crude opium is stored in earthen- pots and dried in the sun to obtain the raw opium of a uniform consistency. The dry produce should be stored in closed vessels. The entire produce goes to the Excise And Narcotics Department which pays according to its cosistency and purity. The average yield of raw opium varics from 13 to 33 kg per hectare, though much higher yields are recorded under good agronomic practices. The crop also yield 3 to 4 quintals of seeds per hectare. The seeds contain up to 50 per cent of a golden-yellow fatty oil which is devoid of narcotic properties.

There are 25 opium alkaloids identified in the raw opium. Of them, morphine, theabine, codeine, narcotine and papaverine are important; morphine is by far the most important. The Indian produce of raw opium contains, on an average, about 20% of the total alkaloids by weight. They, in turn, posses 9 to 14% of morphine, 5-7% narcotine, 1. 25-3. 75% codeine, 0.4-1% papverine and 0. 2-0. 5% theabine. The produce obtained in Turkey and the Balkan countries is collected from one incision only and is therefore rich (10-21%) in morphine; conversely, the Indian opium is richer in codeine and narcotine.

The crop is attacked by the leaf-miner (phyllocnistis sp.), which can be kept under control by spraying with 0. 2% Metasystox or Rogor. Sometimes, cutworms {Agrotis suffura Hubn.) cause damage to the young plants; the flooding of the fields makes these worms float on the water and they are ultimately pickedby birds. Downy mildew (Peronospora arborescens (Berk) formation. It is controlled by the application of 0. 2% Diathane Z-78. Root- rot due to Rhizoctonia is also reported on the crop.

SENNA (Cassia angustifolia Vahl.). Sena is a native of South Arabia and is now naturalized in the Tirunelvelly and Ramnathapuram districts of Tamil Nadu. India is the main producer of this crop in the world and exports senna leaves and pods worth over RS 6 million annually. The leaves and the pod-shell contain the laxative principle (sennocide) which is extensively used as a laxative in medicine.

The crop is grown on marginal red lateritic soils. The growing areas of (Tirunevelly and Ramnathpuram) have no distinct winter season; the average maximum temperature (november to February) is 18.3c and the region is received in autumn from the northeasterly monsoon.

Senna is a small, perennial, branched undershrub, remaining in field for 5 to 7 months. It is grown as a pure crop as well as a mixed crop with gram, gingelly, chilles and cotton. Generally, two sowing seasons are recognised, i.e. February to March (irrigated crop) and November (rainfed crop). The seed-rate is 27 kg per hectare under rainfed conditions and 15 kg per hectare for the irrigated crop. The seeds are broadcast or preferably drilled in lines, 30 cm apart. As soon as the seedlings emerge one to two hoeings are given and the plants close up the rows as they grow. This crop genetrally gets the benefit of residual fertiliser applied to the preceding paddy crop and, therefore, in actual practice it is seldom given fertiliser. The application of 20 kg of N and 40 kg of P per hectare at planting, supplimented with 40 to 60 kg/ha of N in 3 split doses is perferred.

The crop is given 5 to 8 irrigations when grown on garden soils. It flowers in about 2 months after sowing and the first flush of flowering stalks is removed to induce a higher degree of branching. The picking of leaves starts in early May and the leaves are stripped off by hand when fully grown, thick and bluish; the second picking is taken alogwith the plucking of pods. The pods are harvested a little before maturity to maintain their green colour; the second crop of pods is obtained at the end of the season when the plants are uprooted during August or April-May. The leaves and the pods are dried in a thin layer in shade for 4 to 7 days; the pods are lightly beaten during drying to remove the inter seed material.

The careless drying of the harvested crop spoils the colour and lowers its active content. The produce is graded, pressed and finally packed in hessian under pressure for long distance transport. The crop yields 1 to 1. 4 tonnes of leaves and about 1. 5 quintals (about one quintal under rain-fed conditions) of pods per hectare. The produce should contain about 2. 5 per cent of active principles, calculated as anthoquinones. Damping-off is common in the seedling stage. To control the disease, seed treatment with fungicides, e.g. Captain, is recommended. The pods are attacked by a borer during storage, leading to considerable damage.

BELLADONNA (Alropa belladonna Linn) It is European species, presently grown on a small scale in Kashmir. The plant is a small perennial herb which grows up to 1. 5 m in height. It branched freely and produces a large tapering root. The leaves and roots of belladonna constitute the commercial drug which contains atropine, hyocyamine and hyocine, used in pharmacy for their mydriatic, analgesic and antispasmodic properties; the roots are used for external application only. The leaves and roots should contain not less than 0. 3 and 0. 4 percent of the total alkaloids calculated as hyocyamine. A acuminata Royel is a closely related Indian species, found at altitudes between 1800 and 3000 meters in the western Himalayas; its leaves and roots contain similar alkaloids. A part of belladonna alkaloids and their products used in India are imported.

The crop prefers a well-drained slightly acidic, siltyloam to clayey-loam soil, rich in lumus. It cannot stand water-logged conditions. It is a crop of the temperate climate, prefers a sunny location and clear whether, particularly preceding and during the harvesting of the crop; continuous dampness or high humidity favours root-rot.

The crop shows a wide variation in growth and alkaloid content in its plants population. Seeds from selected plants with high alkaloid contents should be used for raising a plantation. Propagation through seed is the easiest and least expensive method, through vegetative methods, such as shoot, root and root-shoot cuttings are also used. The seeds are very small, weighing about 700 per g. They should be treated with ethyl alcohol for 3 minutes or with petroleum either for 6 minutes for improving germination. The treated seeds should be washed in running water for a few hours to remove the adhering chemicals. The seeds are sown in rows in the nursery during early spring. Germination takes place 10 to 21 days and is 15 to 40 per cent. Therefore 4 kg of seed gives enough seedlings to plants in one hectare. The seedling bearing 1 to 3 leaves are planted in the field during august at 45 x 60 cm. or 60 x 60 cm. spacing. Ridge planting is preferred in localities receiving heavy monsoon rains. The land is given about 40 tonnes of farm yard manure, besides 100 kg. of diammonium phosphat and 30 g. of K2O per hectare before planting and 20 kg. of N is given at the time of branching and each time the crop is picked. The plantation is given to 2 to 3 weedings and hoeings before the first leaf crop is obtained and then I or 2 hoeings are usually given before each leaf picking.

The crop is irrigated after every 10 to 15 days during summer. The first picking of leaves is obtained in October; in subsequent years, 3 to 4 leaf crop are obtained for the next three years. Harvesting is done by cutting the plants 20 to 25 cm. on bright sunny days above he ground, except at he time of the autumn harvest when the plants are cut 3 cm. above the ground. The stumps put forth fresh growth during the succeeding spring and bear flowers during June-August and the berries are produced in October. The alkaloids are synthesized in the root and are translocated through the stem to the leaves.

The harvested crop is dried rapidly in the sun for 2-3 days and the leaf-stalks are detached only after the produce is dried. The plants are unrotted after three or four years; the thicker are sliced into 3-4 cm. long pieces and dried. The crop loses 70-80 per cent of its weight during drying. A well dried leaf crop retains its green colour. The average crop yield in the first year is 300 kg. of leaves and thereafter, 750 kg. of leaves per hectare annually. An additional root crop of 2-3 quintals per hectare is obtained when the plants are finally uprooted. Hire average yields of 1-1. 2 tonnes per hectare are reported from European countries. The produce should be stored in cool dry place away from light.

Cutworms (AGROTIS flammatra) attack the tender growing seedling during yearly summer. The application of 5 percent ahe Aldrin dust at 20-25 grammes per square meter of the nursery-bed before sowing protects the crop. The beds may be dranched with 1 : 19 wettable solutions of chlordane, 2-3 times after every 10 days during the attack of the pace. Sometimes damping off of seedlings is caused by pythium sp. and chloropicrin is recommended as a fumigant. Root-rot also damages the crop; the affected plants along with the adhering soil are removed and burnt. Seeds treated with the Agrosan generally protect the seedlings from soil-borne diseases.

RAUWOLFIA (Rouwolfia serpentina Benth) It is an evergreen, perennial indigenous herb found widely distributed in the Himalayan foothills and Peninsular India. The root constitutes the drug and its virtues as an important medicine, were known to the ancient Ayurvedic physicians; it contains 55 alkaloids, reserpine being the most important. The root powder or other preperations containing its alkaloids are prescribed in the treatment of high blood pressure, insomnia, and certain forms of insanity. Roots of rauwolfia and its products command a sizeable market both in India and abroad.

Rauwolfia grows in sandy-loam to clayey-loam acidic soils, rich in humus. It prefers tropical to subtropical climate, receiving heavy monsoon rains between June and August, and the temperatures between 10 and 38 degree centigrades are considered ideal for its growth. The plants sheds its leaves during winter under conditions obtaining in northern India.

It is a one-and-a-half to 2 year crop and can be grown from seeds, root, root-shoot and shoot-cuttings. The seed-crop, however, gives larger (root) yields. The seed rate is 8 to 10 kg per hectare, the average germination being only about 15%. Heavy seeds are selected by floating them in water. They are placed under a moist piece of cloth for 24 hours to soften their hard covering they are sown in well prepared seedbeds in lines, 20cm apart, during April May. The germination is erratic and takes 3 to 8 weeks; the seedlings grow 5 to 8 cm. tall in the next 2 months and are transplanted in well-prepared field at spacing of 45 * 35 cm, 45 * 45 cm, 45*45cm, 45*60 cm or 60*60 cm, depending upon the fertility of the soil and on the intercrops proposed to be grown. The seedlings generally do well and gaps, if any, are filled by fresh planting. The land is preferably mannered with 45 tonnes of farmyard manure per hectare.

The crop is given 90 kg of N; 45 kg of p2o5 and 45 kg of k2o per hectare in all; half of n and the entire quantity of superphosphate and potash is given as basal dose and the remaining N is preferably applied in two split doses, one 75 days after planting and the other during the succeeding spring.

The crop is given monthly irrigation from January to May and after a period of 40-45 days during autumn. Rauwolfia has a deep root-system and is a drought-enduring species; continuous drought, however, reduces its total yield. The crop requires 5 weedings and hoeings during its entire growing period. Whereas a heavy root crop is obtained when rauwolfia is raised as a pure crop, the growing of intercrops, such as maize, cowpea or brinjal, during kharif and radish, wheat or a cole crop, during rabi, gives larger overall profit. The roots are dug-out from November (in northern India) to January February in (southern India). The root bark the thin fibrous roots contain a larger percentage of alkaloids and should not be damaged a loss during digging. The roots are dried in the sun, and 55-60 percent of their weight is lost. The average yield is 950 kg. per hectare.

Adults of Anomalapolita feed on the leaves of rauwolfia during the rainy season and are controlled by spraying 0. 2 percent folidol. Sometimes, mosaic also affects the young growing leaves and inflorescenc. Nematode infestation is restricted to acidic soils. A wilt due to Fusarium sp. and leaf-blight due to Alternaria sp. and reported to cause minor damage. Sometimes a brown leaf spot is found on the lower surface of the leaves caused by Cercospora rauwolfiae. Die-back is caused by Colletotri-chumdematium, particularly under humid growing conditions. The affected branched may be pruned and the plants are sprayed with 0. 2 percent Diathane Z-78 which controls the spread of the disease.

IPECAC (Cephaelis ipecacuanha (Brot.) A. Rich, It is a perennial, evergreen, straggling herb, upto 50 centimetre tall, inhabiting the tropical forest of the south America. It produces slender 10-30 cm. long and 4-10 cm. thick, annulated crockery rhizones. The root bark is the drug of the commerce, used as an expectorant and emetic, mainly in the treatment of amoebic dysentery. The measure world supllies come from Brazil and the neighbouring countries.

India, however, is one of the few countries which grow this crop commercially; its cultivation is done by the West Bengal Cinchona department in the Darjeeling district and to a smaller extent in Sikkim and parts of Assam. The annual production ranges between 25 and 30 tonnes of dry roots and part of the produce, including emetine salts, is exported earning a foreign exchange of 1 million rupees annually.

The crop prefers warm and moist sandy loam forest soil, rich in humus and potash. A high well distributed rail fall (minimum 200 cm.), a temperature range of 10 to 38 degree centigrade and the altitudes of 500 to 600 meters, and sides shelter from strong wind constitute the most suitable environment for ipecac cultivation. The crop could be raised from seeds shoot and root cuttings. The vegetative propagation, however, shortens commercial varieties are known, mainly after the name of the country of origin. Seeds are small and are sown by broad cast by during January and March in well prepared and heavily manuared raised seedbeds of convenient size. About 35 g. of seed is sown per square meter.

The average germination is 30 percent and the seed take 3-5 months to germinate. The seedbeds are shaded during the day and kept moist and free from weeds. Seedlings about 4 cm. tall, are transferred to the rooted nursery, with 5x5 cm spacing between the plants after the monsoon rains are over. They remain there till the following March and April, when they are again transferred to a third side with spacing of 20x20 cm. between the plants. The plants remain there for three year till the roots are dug out.

Ipecac is thus slow growing 4 year crop which is very exacting in its requirement for continues shad, moist beds (but no water logging) and regular interculture. The plants give out dark green elliptical leaves and bear white flowers and small dark-purple globose berries in the second year. The flowers are dimorphic, heterostylous (and therefore cross pollinated) and are formed in group of 6-8. The berries ripen during September-October. The seed is white, plano-convex, 5-6 x 1. 5-2 mm. and is cover with a hard tests. About 1/3 of the seeds are sterile. The growing plants require a good amount of nutrient supply which is mainly added to the soil through heavy organic manuring; information on the use of inorganic fertilizers is not known. Each plant forms 2-3 long rhizomes which are dug out during dry weather; the rhizomes are cleaned of the adhering soil and rapidly dried in the direct sun for 2-3 days. The dry rhizomes are broken into smaller pieces and finally packed in bales for transporting to the extraction sides. The yield varies from 600-1000 kg. of roots per hectare.

The roots contain emetine caphaeline and psychotrine as its main alkaloids; emetine, however is the most important. The average total alkaloid content in the Indian crop is 2. 5 percent of which 1. 3-1. 4 percent is emetine. The alkaloids are extracted in the form of their salts viz. emetine sulphate and emetime hydrocloride, for marketing. According to the Indian pharmacopoeia (1966), the ipecac, of which not less than 50% should consist of nonphenolic alkaloids.

The seed beds are sometimes infested with Fusarium and rhizoctonia spp. causing damage to the plant suitable fungicids may be used to control the infection of the plants.

FOXGLOVE (Digitals lanata Enrh). An exotic biennial herb, cultivated mainly in central and southern Europe for leaves which contain glycosides used for heart stimulation. India imports a major parts of its requirements of this drugs. The crop perfers silty-loam to clayey-loam soils, rich in organic matter and temperate climate (1200-2000 m above the sea-level). The seed-rate used is 500 grammes per hectare. The nursery is raised in early spring and seedlings, when 8-10 weeks old, are transplanted, 30x45 cm to 60x60 cm apart, depending upon the soil fertility. It is an irrigated crop and makes only a moderate demand for nutrients, mainly as nitrogenous and phosphatic fertilzers. The plants flower in the second year, but the flowering stalks are removed to induce a larger leafy growth. In general, one harvest of the leaf crop is obtained in October in the first year, whereas 3 harvests of leaf crop are obtained in the second year. The average yield recorded in India in the second year is 600 kg/hs; higher yield up to 1, 500 kg are reported from elsewhere. Digitalis leaves are thermolabile and hygroscopic and therefore, should be rapidly dried at 40 C immediately after collection. They should contain 0. 1% glycoside (digoxin, digitoxin, gitoxin, etc.) calculated as lanatocide-c and not more than 5% moisture. The leaves could be stored in the form of coarse powder in airtight containers placed in a cool and a dry place.

DILL OR SOWA (Anethum graveolens Linn.). Sowa is a rabi crop grown almost throughout the country for its fresh aromatic leaves used in cooking, and its fruits are marketed as a common condiment.

The fruits contain an essential oil, rich in carvone and is used in pharmacy for the preparation of dill water and similar preperations to treat flatulence, abdominal and colic pain. India exports dill fruits worth about Rs 2 million annually. There are two known varieties, viz. the East Indian Dill (A. graveolens var. sowa) and European Dill (A. graveolens Linn.); the former alone is cultivated in India commercially; its oil possesses superior aroma, but is considered inferior in pharmacy owing to the presence of a toxic substance (dillapiole) which is, however, easily removed.

Dill prefers well-drained fertile loamy soil and can be raised under a wide range of climatic conditions. The seeds are sown direct in the fields in rows or along the bunds in early autumn and the seedlings are thinned after about 40 days of sowing to maintain a spacing of 60 x30 cm. The crop is given 40kg each of N, P and K per ha at planting and another 40kg of N as top-dressing depending upon the fertility status of the field. The crop mature by the end of April in northern India and green mature umbnles are picked in 10-25 days to avoid seed-shattering. The average yield comes to 1 tonne of fruits per ha.

The sowa seeds on distillation yield 2. 5 to 3 per cent of an essential oil rich in arvone which imparts to the oil its characteristic flavour.

Powdery mildew (Erysiphe umbelliferum forma anethi) sometimes causes heavy damage to the crop and is controlled by 2 to 3 sprayings of sulphur at 25 kg/ha during the early flowering stage. Aphids occasionally cause damage; the spraying of Malathion (0. 5%) 2 to 3 times during infection is recommended.

LIQUORICE OR MULHATI (Glycyrrhiza glabra Linn.). Liquorice is a hardy perennial legume, about 0. 6 m tall, found wild in countries of west Asia. Its dried peeled or unpeeled underground stems and roots constitute the drug. It is demucent, mildlu laxative, expectorant and, as such, is an important constituent of all cough and catarrh syrups, throat lozenges and pastilles; its extract containing glycyrrhizin (2. 14%) has a healing effect on peptic ulcers. Large quantities of liquorice root is used in confectionery and tobacco-blending. There are a number of commercial cultivation varieties of liquorice, such as typical Regal and Herd. (Spanish liquorice) which is the sweetest of all and therefore, fetches higher price; var. glandulifera Waldst and Kit. (Russian liquorice) is richer in glycyrrhizin but the sweet taste is accompanied with perceptible but mild, bitterness owing to the presence of liquiritin and isoliquritin; var. violaca Boiss. (Persian liquorice) produces thich, hard and lumpy roots and is considered inferior in quality.

Liquorice grows well in fertile sandy-loamy soils in a warm and dry climate, having a long growing season marked with well-defined winters to induce the translocation of food to the underground perennating rhizomes. Heavy rain or frost affects its growth adversely. Most of the growing areas fall around 14N latitude. The crop is raised from rooted cuttings which are planted in early spring 90 x 60 cm apart in rows. The beds are worked up to a depth of 1 metre and liberally mannered. Seeds are seldom used. Var. typically produces a strong taproot which gives out rhizomes, whereas var. glandulifera sends out rhizomes are ready for harvesting in 3 to 4 years and are dug out in autumn after rains. A portion of the harvested material is decorticated before drying to produce the peeled liquorice of commerce. The material is cut into pieces, 15-20 cm long and 1 to 2 cm in diameter, and are dried alternatelly in shade and the sun. This drying reduces the weight of the material to 50 per cent. Artificial drying can also be done at 30-40 C. The crop yield ranges from 1 to 3 tonnes per hectare, depending upon the soil fertility, the variety, the climate and cultivation practices.

DIOSCOREA. The tubers of a number of non-edible dioecious species of Diocorea provide raw material for the industrial production of corticosteroids is around 300 tonnes, valued at about Rs 3, 000 million. Of the several species, D. composita Hemsl, and D. floribunda Mart. and Gal. (from Central America) and D. deltoidea Wall. ex Kunth. (from western Himalayas) and D. prazeri Prain and Burk. (from Eastern Himalayas) stand out prominently because of the higher percentage of diogenin content in their tubers. Of late, a D.

floribunda clone, developed at the Indian Institute of Horticultural Research, Bangalore, has been found to grow fast and give exploitable tuber yield in about 18 months of the growing period.

The crop of Discorea floribunda is raised from tuber pieces, each weighing 50-70 grammes, treated with a stemic fungicide for protection against soft- rot; these tuber pieces are planted in pits at 60 x45 cm spacing during March-April. The tubers sprout between 30 and 60 days after planting. Each pit is given 1.5kg of farmyard manure or compost along with 30 kg each of N and P per ha at planting, supplemented with similar quantities of fertilizers during the rainy season. Another application of 60 kg of N+40kg of P is given in 2 split doses in the second year. The growing vines are given support for getting the optimum uy\yield. The tubers grow up to 30 cm depth in the soil and, being soft, should be dug out carefully. An average yield of 1 kg of fresh turbers, containing 70 per cent moisture, per plant is reported from Bangalore.

The calculated tuber yield as reported, is 7. 5 tonnes (dry) per ha, containing, on an average, 3 per cent diogenin.

AROMATIC PLANTS

The aromatic plants possess odoriferous and volatile substances which occur as essential oils, gum exudate, balsam and oleoresin in one or more parts, viz. root, wood, bark, foliage, flower and fruit. The chemical nature of these aromatic substances may be due to a variety of complex the chemical compounds. Many of these aromatics are powerful germicides and have anti-bacterial properties, but the bulk of the produce finds use in perfumery and the food-flavouring industries. Amongst the two, the per-fumeru and allied industries consume much larger amounts of the natural fragrant material. According to the UN Word Statistics (1972), the annual world trade (excluding countries in eastern Europe) in essential oils and perfummery aromatics for 1969 was of the order of Rs 2250 million; also, a large quantity of the aromatic material of plant origin is utilized in cosmetics, toiletries and allied industries. Our current volume of foreign trade in the perfumery material, essential oils and aromatic compounds is around Rs 65 million and this amount accounts for 1. 6 per cent of the world trade. Some sixty-two types of essential oils come to the international market with a large and consistent demand. However, our treatment of the aromatic plants is confined to a few more important essential-oil crops grown in the country.

The methods employed to obtain aromatic substances from plants are classified into distillation, enfleurage, maceration, expression and solvent extraction. Expect in the case of flowers crops, such as jasmine and kewara in which the fragrant constituents are likely to be decomposed or destroyed, the essential oils are mostly obtained by distilling the produce; in fact, steam distillation is the oldest method of separation of essential oils. The perfumery material is filled in a large-galvanizediron still over a perforated netal grid. Water is filled in the still below the level of the grid so that it generates a low-pressure steam on heating to pass through the material. The water vapours carry with it the essential oil of the perfumery material. These vapours are passed through a condenser and collected in a vessel where the oil is ecanted with a separating-funnel.

A simple field distillation unit could be fabricated by a skilled blacksmith. For more efficient and quick distillation of the produce; " steam distillation" units are employed. These units are built on the same principle except that live steam at 40-100 1b pressure per inch is injected into the filling-still through perforated coils and the distillation is completed in a shorter period. It has the advantages of handling a larger quantity of the material, besides improving upon the recovery of the essential oil.

As stated earlier, the solvent-extraction method is employed for the extractors are of two types, viz. stationary and rotatory types, and low- bowling solvents, like petroleum either, alcohol or benzen, are used for extracting the odoriferous principles. The stationary type extractors consists of vertical cylinders provided with type extractors consists of vertical cylinders provided with perforated metal grids arranged horizontally around a central vertical shaft. The flower crop is charged over the grids which come into constant with the solvent periodically and the essential oil is removed in successive washings. The rotatory type consists of an iron drum which rotates on a horizontal axis. The interior of the drum is divided with a perforated metal partition of holding floers and the solvent is filled in the lower part of the extractor. While the drum moves, the solvent seeps through the perforations and drips back, so that the essential oil is washed out to the solvent. This extract is than distilled in a vacuum still at a low temperature to recover the disolvant. The floral concentrate, thus obtained, also contains some waxes and plant pigments which are removed by treating with warm alcohol. The filtered solution, so obtained, is either used as such, or is concentrated in vaccum into a viscous oil.

LEMON GRASS (Cymbopogon flexuosus Stapf.). It is a stemless perennial grass, found wild in the southern states of India. The leaves yield an aromatic oil, containing 75-85 per cent citral. The oil is used in soaps, cosmetics and disinfectants and is a raw material for manufacturing ions and vitamin A. The crop is grown on about 390, 000 ha in Kerals and about 90 per cent of the produce is exported, earning about Rs 10 million in foreign exchange annually.

The crop is grown mainly as a rain-fed crop on poor marginal lands. It is a hardy drought-resistant plant and is grown under a wided range of climatic conditions. Two types are recognized : (1) the red-stemmed grass is the true lemon-grass and a selection 'OD-19' made at the Lemon Grass Research Station, Oodakkali (Kerala) is recommended for high yield, (2) the white-stemmed (var. albscens) yields oil or low citral content. The crop is best propagated through seed raised in nurseries; 10kg of the seed produces enough seedlings for planting a hectare. About 2-month-old seedlings are planted in rows, 40 to 15x 10 cm apart, during rains and the first harvest is ready after 90 days. In

Kerala, 3 harvests are obtained in the first year and 4 to 5 harvests during each of the 3 to 5 succeeding years; the crop is cut after every 60 to 65 days, except during the dry season. The fields are mannered liberally with ash and spent grass (obtained after the distillation of the oil); farmers seldom apply inorganic fertilizers. The herbage contains 0. 35% oil on fresh-weight basis. The grass yield ranges from 18 to 25 tonnes per hectare, giving 60-72 kg of oil.

CITRONELLA GRASS (Cymobopogon winteriaruns Jowitt). It is a stemless perennial grass. The oil is mainly used in soaps, Cosmetics, deodorants and mosquito-repellent creams. It is a recent introduction into India and its cultivation. mainly in the lower hills of Assam, in Karnataka and southern Gujrat, covers about 2, 000 hectares. A part of out requirement is still met by imports, Java citronella is grown up to 1, 000 m above sea level on well-drained sandy-loanto clayey-loamy soils with pH varying from 5 to 7. 5 As a rainfed crop, it is propagated by using rooted slips, and is planted during the rainy season in rows, 60 to 45 cm x 45 to 30 cm apart, depending on the rate of growth and the soil fetility. Usually, the leafy portion is removed at planting during the monsoon season and the plants begin to tiller in 30 days after planting.

A healthy one-year-old clump yields 60 to 80 slips. The crop needs a large quantity of nitrogenous fertilizers, When grown on medium soils, it is given 60 kg of P, 40 kg of K and 20 kg of N per ha at planting, supplemented with 80 to 100 kg of N per hectare annually as top-dressing in 3 to 4 split doses.

The crop is irrigated after every 10-15 days during the dry season and the first harvest is count 20 cm above the ground after 90 days of planting; usually 3 cuttings are obtained annually (4 under Assam conditions) for 3 to 5 year after planting.

CELERY (Apium graveolens Linn). Celery is a native of the Mediterranean region, introduced into India during late nineteenth century. India is now the principal grower (of the annual type) and exports large quantities of celery seeds (worth 17. 5 millions to the American and European markets. About 8000 ha is put under this crop, mainly in the Amritsar, Gurdaspur and Jallundhar districts of the Punjab State and to a smaller extent in the Saharanpur district of Uttar Pradesh. The clery seed is used in ground form as a dry seasoning powder and for the extraction of an oleoresin used to flavour a large variety of canned food products. The celery seed oil commands a larger market mainly in the confectionery industry. Whereas the bulk of celery seed is exported, a few local firms also produce its essential oil and olioresin on a small scale.

Celery is an erect, branchin herb, about 100 cm tall. it is a rabi crop which remains for 2 months in the nursery and for another 4 to 4 1/2 months in the field. Nursery is raised during early November. The seed-rate used is 2 kg. per hectare. The nursery-beds are kept moist and free from weeds through periodic irrigation followed by interculture. The seedlings grow up to 10 cm tall by the end of December and are ready for transplanting. The seedlings are usually planted 45 cm x 20 cm apart in early January in well-prepared fields, to which 30-50 tonnes of farmyard manure per ha is added during the preparatory tillage. On medium soils, about 80 Kg N, 40 Kg of P and 20 Kg of K per ha is applied to the crop; half of N along with the entire quantity of P and K is given to the rows at the time of planting and the remaining N is given as a top-dressing after one month. The crop requires 10-12 irrigations, each about 5 cm deep. Once established the crop requires 3 to 4 hoeings to keep down weeds. The plants bear flowers in umbels during early March and the fruits mature in late April. The Crop is harvested when about 80 per cent of the umbels begin to turn light brown. The harvested crop as stacked in the field for few days and is then threshed to obtain the seeds. The average grain yield ranges from 10 to 12 quintals per ha.

The celery (seed) on distillation yields to 2. 1 to 2. 3% of an essential oil containing selinene, d-limonene and sesquiterpenes. Oleoresin is prepared by using the method of the solvent extraction of the seeds. The seeds yields glycoside opiin. The crop remains remarkably free from pests and diseases.

Rose geranium (Pelargonium graveolens L'Herit) Pelargonium is a native of the hilly tracts of Cape Colony (South Africa). The highly aromatic 'Rose Geranium' is a hybrid (P. graveolens x P. radens), introduced by two Frenchmen-Earnest Sen and J. Priors in Yercaud in the Sheraroy Hills (Salem district) in Tamilnadu. It is now grown in a limited areas around Bangalore, Yercaud and in the Nilgiri Hills. The major world supplies of the oil come from Malagasy Republic. The oil of geranium has a refreshingly delicate rose-like aroma containing 66-78 per cent of alcohols calculated as geraniol. As such also, it itself is a perfume; it blends well with a wide range of floral and oriental perfumes. It is used for scenting oinments, pharmaceutical and tobacco products. It is suitable in a slightly alkaline medium and, therefore, it is widely used in the manufacture of high-grade soaps and cosmetic products. Our total annual production of the oil is around 12 tonnes and, therefore, a sizeable quantity of the oil is annually imported.

Two plant types of 'Rose Geranium' are recognized in India, Viz. the Algeriaan type from the slender plants, with dark pink flowers. It is less suitable for humid conditions; the other is Bourbin type which produces more leafy growth and bears light pink flowers. It is a perennial crop and about two to three harvests of leaves are taken annually in the second and third years. It can be grown as a catch crop in newly planted orchards.

'Rose Geranium' flourishes well in deep well-drained, preferably sandy loam to clayey-loam soils. It grows luxuriantly in a mild subtropical climate; locality receiving excessive heat in summer or very low temperatures in winter are unsuitable. The 'Rose Geranium' can withstand drought but its yield is reduced. It is raised in nursery during early spring from 8-15 cm long stem cutting each with 2 to 4 nodes. Sandy beds are preferred for the nursery to avoid excessive moisture which damages the young sprouts. Under a favourable day temperature of 10 to 15 degree Centigrade, about 80 per cent cuttings sproute in 3 weeks and are ready for field planting at 50 x 100 cm spacing with the onset of the monsoon rains in May-June. The field are brought to a fine tilth, are mixed with 45 tonnes of farmyard manure per hectare. In the Nilgiris the crop is given a basal application of a fertilizer mixture, containing 35, 45 and 17 kg of N, P and K per hectare; therefore, another 35 kg of N may be applied in two split applications annually. Initially, the crop is given 1 to 2 hoeings and weedings and the rows close up. The pruning of branches after the rains helps to induce bushy growth. The crop is irrigated at intervals of 10 to 15 days during summer depending upon the soils texture and the atmospheric humidity. Too moist or continued dry conditions lowers the crop yield. Generally, the first crop is obtained 6 to 8 months after planting and the average oil yields 8 kg; two or three crop are received in subsequent years, yielding 8 to 18 kg. of oil per hectare. In countries, e.g. Algeria and Malagasy Republic, the oil yields is reported to range from 30 to 35 kg. per hectare. The fresh leaves contain 0. 12 to 0. 2% (w/w) volatile oil and semi-dry or even dry leaves can be distilled. The oil improves in odour on ageing.

Fusarium sp. serious damages the geranium crop; the diseases is favoured by continued misty weather and excess soils moisture. The removal of diseased parts arrests the spread of the diseases and the spraying of the crop with 5% Bordeaux mixture periodically is recommended to control the diseases. However, when the roots are attacked, the plant dies and such infected plants should be pulled out along with the adhering soils and burnet.

PATCHOULI (Pogostemon cablin Benth) Patchouli is a native of humid Indo-Malayan tropics. The plant is small bushy herb which yields fragrant leaves containing a very sweet smelling oil. It is grown in small pockets mainly in Karnataka and Tamil Nadu. The oil of Patchouli is used to manufacture soap, cosmetics and incense and for imparting lasting oriental perfumery notes to many fancy products.

Two plants types of Patchouli are mainly recognized, viz. Jahore type which yields a poor leafy growth but produces a superior quality of oil; the other is Singapore type that gives more foliage and, therefore, more oil. It is a perennial crop, remaining in the field for about 3 years and gives 2 to 3 crops of leaves annually. It is a good catch crop for young orchards and can be raised as an intercrop in plantations where the over head shade is not heavy.

Patchouli requires deep, well-drained, fertile, slightly acidic soils, rich in humus; its growth is luxuriant in regions experiencing mild summer (24-280C), and a good rainfall ranging from 150 to 300 cm. Its sursery is raised in shade by planting 10-12 cm-long cuttings at 10 x 10 cm spacing during the rainy season and the beds are kept continuously moist. Under favourable conditions, about 85-90 per cent cutting per forth roots in a fortnight and they are ready for planting in the field in six to eight weeks at 90 x 90 cm spacing. The crop requires a liberal amount of organic matter and fertilizers; usually 10-12 tonnes of farmyard manure with 100 kg of P per ha is incorporated into the soil at the planting time, followed by 80 to 100 kg of N per hectare to the crop annually as top dressing in two split applications. The first crop is ready for harvesting in the next 4 to 6 months as indicated by the browning of the lower leaves, and the herbage is cut 10-25 cm below the apex in the morning hours. Usually, one or two growing branches are left unplucked to ensure a better growth of the succeeding harvest. The harvested leaves are dried in thin layers in sgade for 3-4 days and they develop their characteristic odour.

Mature stalks are removed before distillation. Ageing improves the odour and the dry HA-77 leaves are therefore stored for a few months before distillation.

A good crop stand yields about 2 tonnes of dry leaves (with 3 to 3. 5% oil) per annum, yielding about 50-60 kg of oil per hectare.

Golden nematode (Meloidogyne incognito) seriously damages this crop. No effective measure to control the nematode are known.

VETIVER OR KHUS (Vetiveria zizanioides (Linn Nash). Khus is a tall perennial grass found wild in the drier tracts of western India. Its spongy, much-branched fine root lets contain a fragrant oil, which is a perfume by itself. The dry aromatic roots are made into curtains, mats, fans, etc. to emit scented cool aroma when moistened. The oil is used as a valuable fixative for blending perfumes and socmetics. A large bulk of the oil is produced by distilling the wild-growing plants found in Bharatpur (Rajasthan), Musanagar, Biswan and Nawabganj etc. in western Uttar Pradesh. The cultivation of khus is scattered over small areas in the Trichur, Palghat, Kozikode, Wynad and Trivandrum district of Kerala, in the Tirunelvelly, Madhrai and Coimbatore districts of Tamil Nadu and in the kurnool and East Godavari districts of Andhra Pradesh.

In southern states, khus is grown as a rainfed crop in well-drained sandy-loam soils in moderately humid localities which received 100-200 cm of rainfall annually. However, a luxuriant growth of healthier roots is obtained from plants growing under warm and damp conditions on rich, partially inundated, masrshy land (Bharatpur). The field are laid out into beds of convenient size and 15-20 cm-long rooted slips are planted. With the onset of the monsoon rains on both the sides of the ridges, made 45 cm apart. The planting of 2 to 3 slips is done in spring in pits when the crop is raised under irrigation. The crop is given 10-12 tonnes of farmyard manure or compost at planting, supplemented with ash and groundnutcake or ammonium sulphate, one month after planting to stimulate growth.

Khus is a 12 to 18 month crop and the roots are dug out during dry months before autumn. The aerial parts are first cut at a height of 15 to 20 cm and are removed, the clumps are then dug out and beaten. The soil is further dug out up to a depth of one metre to remove the remaining rootlets. The roots are light to yellowish brown containing usually 0. 6 to 0. 8 per cent of dark brown viscous, persistently fragrant oil. The yield is 3 to 5 tonnes of fresh root, yielding about 20 kg of oil per hectare.

JASMINE. Among the perfume yielding jasmines, juhi (Jasminum curiculatum Vahl) and chameli (J officinale Linn) are commonly used for producing attars which sell at fancy prices. Jasmine ' concrete' and absolutes' are used to impart a gentle pleasing aroma to innumerable high-grade preparations. In the Western countries, Spanish (alsocalled French) jasmine (J. officinale Linn var grandiflorum Bailey) is largely cultivated; it has 7 to 11 leaflets and the flower bud has a dull creamy to punish spot on the posterior most petal. A high yelding clone of the Spanish jasmine has been recently developed at the Tamil Nadu Agricultural University, Coimbatore.of fresh flowers per hectare annually against 1. 6 to 3 tonnes of flowers obtained from the Spanish jasmine in India. The crop remains in the field for 10 to 15 years.

The jasmines prefer well drained, rich sandy-loam to clayey-loam soils and remain in loom longer in a mild climate; the var. grandiflorum is more sensitive to fros. It is raised from 20 cm long stem cutting prepared from near mature wood and planted in deep pits at 1.5 x 1 m spacing during the rainy season. The growing plants are pruned during January February and July to induce lateral branching and flowering, and are given farmyard manure liberally. The plantation needs fortnightly irrigation during dry months. Picking is done during the early morning hours and the percentage recovery of the concrete ranges from 0. 24 to 0. 38 by using the solvent extraction method. Fresh flowers lose their fragrance soon, and it is essential that the solvent extraction apparatus as available at the site where the jasmine plantation is raised for perfumery aromatics.

KEWARA (Pandanus odoratissimus Linn) Kewara is a large indigenous shrub, 3 to 6 m tall, bearing white or creamy dioecious flowers including its enclosing spathe contains a fragrant oil. The kewara attar and kewara water are commonly used at ceremonial functions in perfuming aerated waters, other drinks and confectionery products. Most of the cultivation is confined to the Ganjam district (400 ha) in Orissa where it is drains and ponds. The plant thrives in clayey loam soil in the tropical climate, usually receiving heavy rainfall.

Kewara is propagated from shoots, branches and leaves which readily from roots during the rainy season. It bears flowers in the fourth or fifth year and has an economic life of 20 years. The crops needs no special care, except periodic pruning. The flowers are borne from June to September. A plant may produce 15 to 40 flowers in a season. A flower takes 15 days to mature and grows grammes. The blossom contains 0. 1 to 0. 3 per cent oil. The attar is mosly produced over sandalwood oil or paraffin base.

PRINCIPLES OF BIODYNAMIC CULTIVATION

Quality or Quantity

The main aim of biodynamic cultivation is to improve the quality of either food, fiber or medicinal plants. Of course, it also aims at improving the yields but, most importantly, it concentrates on quality.

In this century, more and more chemical fertilisers have been developed to produce maximum yields. The main objective has been to increase the yields. The reason is simple: bigger yields bring more money. Most vegetable producers have been cheating the consumer by selling them water for the price of vegetables. For example, dried carrots which have been chemically fertilised show less weight than organic carrots.

Adding fertilisers, which are salts, to plants, means that the plants draw more water from the soil in order to balance the ratio of fiber to salt inside. Consequently, as the plant cells expand and swell with water, the ratio of proteins and even vitamins decreases, and the essential oils, which have important medicinal properties, deteriorate. It has been scientifically proven that the amount of vitamins is less in chemically fertilised products. There is an imbalance of vitamins because the fertilised plants draw only one kind of nutrient and not all the trace elements. Hence, it does not produce the entire range of vitamins, and its whole value changes.

Quality of Medicinal Plants

What we want to achieve in biodynamic farming of medicinal plants, is the cultivation of the inherent quality of the plant. That is the very subtle active principle, which the plant has in very minute quantities. Instead of substance, here we are dealing with essential oils, which are almost not substantial, sometimes present only in parts per million. What is quality, and how can we provide quality in food or in medicinal plants? What are the indicators for quality in medicinal plants? Quality comprises certain active principles, such as taste, juice, colour, seed content in the fruits, nutritional value, the vitamin and protein content. The question is, do we know how to evaluate subtle medicinal properties?

How do we define the taste, the aroma, the smell of flowers? How do we increase the scent of a rose, and how do we make oranges more sweet? How do we increase the content of active principles in medicinal plants? Does science know how to produce the best quality of food?

Modern agricultural sciences are based on how to work with yields. We know how to produce quantity but we don't know how to produce quality. We are facing the tragedy that roses don't have any smell any more; oranges have lost their taste; tomatoes are not sweet any more; carrots are bitter, and cultivated medicinal plants have less active principles.

Characteristics of the Himalayan Flora and Fauna

Each plant develops in a particular ecological zone. Here in the Darjeeling Hills we meet with this fantastic possibility of having land from very low elevations up to very high summits. Additionally the climate provides a lot of warmth and moisture. This combination of moisture and warmth creates very specific kinds of chemicals in the plants a lot of light. In contrast, the valleys are full of moisture, heat with a lot of vegetation and rather dark forests. Those extremes produce substances that are very different from each other.

In the higher regions of the Himalayas plants grow on very dry alpine soils. These, in many cases, are sandy and not very fertile. The cold climate limits the plants' growth. On lower elevations, the plants produces a lot of leaf, and in higher altitude they prominent with the flowers.

Polarities in Biodynamics

There is a polarity between yields and quality, between substance and un-substance, between big quantity of products and very small quantities of subtle ethereal oils. Regarding the definition of quality, a polarity can be observed between something very physical, such as the weight, substance-and something very subtle, such as ethereal oils.

In biodynamic farming we are trying to rediscover what is important in agriculture.

EARTH AND SUN

The entire plant life is a product of the earth and the sun-as some people say, the Mother Earth, and the Father Sun. In many cultures, the sun is masculine and the earth is feminine.

Sun	Earth
Warmth, Heat	Coolness, minerals,
Seasonal Rhythm	Gravity, Water
Space	Soil
Light	Darkness

The Principle of Light

The colours of the beautiful high altitude flowers are a powerful manifestation of light. Colour is the resistance of substances to light, the tension between the light and the earth. The alpine regions are full of light.

This leads to very special structures of medicinal plants: the flowers are very colourful and bright, the leaves are very delicate-and with a lot of medicinal value. With hardly any substance alpine medicinal plants tend to be small but very powerful. The light that they accumulate is all transformed into essential oils. The more light, the more essential oils are produced. These medicinal plants pass through the whole winter with very little water. They are processing all this light, and they have to concentrate everything into essential oils.

The tannin in the tea leaf, for example, is nothing but concentrated sunlight. It is this sunlight which activates our senses, working on very subtle principles.

Using Polarity Principles in Biodynamic Agriculture

An example: Curcure (Equisetum arvense L.) is a plant without leaf. It consists only of stem. It grows in shady places, and is very rich in silica. The amount of silica, almost 90%, is one of the highest in the plant world. Silica is a mineral, belonging to the earth, but it lets the light go through.

Where do we find silica? In sand. Sixty or seventy per cent of the earth's crust is silica. And if you want to know how silica is connected to life, just look at a window: the glass is pure silica. There is silica in spectacles, silica in the eyes and skin, in the hair-and in leaves. Silica has an affinity to light. In fact, it draws light.

With silica as a carrier of light, we can make use of the polarity of light and darkness in agriculture. Equisetum arvense contains a lot of silica, and therefore belongs to the realm of light. On the contrary, fungus belongs to the realm of cold, moisture and darkness. We can use a product from one realm to control an imbalance in another. Equisetum arvense is an excellent fungicide.

Biodynamic Preparations

Out of his own insight, Rudolf Steiner introduced what is known as biodynamic preparations. Naturally occurring plant and animal materials are combined in specific recipes in certain seasons of the year and then placed in compost piles. These preparations bear concentrated forces within them and are used to organise the chaotic elements within the compost piles. When the process is complete, the resulting preparations are medicines for the Earth which draw new life forces from the cosmos. Effects of the preparations have been verified scientifically.

One of the preparations is made from silica powder, processed in a special way. It is applied to the plants at the time when they are producing the part that shall be harvested. In case of medicinal plants, if, for example, the root is harvested for medicinal purposes, silica is applied when the root is forming. The same applies for the flower, leaf, etc.

This silica powder preparation helps to increase the concentration of silica in the plant. With silica, the plant increases its rate of photosynthesis, draws more light, and produces more of those finer aspects. The medicinal value of plants cultivated under such conditions will be naturally higher and their pests lesser.

Silica is an excellent remedy for the foggy Darjeeling climate. The monsoon mists hold back the plant, whereas silica will activate the plant growth. Too this way one can balance an unfavourable climatic situation with biodynamic preparations.

One of the biodynamic preparation is made from quartz crystals: the crystal form of silica. These crystals have geometric forms, perfect hexagonal shapes. The geometry shows another polarity of form and formlessness: in silica we have these beautiful shapes, and in fungus we have amorphous shapes, without form.

Geometric Principles and Medicinal Values

Alpine flowers are of the most perfect shapes, like stars: they have the most beautiful, artistic quality. The same applies for this quartz. These perfect shapes are based on the same geometric principle. It belongs to the heights, near the light, close to the stars. In pentagonal and hexagonal flowers we find the same geometrical principles as in crystals.

The differences between the root and the flower of such alpine medicinal plants reveal the polarity that we are talking about. The flower is very nicely shaped, though every species is different. But why do we not study the roots to differentiate those plants?

Because they are all more-or-less the same. There is no differentiation at the root level, and yet there is this high differentiation at the flower level.

How do these plants know that they have to grow like this? Why are they shaped and coloured like this? For example, this plant has five petals, five sepals, five stamens, so it is shaped by the principle of five, but where does it come from? It is these principles that form the plant, and along with it its medicinal values.

We can release this formative principle in our plants and understand how it starts shaping them and bringing forth these fine aspects of scent, aroma, taste, colour and medical properties.

In comparison, in tropical plants the principle of flower has been pushed into the leaf. Tropical climate produces fleshy plants that would never grow in the Alpine regions. These plants need moisture. It is warmth, which, combined with light, manifests in these plants in the leaves instead of in the flower.

Many plants, where this principle of warmth pushing into the leaf operates, develop a lot of poison. When this principle, that belongs to the flower, has been pushed as far as into the root, it colours even the roots. Colour at the root level means that what belongs to the flower has been pushed deep inside the plant.

COSMIC INTEGRATION

The Zodiac Principles

The ultimate fine-tuning of biodynamic principles lies in harnessing cosmic influences for cultivation. Only at particular times of the month or year are the cosmic influences are most supportive to the growth of a particular part of the plant.

The cosmic factor that determines a month is the moon. The movement of the moon in relation to the Zodiac is most interesting. The Zodiac symbols are Greek in origin. The Chinese developed a different system, and the Tibetans created their own amalgamation of the Indian and Chinese systems.

All the different systems have twelve constellations, though represented by different archetype figures and animals. Within these twelve signs there are four groups of three constellations each which have the same qualities. They are related to the four elements, earth, water, fire, air. These four elements can be placed in relation to the four parts of the plant: the root, the leaf, the flower and the fruit.

- The roots are associated with the earth: there is no base and ground without earth.
- The leaves relate to the water element: the more water, the more leaf.
- The flower corresponds to air and light: there is no light without air. (There is no light on the moon because there is no atmosphere.)
- Fruits are associated with fire: there is no ripening without warmth.\

Cultivating the soil on specific days means harnessing the cosmic influences for the particular plant. Recent research has shown that in one month there are three periods which are variously beneficial for the root, the leaf, the flower and the fruit. These period are governed by the moon cycle. The different parts of the plant are stimulated, one at a time, three times in a month. Researchers discovered this by planting radishes every day and then observing their growth. Radishes from one day would be of very of good quality while those from another day would be smaller and less healthier. In between would be radishes with shrivelled roots or too much leaf. Anybody can try this experiment. The researchers found that the yields can be increased 20 to 30% just by cultivating at the right time.

Re-presenting Traditional Knowledge

When I was working in Peru, in the Andes, at 4000 metres above sea level, the farmers there told me that they always plant their seeds according to the moon. Farmers all over the world observe these natural laws. Farmers in Africa, America and Asia: they all have some knowledge about how to harness the position of the moon. But nowadays a lot of such traditional knowledge has been lost. A farmer in Peru told me: "If we use fertilisers, the moon doesn't matter. " In his simple words he clearly stated that if we use fertilisers, we cut off the cosmic influences. Another farmer in a village, at 4, 000 metres altitude, told me: "We want to produce food that in itself has medicinal value."

There is a clearly palpable loss of traditional knowledge. Children are not trained in going back to the countryside and asking the elder people:

'What do you know about our environment?' Instead of learning from the old people about the medicinal plants, etc., they generally say: 'Oh, the old people don't know how to read, so they are ignorant'. That is the tragedy in which a lot of traditional knowledge is lost.

We can observe that the younger generation rejects the oral traditions because they clash with modern knowledge presented in writing. When I worked in the Andes, we tried to present traditional knowledge in a modern language. There is a psychological aspect to it. When a young person reads his grandfather 's knowledge in a nicely-presented, logically-written paper, he considers it to be important. And if he sees it on the TV, then it is even more important!

If traditional knowledge is presented in a format that young people can understand, they re-evaluate it. So, we produced a magazine with a picture of the grandfather and an article about the elaborate cultivation system that he had developed. This magazine was presented to all the farmers. Only then did they have the courage to go to that farmer and ask him questions. He finally became their teacher. He could only become their teacher because his insightful tradition was validated by a written system of knowledge.

❐

Ayurvedic Medicine

INTRODUCTION

Ayurveda Ayurvedic medicine is a system of traditional medicine native to the Indian subcontinent and practiced in other parts of the world as a form of alternative medicine. In Sanskrit, the word ayurveda consists of the words âyus, meaning "longevity", and veda, meaning "related to knowledge" or "science". Evolving throughout its history, ayurveda remains an influential system of medicine in South Asia. The earliest literature on Indian medical practice appeared during the Vedic period in India. The Sucœruta Sanhitâ and the Charaka Sanhitâ were influential works on traditional medicine during this era. Over the following centuries, Ayurvedic practitioners developed a number of medicinal preparations and surgical procedures for the treatment of various ailments and diseases.

In Western medicine, Ayurveda is classified as a system of complementary and alternative medicine (CAM) that is used to complement, rather than replace, the treatment regimen and relationship that exists between a patient and their existing physician.

Overview

Ayurveda is grounded in a metaphysics of the "five great elements"— all of which compose the Universe, including the human body. Chyle or plasma (called rasa dhatu), blood (rakta dhatu), flesh (mamsa dhatu), fat (medha dhatu), bone (asthi dhatu), marrow (majja dhatu), and semen or female reproductive tissue (shukra dhatu) are held to be the seven primary constituent elements— saptadhatu of the body. Ayurveda deals elaborately with measures of healthful living during the entire span of life and its various phases. Ayurveda stresses a balance of three elemental energies or humors: vata (air & space – "wind"), pitta (fire & water– "bile") and kapha (water & earth – "phlegm"). According to ayurveda, these three regulatory principles— Doshas —are important for health, because when they are in balanced state, the body is healthy, and when imbalanced, the body has diseases. Ayurveda holds that each human possesses a unique combination of Doshas. In ayurveda, the human body perceives attributes of experiences as 20 Guna. Surgery and surgical instruments are employed. It is believed that building a healthy metabolic system, attaining good digestion, and proper excretion leads to vitality. Ayurveda also focuses on exercise, yoga, meditation, and massage.

Thus, body, mind, and spirit/consciousness need to be addressed both individually and in unison for health to ensue.

The practice of Panchakarma is believed to eliminate toxic elements from the body. Eight disciplines of ayurveda treatment, called ashtangas, are given below:

- Internal medicine *(Kaaya-chikitsa)*
- Paediatrics *(Kaumarabhrtyam)*
- Surgery *(Shalya-chikitsa)*
- Eye and ENT *(Shalakya tantra)*
- Demonic possession *(Bhuta vidya)* : Bhuta vidya has been called psychiatry.
- Toxicology *(Agadatantram)*
- Prevention diseases and improving immunity and rejuvenation *(rasayana)*
- Aphrodisiacs and improving health of progeny *(Vajikaranam)*

In Hindu mythology, the origin of Ayurveda medicine is attributed to the physician of the gods, Dhanvantari.

Practices

Balance

Hinduism and Buddhism have been an influence on the development of many of ayurveda's central ideas — particularly its fascination with balance, known in Buddhism as Mâdhyamaka. Balance is emphasized; suppressing natural urges is seen to be unhealthy, and doing so may almost certainly lead to illness. However, people are cautioned to stay within the limits of reasonable balance and measure. For example, emphasis is placed on moderation of food intake, sleep, sexual intercourse, and the intake of medicine.

Diagnosis

The Charaka Samhita recommends a tenfold examination of the patient. The qualities to be judged are:

- constitution
- abnormality
- essence
- stability
- body measurements
- diet suitability
- psychic strength
- digestive capacity

- physical fitness
- age.

In addition, Chopra (2003) identifies five influential criteria for diagnosis:

- origin of the disease
- prodrominal (precursory) symptoms
- typical symptoms of the fully developed disease
- observing the effect of therapeutic procedures
- the pathological process'.

Ayurvedic practitioners approach diagnosis by using all five senses. Hearing is used to observe the condition of breathing and speech. The study of the vital pressure points or marma is of special importance.

Hygiene

Hygiene is an Indian cultural value and a central practice of Ayurvedic medicine. Hygienic living involves regular bathing, cleansing of teeth, skin care, and eye washing. Occasional anointing of the body with oil is also prescribed.

Treatments

Ayurveda stresses the use of plant-based medicines and treatments. Hundreds of plant-based medicines are employed, including cardamom and cinnamon. Some animal products may also be used, for example milk, bones, and gallstones. In addition, fats are used both for consumption and for external use. Minerals, including sulfur, arsenic, lead, copper sulfate and gold are also consumed as prescribed. This practice of adding minerals to herbal medicine is known as rasa shastra.

In some cases, alcohol is used as a narcotic for the patient undergoing an operation. The advent of Islam introduced opium as a narcotic. Both oil and tar are used to stop bleeding. Traumatic bleeding is said to be stopped by four different methods ligation of the blood vessel; cauterisation by heat; using different herbal or animal preparations locally which facilitate clotting; and different medical preparations which constrict the bleeding or oozing vessels. Different oils may be used in a number of ways including regular consumption as a part of food, anointing, smearing, head massage, and prescribed application to infected areas.

Shrotas

Ensuring the proper functions of channels (shrotas) that transport fluids from one point to another is a vital goal of Ayurvedic medicine, because the lack of healthy shrotas is thought to cause rheumatism, epilepsy, paralysis, convulsions, and insanity. Practitioners induce sweating and prescribe steam-based treatments as a means to open up the channels and dilute the Doshas that cause the blockages and lead to disease.

History

Around 1500 BC, ayurveda's fundamental and applied principles got organised and enunciated. Ayurveda traces its origins to the Vedas, Atharvaveda in particular, and is connected to Hindu religion. Atharvaveda (one of the four most ancient books of Indian knowledge, wisdom and culture) contains 114 hymns or formulations for the treatment of diseases. Ayurveda originated in and developed from these hymns. In this sense, ayurveda is considered by some to have divine origin. Indian medicine has a long history, and is one of the oldest organised systems of medicine. Its earliest concepts are set out in the sacred writings called the Vedas, especially in the metrical passages of the Atharvaveda, which may possibly date as far back as the 2nd millennium BC. According to a later writer, the system of medicine was received by a man named Dhanvantari from Brahma, and Dhanvantari was deified as the god of medicine. In later times his status was gradually reduced, until he was credited with having been an earthly king. The Sushruta Samhita of Sushruta appeared during the 1st millennium BC. Dwivedi & Dwivedi (2007) – on the work of the surgeon Sushruta – write:

"The main vehicle of the transmission of knowledge during that period was by oral method. The language used was Sanskrit — the vedic language of that period (2000–500 BC). The most authentic compilation of his teachings and work is presently available in a treatise called Sushruta Samhita. This contains 184 chapters and description of 1, 120 illnesses, 700 medicinal plants, 64 preparations from mineral sources and 57 preparations based on animal sources. "

Underwood & Rhodes (2008) hold that this early phase of traditional Indian medicine identified 'fever (takman), cough, consumption, diarrhea, dropsy, abscesses, seizures, tumours, and skin diseases (including leprosy). Treatment of complex ailments, including angina pectoris, diabetes, hypertension, and stones, also ensued during this period. Plastic surgery, cataract surgery, puncturing to release fluids in the abdomen, extraction of foreign elements, treatment of anal fistulas, treating fractures, amputations, cesarean sections, and stitching of wounds were known. The use of herbs and surgical instruments became widespread. The Charaka Samhita text is arguably the principal classic reference. It gives emphasis to the triune nature of each person: body care, mental regulation, and spiritual/consciousness refinement.

Other early works of ayurveda include the Charaka Samhita, attributed to Charaka. The earliest surviving excavated written material which contains the works of Sushruta is the Bower Manuscript, dated to the 4th century AD. The Bower manuscript quotes directly from Sushruta and is of special interest to historians due to the presence of Indian medicine and its concepts in Central Asia. Vagbhata, the son of a senior doctor by the name of Simhagupta, also compiled his works on traditional medicine. Early ayurveda had a school of physicians and a school of surgeons. Tradition holds that the text Agnivesh tantra, written by the sage Agnivesh, a student of the sage Bharadwaja, influenced the writings of ayurveda.

The Chinese pilgrim Fa Hsien (ca. 337–422 AD) wrote about the health care system of the Gupta empire (320–550) and described the institutional approach of Indian medicine, also visible in the works of Charaka, who mentions a clinic and how it should be equipped. Madhava (fl. 700), Sarngadhara (fl. 1300), and Bhavamisra (fl. 1500) compiled works on Indian medicine. The medical works of both Sushruta and Charaka were translated into the Arabic language during the Abbasid Caliphate (ca. 750). These Arabic works made their way into Europe via intermediaries. In Italy, the Branca family of Sicily and Gaspare Tagliacozzi (Bologna) became familiar with the techniques of Sushruta. British physicians traveled to India to see rhinoplasty being performed by native methods. Reports on Indian rhinoplasty were published in the Gentleman's Magazine in 1794. Joseph Constantine Carpue spent 20 years in India studying local plastic surgery methods. Carpue was able to perform the first major surgery in the western world in 1815. Instruments described in the Sushruta Samhita were further modified in the Western World.

Current status

Within India

In 1970, the Indian Medical Central Council Act which aims to standardize qualifications for ayurveda and provide accredited institutions for its study and research was passed by the Parliament of India. In India, over 100 colleges offer degrees in traditional ayurvedic medicine. The Indian government supports research and teaching in ayurveda through many channels at both the national and state levels, and helps institutionalize traditional medicine so that it can be studied in major towns and cities. The state-sponsored Central Council for Research in Ayurveda and Siddha (CCRAS) is the premier institution for promotion of traditional medicine in India. The studies conducted by this institution encompass clinical, drug, literary, and family welfare research.

To fight biopiracy and unethical patents, the Government of India, in 2001, set up the Traditional Knowledge Digital Library as repository of 1200 formulations of various systems of Indian medicine, such as Ayurveda, Unani and Siddha. The library also has 50 traditional Ayurveda books digitized and available online.

Central Council of Indian Medicine (CCIM) a statutory body established in 1971, under Department of Ayurveda, Yoga and Naturopathy, Unani, Siddha and Homoeopathy (AYUSH), Ministry of Health and Family Welfare, Government of India, monitors higher education in Ayurveda. The Bachelor of Ayurveda, Medicine and Surgery (BAMS) degree is the basic five-and-a- half year course of graduation. It includes eighteen different subjects comprising courses on anatomy with cadaver dissections, physiology, pharmacology, pathology, modern clinical medicine & clinical surgery, pediatrics, along with subjects on ayurveda like Charaka Samhita, history and evolution of ayurveda, identification and usage of herbs (dravyaguna), and ayurvedic philosophy in diagnostics and treatment. Many clinics in urban and rural areas are run by professionals who qualify from these institutes. Mukherjee & Wahile cite World Health Organization statistics to demonstrate the popularity of traditional medicine as the primary system of health care.

Outside India

Academic institutions related to traditional medicine in India have contributed to ayurveda's international visibility. Kurup (2003) comments on the role of Gujarat Ayurved University:

Several international and national initiatives have been formed to legitimize the practice of Ayurvedic medicine as CAM in countries outside India:

- WHO policy of traditional medicine practice
- The US National Centre for Complementary and Alternative Medicine
- The National Ayurvedic Medical Association
- The European Federation for Complementary and Alternative Medicine
- The European Ayurveda Association

In 2009, the United States of America National Centre for Complementary and Alternative Medicine (NCCAM) of the National Institutes of Health expended $1. 2 million of its $123 million annual budget on ayurvedic medicine- related research.

Due to different laws and medical regulations in the rest of the world, the unregulated practice and commercialization of Ayurvedic medicine has raised ethical and legal issues; in some cases, this damages the reputation of Ayurvedic medicine outside India.

Journals

A variety of peer reviewed journals focus on the topic of ayurvedic medicine:

- Ancient Science of Life
- Theoretical and Experimental Journal of Ayurveda and Siddha
- Journal of Research & Education in Indian Medicine (JREIM),
- AYU
- The International Journal for Ayurveda Research

None of the journals except IJAR are PubMed indexed. The first subspeciality journal for the field of Ayurvedic medicine was launched in July 2010. It's focus is rheumatology and it is titled the Journal of Clinical Rheumatology in Ayurveda.

Patents

In December 1993, the University of Mississippi Medical Centre had a patent issued to them by United States Patent and Trademark Office on the use of turmeric for healing. The patent was contested by India's industrial research organization, Council for Scientific and Industrial Research (CSIR), on the grounds that traditional ayurvedic practitioners were already aware of the healing properties of the substance for centuries, and that this prior art made the patent a case of bio-piracy.

The Government of India had become involved in promoting traditional medicine by 1997. R A Mashelkar, director-general of the Indian Council of Scientific and Industrial Research, made the following observation:

"This is a significant development of far-reaching consequences for the protection of the traditional knowledge base in the public domain, which has been an emotional issue for not only the people of India but also for the other third world countries. "

Scientific evidence

As a traditional medicine, many ayurveda products have not been tested in rigorous scientific studies and clinical trials. In India, research in ayurveda is largely undertaken by the statutory body of the Central Government, the Central Council for Research in Ayurveda and Siddha (CCRAS), through a national network of research institutes.

A systematic review of ayurveda treatments for rheumatoid arthritis concluded that there was insufficient evidence, as most of the trials were not done properly, and the one high-quality trial showed no benefits. A review of ayurveda and cardiovascular disease concluded that while the herbal evidence is not yet convincing, the spices are appropriate, some herbs are promising, and yoga is also a promising complementary treatment.

Some ayurvedic products, mainly herbs used for phytotherapy, have been tested with promising results. Studies suggest that Turmeric and its derivative curcumin are antioxidants. Tinspora cordifolia has been tested.

Among the medhya rasayanas (intellect rejuvenation), two varieties of Salvia have been tested in small trials; one trial provided evidence that Salvia lavandulifolia (Spanish sage) may improve word recall in young adults, and another provided evidence that Salvia officinalis (Common sage) may improve symptoms in Alzheimer 's patients. In some cases, ayurvedic medicine may provide clues to therapeutic compounds. For example, derivatives of snake venom have various therapeutic properties. Many plants used as rasayana (rejuvenation) medications are potent antioxidants. Neem appears to have beneficial pharmacological properties.

Mitra & Rangesh (2003) hold that cardamom and cinnamon stimulate digestive enzymes that break down polymeric macromolecules in the human body. Research suggests that T. arjuna is useful in alleviating the of angina pectoris and in treating heart failure and coronary artery disease. T. arjuna may also be useful in treating hypercholesterolemia.

Safety

Rasa shastra, the practice of adding metals, minerals or gems to herbs, is a source of toxic heavy metals such as lead, mercury and arsenic. Adverse reactions to herbs due to their pharmacology are described in traditional ayurvedic texts, but ayurvedic practitioners are reluctant to admit that herbs could be toxic and the reliable information on herbal toxicity is not readily available.

A 2004 study found such toxic metals in 20% of ayurvedic preparations that were made in South Asia for sale around Boston and extrapolated the data to the United States more broadly. It concluded that excess consumption of these products could cause health risks. A 2008 study of more than 230 products found that approximately 20% of remedies (and 40% of rasa shastra medicines) purchased over the Internet from both US and Indian suppliers contained lead, mercury or arsenic.

Traditionally the toxicity of these materials are believed to be reduced through purification processes such as samskaras or shodhanas (for metals), which is similar to the Chinese pao zhi, although the ayurvedic technique is more complex and may involve prayers as well as physical pharmacy techniques. One medical journal reported:

"Crude aconite is an extremely lethal substance, yet ayurveda looks upon it as a therapeutic entity. Crude aconite is always processed, i.e. it undergoes 'samskaras' before being utilised in the Ayurvedic formulations. This study was undertaken in mice, to ascertain whether "processed" aconite is less toxic as compared to the crude or unprocessed one. It was seen that crude aconite was significantly toxic to mice (100% mortality at a dose of 2. 6 mg/mouse) whereas the fully processed aconite was absolutely non-toxic (no mortality at a dose even 8 times as high as that of crude aconite). Further, all the steps in the processing were essential for complete detoxification. "

Following concerns about metal toxicity, the Government of India ruled that ayurvedic products must specify their metallic content directly on the labels of the product. The harmful effects of the samples is attributed in part to the adulterated raw material and lack of workers trained in traditional medicine. In a letter to the Indian Academy of Sciences, director of the Interdisciplinary School of Health Sciences, University of Pune Patwardhan Bhushan stated that the metal adulteration is due to contamination and carelessness during the much faster modern manufacturing processes, and does not occur with traditional methods of preparation.

HERBALISM

Herbalism, also known as medicinal Botany (a neologism by Dr. K. Seshagirirao, University of Hyderabad, India), medical herbalism, herbal medicine, herbology, botanical medicine and phytotherapy, is a traditional medicinal or folk medicine practice based on the use of plants and plant extracts. The bio-informatics related to this subject could be referred to as MedBotanics (Seshagirirao).

Utilizing the healing properties of plants is an ancient practice. People in all continents have long used hundreds, if not thousands, of indigenous plants for treatment of various ailments dating back to prehistory.

There is evidence that suggests Neanderthals living 60,000 years ago in present-day Iraq used plants for medicinal purposes (found at a burial site at Shanidar Cave, Iraq, in which a Neanderthal man was uncovered in 1960. He had been buried with eight species of plants) These plants are still widely used in ethnomedicine around the world.

The first generally accepted use of plants as healing agents was depicted in the cave paintings discovered in the Lascaux caves in France, which have been radiocarbon dated to between 13,000 - 25,000 BC. Anthropologists theorize that over time, and with trial and error, a small base of knowledge would have been acquired within early tribal communities.

As this knowledge base expanded over the generations, the specialized role of the herbalist emerged. The process would likely have occurred in varying manners within a wide diversity of cultures.

Plants have an almost limitless ability to synthesize aromatic substances, most of which are phenols or their oxygen-substituted derivatives such as tannins. Most are secondary metabolites, of which at least 12,000 have been isolated, a number estimated to be less than 10% of the total. In many cases, these substances (esp. alkaloids) serve as plant defense mechanisms against predation by microorganisms, insects, and herbivores. Many of the herbs and spices used by humans to season food yield useful medicinal compounds.

The use of and search for drugs and dietary supplements derived from plants have accelerated in recent years. Pharmacologists, microbiologists, botanists, and natural-products chemists are combing the Earth for phytochemicals and leads that could be developed for treatment of various diseases. In fact, approximately 25% of modern drugs used in the United States have been derived from plants.

The use of herbs to treat disease is almost universal among non-industrialized societies. A number of traditions came to dominate the practice of herbal medicine in the Western world at the end of the twentieth century:

- The Western, based on Greek and Roman sources,
- The Ayurvedic from India, and
- Chinese herbal medicine (Chinese herbology).
- Shamanic Herbalism
- Simple Herbalism.

Many of the pharmaceuticals currently available to Western physicians have a long history of use as herbal remedies, including opium, aspirin, digitalis, and quinine. The World Health Organization (WHO) estimates that 80 percent of the world population, presently use herbal medicine for some aspect of primary health care. Herbal medicine is a major component in all traditional medicine systems and a common element in Ayurvedic, homeopathic, naturopathic, traditional Chinese medicine, and Native American Indian medicine.

According to the WHO, 74% of 119 modern plant-derived pharmaceutical medicines are used in ways that correlated directly with their traditional uses. Major pharmaceutical companies are currently conducting extensive research on plant materials gathered from the rainforests and other places for possible new pharmaceuticals.?

Biological Background

All plants produce chemical compounds as part of their normal metabolic activities. These can be split into primary metabolites, such as sugars and fats, found in all plants, and secondary metabolites found in a smaller range of plants, some only in a particular genus or species.

The autologous functions of secondary metabolites are varied. For example, as toxins to deter predation, or to attract insects for pollination. It is these secondary metabolites which can have therapeutic actions in humans and which can be refined to produce drugs. The word drug itself comes from the Swedish word "druug", which means 'dried plant'. Some examples are inulin from the roots of dahlias, quinine from the cinchona, morphine and codeine from the poppy, and digoxin from the foxglove. The active ingredient in Willow bark, once prescribed by Hippocrates, is salacin, or salicylic acid alpha-hydroxybenzoic acid, C6H4(OH)(COOH). S.A. led to the development of Aspirin, acetyl-salicylic acid, originally a trade name, patented by Bayer.

In 2004 the National Centre for Complementary and Alternative Medicine began funding clinical trials into the effectiveness of herbal medicine.

Surveys of a scientific approach to herbal medicine can be found in the books Evidence-based herbal medicine, and Herbal and traditional medicine: molecular aspects of health.

Popularity

A survey released in May 2004 by the National Centre for Complementary and Alternative Medicine focused on who used complementary and alternative medicines (CAM), what was used, and why it was used. The survey was limited to adults age 18 years and over during 2002 living in the United States. According to this survey, herbal therapy, or use of natural products other than vitamins and minerals, was the most commonly used CAM therapy (18.9%) when all use of prayer was excluded.

Herbal remedies are most common in Europe. In Germany, the term apothecary (Apotheke) is still used, and next to prescription drugs one can order essential oils, herbal extracts, or herbal teas. It is even seen as a preferred treatment over the unnecessary overuse of industrialized production of chemical medication.

In the United Kingdom, the training of medical herbalists is undertaken in private colleges. Recently, Bachelor of Science degrees in herbal medicine are offered at Universities such as University of East London, Middlesex University, University of Central Lancashire, University of Westminster, University of Lincoln and Napier University in Edinburgh.

At UCLAN the training of medical herbalists is extensive, and involves the study of anatomy, physiology, biochemistry, pathology, differential diagnosis etc. This enables the herbalist to be able to talk on equal terms with conventional medical practitioners. They learn about when they can treat, and when they should refer. They study the biochemistry of the body and the chemistry and structure of plants. Alongside this, they study traditional herbal medicine: Indications and Actions, and Energetics. They learn to recognise where conventional medical opinion diverges from traditional herbal medicine doctrine. They look at lots of different models for health care. A significant amount of self reflection is required. A medical herbalist is trained to view a situation from multiple perspectives in a non-dogmatic way.

Types of Herbal Medicines

Medicinal plants can be used by anyone, for example as part of a salad, an herbal tea or supplement, although some herbs considered dangerous are restricted from sale to the public. Sometimes such herbs are provided to professional herbalists by specialist companies. Many herbalists, both professional and amateur, often grow or wildcraft their own herbs. Many common weeds have medicinal properties (e.g. dandelion).

In the herbal "Healing Wise" by Susun S Weed, the three traditions of healing include" the Wise Woman Tradition, the Heroic Tradition, and the Scientific Tradition. The Scientific tradition relies on use of herbal medicines in the form of isolating the active ingredients in herbs, many modern pharmaceuticals are derived from isolating active ingredients from herbs. The Heroic Tradition relies on the belief that the body is dirty and must be cleansed, it promoted the use of purifying herbs and diuretics.

The Wise Woman Tradition uses herbs to nourish and tonify the body, herbs are used in the most natural forms possible, and they are used to support the body in healing itself. Learn more about the Wise Woman Tradition of healing with Herbal Medicine from this article, which includes the Six Steps of Healing by Susun Weed Medicinal herbs can be used in various forms:

Herbal Teas

There are two methods of making herbal teas, infusion and decoction. Infusion is steeping lighter parts of the plant (leaves, flowers, light stems) in boiled water for four to eight hours. Decoction is boiling tougher parts, such as roots or bark for a longer period of time. Herbal teas are often used as a home remedy, and as an alternative to tea and coffee.

Some popular herbal teas include borage, chamomile, dandelion, elderflower, hibiscus, nettle, and various species of mint. Each herb has unique medicinal properties, and a range of secondary effects; and this is linked to its use as a casual drink. For instance, Borage can be used medicinally (amongst other things) as an aid against depression; and it may be drunk more casually to lift the spirits. It was traditionally served as a pep drink for weary travellers. Secondary effects include use as an anti-inflammatory or balsam; and hormonal and metabolic regulation. Other herbs may have similar side-effects, but in different proportions and are used in different ways.

Mixing Herbs: To counteract the various complications and side-effects of an ailment, or to produce a more rounded taste, a number of herbs may be mixed. A well-known mixture used against a cold includes eucalyptus leaf, mint leaf (which contains Menthol) and juniper berry. Another is the age-old favourite "dandelion and burdock", from which the popular fizzy drink was derived.

Fresh or Dried? Many flower and leaf herbs lose volatile compounds within a few hours, as the juices and oils evaporate, the scent leaks away, and the chemicals change their form. Drying concentrates other compounds as water is removed. Most herbal traditions use dried material and the reported effects for each herb tend to be based upon dried herbs unless otherwise specified.

If you are using fresh herbs, you will need more of them, and the tea will have a somewhat different effect. Finely chop the leaf immediately before using it.

Generic Western Tea is usually the leaf of one specific plant, Camelia Sinensis, which grows mainly in India and China. It can be seen as just one of many herbal teas. It is a stimulant, and its main property is to increase alertness, along with a slightly sedative or calming effect. But unlike a fresh herbal tea, it may include artificial additives to enhance the taste and to preserve it in the shops. More expensive recipes include Darjeeling (from Darjeeling in India) and Earl Grey (which has bergamot added).

Making a Nourishing Herbal Infusion

Typically, one ounce by weight (about a cup by volume) of dried herb is placed in a quart jar which is then filled to the top with boiling water, tightly lidded and allowed to steep for 4-10 hours. After straining, a cup or more is consumed, and the remainder chilled to slow spoilage. Drinking 2-4 cups a day is usual. Since the minerals and other phytochemicals in nourishing herbs are made more accessible by drying, dried herbs are considered best for infusions.

Stinging nettle (Urtica dioica) builds energy, strengthens the adrenals, and is said to restore youthful flexibility to blood vessels. A cup of nettle infusion contains 500 milligrams of calcium plus generous amounts of bone-building magnesium, potassium, silicon, boron, and zinc. It is also an excellent source of vitamins A, D, E, and K. For flexible bones, a healthy heart, thick hair, beautiful skin, and lots of energy, make friends with sister stinging nettle. It may make you feel so good you'll jump up and exercise.

Oatstraw (Avena sativa) reduces high cholesterol, increases libido, and strengthens the nerves. A cup of oatstraw infusion contains more than 300 milligrams of calcium plus generous amounts of many other minerals. Its steroidal saponins nourish the pancreas and liver, improving digestion and stabilizing moods. Oatstraw is best known however for its ability to enhance libido and mellow the mood. Do be careful whom you share it with, or you may find yourself sowing some wild oats. In Auryuvedic medicine, oatstraw is considered the finest of all longevity tonics.

Red clover (Trifolium pratense) is better in every way than its cousin soy. It contains four phytoestrogens; soy has only one (isoflavone). Red clover infusion has ten times more phytoestrogens than soy "milk," fewer calories, more calcium, and no added sugars.

Red clover is the world's leading anti-cancer herb; soy isoflavone encourages the growth of breast cancer cells in the lab. Red clover improves the memory; Japanese men who ate tofu twice a week doubled their risk of Alzheimer's disease. Soy beverage can contain up to 1000 times more aluminum than milk, according to Sally Fallon, lipid researcher and fat specialist. She believes that "the highly processed soy foods of today are perpetuating. .. nutrient deficiencies... ."

Comfrey (Symphytum) leaf is free of the compounds (PAs) found in the root that can damage the liver. I have used comfrey leaf infusion regularly for decades with no liver problems, ditto for the group of people at the Henry Doubleday Research Foundation who have eaten cooked comfrey leaves as a vegetable for four generations. Comfrey is also known as "knitbone," and no better ally for the woman with thin bones can be found. And, don't forget, comfrey contains special proteins used in the formation of short-term memory cells. Its soothing mucilage adds flexibility to joints, eyes, vagina, and lungs.

Learn more about Tea and Infusions in the article series Be Your Own Herbal Expert - Tea for you, Infusion for me.

AYURVEDA IN INDIA

Ayurveda in India—the science of life, the origin of most forms of natural and alternative medicine—has its mention in one of the oldest (about 6, 000 years) philosophical texts of the world, the Rig Veda. The Sutrasthana of Charaka Samhita, a much referred ayurvedic text, says; "The three—body, mind and soul—are like a tripod, the world stand by their combination; in them everything abides. It is the subject matter of ayurveda for which the teachings of ayurveda have been revealed. "

In its broader scope, ayurveda in India has always sought to prepare mankind for the realization of the full potential of its self through a psychosomatic integration. A comprehensive health care is what this natural and alternative medicine prescribes for the ultimate self-realization. "Life (ayu) is the combination (samyoga) of body, senses, mind and reincarnating soul. Ayurveda is the most sacred science of life, beneficial to humans both in this world and the world beyond. " —Charaka Samhita, Sutrasthana, 1. 42-43.

The verses of Rig Veda, the earliest source of ayurveda, refer to panchamahabhut (five basic elements of the entire creation), and the three doshas or primary forces of prana or vata (air), agni or pitta (fire) and soma or kapha (water and earth) as comprising the basic principles of ayurveda. One branch of Indian philosophy—Sankhya states that there are 24 elements, all of which constitute the foundation of the gross world: earth, water, fire, air and ether. These five elements in different combinations constitute the three body types/doshas—vata dosha (air and ether), pitta dosha (fire) and kapha dosha (earth and water). The panchamahabhut and the dosha theories are the guiding factors of ayurveda as a therapeutic science. The Rig Veda also mentions organ transplants and herbal remedies called soma with properties of elixir.

This science or knowledge of healing, as mentioned in the Rig Veda, was revealed to Rishi Bharadvaja from the great Cosmic Intelligence. The knowledge consists of three aspects known as the Tri-Sutras of ayurveda, which are— etiology or the science of the causes of disease, symptomatology or the study and interpretation of symptoms and medication and herbal remedies. Approximately, during 4, 000 to 3, 000 BC, Sam Veda and Yajur Veda, the second and third Vedas came into being. Chanting of mantras and performance of rituals were, respectively, dealt in these two Vedas. And, during 3,000 to 2,000 BC Atharva the fourth Veda was authored, of which ayurveda is an upaveda (subsection). Though it had been practiced all along, it was around this time that ayurveda in India, was codified from the oral tradition to book form, as an independent science. It enlists eight branches/divisions of ayurveda: Kayachikitsa (Internal Medicine), Shalakya Tantra (surgery and treatment of head and neck, Ophthalmology and Otolaryngology), Shalya Tantra (Surgery), Agada Tantra (Toxicology), Bhuta Vidya (Psychiatry), Kaumarabhritya (Pediatrics), Rasayana (science of rejuvenation or anti-aging), and Vajikarana (the science of fertility). The oldest treatise available on this codified version is Atreya Samhita.

The most fascinating aspect of ayurveda is, it was using almost all methods of healing like lifestyle regimen, yoga, aroma, meditation, gems, amulets, herbs, diet, jyotishi (astrology), colour and surgery etc. in treating patients. Though ayurveda came into being as an independent upaveda of Atharva Veda, it has close links with other Vedas also. The Yajur Veda, which recommends rituals to pacify the panchamahabhuts in a view to heal both the Cosmic Being and the individual soul, is related to ayurveda in its principles and regulations of lifestyle. The upaveda called Dhanur Veda or the martial arts and ayurveda both refer to each other in the treatment of marmas or sensitive points in the body. Ayurveda recommends specific ayurvedic massages, exercises and bodywork for this purpose.

Around 15, 00 BC ayurveda was delineated into to two distinct schools: Atreya—The School of Physicians, and Dhanvantari—The School of Surgeons. This made ayurveda a more systematically classified medical science, hereafter. Dhanvantari, who is considered to be a reincarnation of Lord Vishnu, was the guiding sage of ayurveda. He made this science of health and longevity popular and widely acceptable. In fact, these two schools of thought led to the writing of two major books on ayurveda—Charaka Samhita and Susruta Samhita.

These two Samhitas were written in the early part of 1000 BC. The great sage-physic in Charaka authored C haraka Samhita revising and supplementing the text written by Atreya, which has remained the most referred ayurvedic text on internal medicine till date. Susruta, following the Dhanvantari School of Thought, wrote Susruta Samhita, comprising the knowledge about prosthetic surgery to replace limbs, cosmetic surgery, caesarian operations and even brain surgery. He is famed for his innovation of cosmetic surgery on nose or rhinoplasty. Around 500 AD, Vagbhatt compiled the third major treatise on ayurveda, Astanga Hridaya. It contained knowledge comprising the two schools of ayurveda.

From 500 AD to 1900 AD, sixteen major Nighantus or supplementary texts on ayurveda like Dhanvantari Bhavaprakasha, Raja and Shaligram among others were written incorporating new drugs, expansion in applications, discarding of old drugs and identification of substitutes. These texts mention about 1814 varieties of plants in vogue.

Evidences show that ayurveda had nurtured almost all the medical systems of the world. The Egyptians learnt about ayurveda long before the invasion of Alexander in the 4th century BC through their sea-trade with India. Greeks and Romans come to know about it after the famous invasion. The Unani form of medical tradition came out of this interaction. In the early part of the first millennium ayurveda spread to the East through Buddhism and greatly influenced the Tibetan and Chinese system of medicine and herbology. Around 323 BC, Nagarjuna, the great monastic of Mahayana Buddhism and an authority on ayurveda had written a review on Susruta Samhita. In 800 AD ayurveda was translated into Arabic. The two Islamic physicians Avicenna and Razi Serapion, who helped form the European tradition of medicine, strictly followed ayurveda. Even, Paracelsus, considered to be the father of the modern western medicine toed the line of ayurveda, as well.

In the postmodern age, the popularity of this vibrant tradition of ayurveda lies in its, subtle yet scientific, approach to heal a person in its totality. It aims, not only at healing the body, but also the mind and spirit, at one go. Its unique understanding of the similarities of natural law and the working of human body, as well as its holistic treatment methods, help it to strike a balance between the two. This gives ayurveda an edge over other healing systems.

Perhaps that's the reason behind ayurveda being the longest unbroken medical tradition in the world, today.

Charaka Samhita

Charaka Samhita is considered to be the most ancient and authoritative writing on ayurveda available today. It also explains the logic and philosophy on which this system of medicine is based. The detailed biography of the composer of this treatise—that is, sage Charaka—is not known to the posterity. Interestingly, it is not an original writing of a single person rather like all Vedic knowledge it is a continuation and renewal of that ancient knowledge system. In fact, Charaka had redacted the Agnivesa Samhita (an edited version of Atreya Samhita). The available form of Charaka Samhita was again worked upon by Drdhabala (living in about 400 AD) long after sage Charaka.

According to Charaka, science is dependent upon yukti—a quality of the intellect that enables it to perceive phenomena brought into existence by a multiplicity of causes. Thus, it's not surprising that much of the treatise of Charaka Samhita is in the form of a symposium wherein groups of ayurvedic scholars take up a series of topics for discussion. This gives indication that the science of ayurveda is a product of constant verification, fine-tuning and authentication by an active community of physicians. The samhita mentions about the gradual development of the fetus within the womb in minutes that equals the modern medical version in accuracy.

The language is Sanskrit and is written in verse form. The style is in keeping with the Vedic oral tradition of conserving knowledge. The samhita contains 8, 400 metrical verses.

Charaka followed the Atreya School of Physicians, which predominantly deals with treatments through internal and external application of medicine. Though the samhita contains all the theoretical knowledge of ayurveda it's focus is on healing the body, mind and soul of a patient in the minimum invasive manner that's Kayachikitsa. Hence, he placed great emphasis on the diagnostic part of the treatment. So much so that he classified everything from solar calendar to topography to the timing of the birth of a child. He identified eight stages of a disease from its inception to the culmination. Charaka also laid great emphasis on the timing and manner of the collection of medicinal plants.

Charaka sought to correct the element of fire or the digestive function in a body. It sought to alter the chemical processes in the cells by purification methods and medicinal application. From a greater perspective Charaka laid emphasis for health and longevity to strike a balance between one's corporeal and spiritual being. That is the reason why Charaka went so detail into the diagnosis of a disease's origin.

Susruta Samhita

Susruta wrote his samhita, the most authentic text on the practice of ayurvedic surgery around the sixth century BC Susruta is, also, renowned as the father of plastic surgery. He represents the Dhanvantari School of surgeons. His samhita discussed in minute details on how to perform prosthetic surgery to replace limbs, cosmetic surgery on nose and on other parts of the body, cesarean operations, setting of compound fractures, and even brain surgery. Susruta's original work seems to have been revised and supplemented by Nagarjuna between the third and fourth centuries AD.

This branch of medicine is believed to have arisen in part from the exigencies of dealing with the effects of war. Epic Ramayana, mentions remarkable feats of surgery having taken place in the past. We have reference to the transplantation of an eyeball and a head in epics.

The style Susruta Samhita is both prose and poetry with poetry being the greater portion. This work, also, is said to be a redaction of oral material passed down verbally from generation to generation.

This work is unique in that it discusses blood in terms of the fourth doshic principle. This work is the first to enumerate and discuss the pitta subtypes. Susruta details about 125 surgical instruments used by him mostly made of stones, wood and other such natural materials. The Susruta Samhita presents many innovations in ayurvedic surgery. Use of shalaka—meaning foreign body (here, rods or a probe etc.) is mentioned by Susruta. Some of the classifications found in the Susruta Samhita are not even traced by the modern medical science. It described five types of pterygium, and the prognosis it made about glaucoma has not been improved since. In fact he is the first surgeon in medical history who systematically and elaborately dealt with anatomical structure of eye. Susruta has discussed about 72 diseases of the eye. He has stipulated drug therapy for various types of conjunctivitis and glaucoma along with surgical procedures of the removal of cataract, pterygium, diseases of ear, nose and throat. The Susruta Samhita, besides being the most authentic text on practice and theory of surgery, is also the most commonly quoted text on health.

Astanga Hridaya

Astanga Hridaya is accepted as the third major treatise on ayurveda. Around 500 AD, Vagbhatt compiled this samhita. It contained knowledge comprising the two schools of ayurveda—the school of surgery and the school of physicians.

There is another similar work called the Astanga Sangraha belonging to the same period. It is slightly bigger in size than the Astanga Hridaya, and is written in verse form whereas the later text was in prose form. It is believed either there are two works by a person or two persons with the same name. However, both the works came into being after the Charaka and Susruta Samhitas.

The Astanga Hridaya primarily deals with kayachikitsa besides, discussing in detail about various surgical treatments. The kapha subtypes are first listed and described in this samhita, completing exhaustive explanation of vata, pitta, kapha with their five subtypes.

Astanga Hridaya seems to emphasize on the physiological aspect of the body rather than the spiritual aspects of it like its counterparts—Charaka and Susruta Samhitas. Despite that, the quality and range of its discussions about ayurveda makes it a work to reckon with.

❒

Herbal Plants

Consumption Pattern

Americans are consuming ever increasing amounts of fresh, frozen, processed and dried culinary herbs and spices, and this trend appears to be here to stay. The same trend is true for specially fruits and vegetables (Fielding 1988). Factors accounting for increased consumption include interest in new foods and tastes, availability of more fresh herbs, advertising and promotion to food services and institutional food chains, and expanding ethnic populations demanding foods and flavourings of their homeland.

Who will be supplying these herbs and are there opportunities for commercial growers in the production of dried and fresh herbs? Much of the dried herbs produced domestically are produced in California by well-established food companies that own and operate drying and processing facilities and already package, transport and market these products. Growth in this area will continue as long as increased demand and consumption of these herbs continue. Additional growth is likely to occur in the contract growing of herbs by private growers to supply raw product to drying and processing companies.

Some companies both grow and process their own product, but most contract practically all of their raw material needs to growers. Processing companies that are now procuring most of their dried herbs abroad may be more willing to obtain some of the same materials domestically Growth in the dried herbal market will also probably occur with an increasing number of spice companies and natural food wholesalers and retailers catering to specialized markets (e.g. organic or pesticide free-herbs and spices, specially restaurants) and which unlike many of the larger food and flavor houses produce specialized herb and other food products.

There has been tremendous growth in the fresh herb market as evidenced by the increased variety of herbs available both in the larger supermarkets,the smaller grocery outlets, farmers markets, and roadside farm markets (Simon

1986, Simon et al. 1989, Simon and Clavio 1989, Simon and Grant 1987a, b). Herbs that were only available dried, or fresh during a few months of the year, are now being marketed fresh cut and more recently, as live potted herbs in the produce sections of supermarkets all year long. Recognizing this growth, the USDA (1989c) now lists weekly prices for herbs sold in nineteen major wholesale markets plus the type of container, package, and weight count, and quality of each unit in the National Market News Report. The herbs now covered include anise, arrugala, basil, borage, chervil, chives, cilantro, dill ginger root horseradish, parsley lemongrass, marjoram, mint, oregano, rosemary savoury, sage, sorrel tarragon, thyme, and watercress.

The successful introduction of new culinary herbs into commercial production requires a purposeful strategy and a solid information base. Unfortunately culinary herbs and essential oil crops have been studied little compared to all other food and fiber crops (Craker et al. 1986). While several extension guides have been published on herbs, few guides based on research are available in this country In a bibliographic review of the scientific literature from 1971-1980 (Simon et al. 1984), over 10,000 authors are listed with published research articles on the major economical herbs of the temperate zone involving horticultural research (38%), botany (17%), chemistry (14%), pharmacology (11%), ecology and germplasm (8%). With the exception of peppermint and spearmint most all crop research on herbs was conducted outside of the United States. Although the United States is the principal world producer of mint oils, only 10% of all published mint research from 1971-1980 originated in the U.S. (Craker et al. 1986).

Promising Herbs

There is a wide range of culinary herbs that can be grown in the continental United States and which may offer potential for production. Many herbs are already being commercially produced, albeit in small quantities, often in relatively small farms. Those herbs which show promise for the fresh market are listed. Three examples of culinary herbs with great promise are discussed below.

Coriander (Coriandrum sativum L): This annual herb native to the eastern Mediterranean and southern European region has long been prized for its spicy aromatic seeds which are used either whole or in ground form as a main ingredient in curry and other food and flavor products. Coriander can be grown as a seed crop in the U.S. using existing mechanization and production technology but seeds ripen unevenly and the mature seeds shatter from the plant. Present demand for coriander seed is met by existing foreign suppliers and although the yield of coriander seed is moderately high (1,100-1,700 kg/ ha) and the cost of production relatively low, there is still a question whether domestic commercial opportunities exist for coriander seed production as a spice. The profit margin of coriander would at best match the more traditional cash crops (maize, soybeans). Postharvest costs of cleaning the seed, handling and shipping can be major factors determining the profitability of this seed spice crop. Coriander seed is also processed via steam distillation for the extractable essential oil of which d-linalool is the major constituent. The oil is then used in the food and perfume industries.

Recently, American consumers have witnessed the introduction of coriander leaves into the marketplace. This fresh product, known as cilantro, is marketed in bunches as a leafy green spice. While new to American cuisine, cilantro has long been a popular herb in Oriental, Middle Eastern and Latin American cooking.

Coriander, a cool season crop, is easy to grow as a culinary herb and is most suited to fertile loam soils. The plant is direct seeded with a seed drill at rates of 13-18 kg/ha in very early spring. In Florida and New Jersey, coriander is often planted weekly At harvest, the whole plant is manually cut and bunched in the field.

One of the major problems in producing cilantro is premature flowering. Bolting becomes acute as the days get hotter and longer. A number of seed companies now offer slow-to-bolt (long-standing) cultivars. There are significant differences among coriander cultivars regarding the response to premature flowering, and while some are less susceptible, none are totally unresponsive to high temperatures and long days (Simon et al. 1989). Thus, cilantro is planted as a spring, early summer, or fall crop.

The aroma of cilantro is also due to an extractable essential oil, although its composition is distinctly different from the seed oil. Quality of fresh cilantro is based upon strong green colour, strong aroma, and visual appearance (i.e. freedom from insects, discolorations). To the grower, yield and the cultivars' resistance to bolt are additional factors to be considered. Cilantro has a relatively short shelf life and requires refrigeration. Cilantro can be kept for 3 to 4 weeks at 0°C, but only 2 to 3 weeks when stored at 5°C (Cantwell 1989).

Cilantro is routinely iced after harvest. Cilantro is expected to become increasingly important in the U.S. due in part to the expanding Hispanic and Arabic populations, its unique flavor, and increasing familiarity in the marketplace.

Sweet Fennel (Foeniculum vulgare Mill.): Sweet fennel has highly aromatic leaves and attractive green fern-like foliage but is best known for its seeds which are sold commercially as a spice. Limited domestic production for seed has occurred periodically, but demand is relatively small and adequate supplies can be obtained abroad. Successful domestic production of fennel for the seed as a spice will probably not occur unless the yields can be significantly improved, supplies from abroad become limited, or a government programme makes the production of new crops more beneficial.

Fennel is a perennial but grown as an annual. It is most suited to well drained light loam soil. The plant is easy to grow and is typically direct seeded (3.5-5 kg/ha seed/acre) into the ground in beds with a specialized planter adapted to small-seeded crops. Plant spacing varies significantly with rows in the beds 60-1 00 cm apart and with final plant stands of 10-3 cm apart in the row. Fennel is a cool-season crop, seeds are sown in early spring and germinate at temperatures >7°C (optimum soil temp. approx. 16-18°C). Yields of up to 2,240 kg/ha have been achieved, although earlier USDA estimates were only in the range of 650-900 kg/ha (Sievers 1948). The plant requires 100-115 days to mature before harvest.

The production of fennel as a culinary herb, cultivated both for its aromatic leaves and enlarged leaf stalk is on the rise. This type, called Florence fennel or finocchio fennel, is a different subspecies than regular fennel produced as a seed spice. Very popular in Europe as a specially vegetable in many culinary dishes, it is commonly consumed raw in Italy and cooked in France. Finocchio is becoming commonplace in U.S. supermarkets and consumer interest and familiarity is increasing. One of the limiting factors to increased consumption is the public's unfamiliarity with it's preparation, use and taste. Unfortunately finocchio fennel is often marketed under the misnomer of anise, another culinary herb (Pimpinella anisum L.), which has led to market and consumer confusion. Both plants contain high amounts of anethole in the essential oil, imparting the licorice-like aroma and taste.

The time to harvest fennel bulbs is difficult to assess because the thickened leaf stalk continues to grow and develop until flowering takes place. Care in harvesting, grading and packing fennel must be taken to ensure a high quality fresh pack. Harvesting, cleaning, trimming and packing is done by hand. The foliage must be dark green and fresh in appearance and the stalk and bulb (enlarged base of leaf stalk) a lighter greenish-white colour. The bulb must be firm and the product free from insects and discolorations. Once harvested, fennel should be kept at 0 to 2°C (Seelig 1974). The plants are retailed individually, either wrapped in plastic or simply displayed like celery.

Great variability (in growth and aroma) in commercially available cultivars of fennel and finocchio fennel exist (Simon et al. 1989) making the proper selection of cultivars for spring and fall production important. Finocchio fennel shows excellent potential for future growth in the U.S.

Oregano (Origanum spp.): Their has been a significant increase in the consumption of oregano for both the fresh and processed market (Tucker 1987). Oregano, the common name for a wide number of plant species with a characteristic aroma and flavor, is a perennial aromatic plant native to the dry calcareous soils of southern Europe, southwest Asia, and the eastern Mediterranean (Simon et al. 1984). A major problem which has limited domestic production was in the difficulty in distinguishing the many plant species and types of oregano imported and marketed as oregano. Imported oregano was found to be derived from 16 plant genera and more than 40 plant species (Calpouzos 1954), resulting in oregano being described as a flavor and aroma rather than an individual plant. Taxonomic work by Tucker (1986, 1989) has identified the major types of commercial cultivars and cultivated taxa in this country and the major types of imported oregano. Yet much of the imported oregano arrives as a blend of plants. Selection of an individual line for domestic production, particularly for the dried leaf or as an essential oil, remains difficult.

The European type of oregano comes mainly from subspecies of O. vulgare L. including ssp. hirtum (Link) Ietswaart, ssp. virens (Hoffmanns. & Link) Ietswaart and ssp. viride (Boiss.) Hayek (Tucker 1989). In contrast Mexican oregano, also called Mexican sage, is principally gathered from the small Mexican shrub, Lippia graveolens H.B.K. (Simon et al. 1984), although leaves from other species are collected.

The essential oil of European oregano is composed mainly of carvacrol and thymol. The range of each can be very wide and many chemotypes are available. The herb or the extracted oil is used in a variety of meat and sausage products, salads, stews, sauces and soups. European oregano and to a larger extent Mexican oregano, are used in flavoring Mexican foods, pizza, and barbecue sauces.

Oregano is generally transplanted to the field and grown on light, dry well-drained soils for periods of 3 to 6 years. Domestic horticultural studies on this species are limited. Although yields of more than 14 tonnes fresh herb/ ha or almost 4 tonnes dried herb/ha were obtained from one commercial line by a single annual harvest (Simon et al. 1989), typically yields are much lower (1.5-3 tonnes dried herb/ha). Plants can be harvested multiple times each year (from 2 to 6) depending upon the location and end-use. Opportunities exist for dried product as well as for the fresh market. Once harvested for the fresh market oregano should be kept at 0deg.C to maximize shelf-life (Cantwell 1989).

Prospects

Production of culinary herbs for the fresh, frozen processed and dried market will likely increase. The large growth in the production of fresh culinary herbs provides opportunities to growers that either develop a market niche or cooperate closely with a broker or specialist in marketing. It is likely that the large volume herbs will continue to come from areas of intensive vegetable production such as Florida, New Jersey and California. Herbs can be expected to become fully integrated with fresh market vegetables in packaging, cooling, transport, and marketing operations. Unless governmental regulations change, there will be strong competition from Mexico, the Caribbean, and other areas to supply fresh herbs to the American public. Overproduction of specific herbs within a limited marketplace can result in significant decreases in the wholesale market prices. Greater opportunities for small producers maybe in the development of specialized markets, rather than for the wholesale trade.

SUPERCRITICAL FLUID EXTRACTION (SFE)

The supercritical fluid extraction (SFE) has been applied only recently to sample preparation on an analytical scale. This technique resembles Soxhlet extraction except that the solvent used is a supercritical fluid, substance above its critical temperature and pressure. This fluid provides a broad range of useful properties. One main advantage of using SFE is the elimination of organic solvents, thus reducing the problems of their storage and disposal in the lipidologist laboratory. Furthermore, several legislative protocols (such as the EPA Pollution Prevention Act in the USA) have focused on advocating a reduction in the use of organic solvents which could be harmful to the environment.

Besides ecological benefits, one of the most interesting properties of SFE is the high diffusion coefficients of lipids in supercritical fluids, far greater than in conventional liquid solvents. Thus, the extraction rates are enhanced and less degradation of solutes occurs.

Several studies have shown that SFE is a replacement method for traditional gravimetric techniques. In addition, carbon dioxide, which is the most adopted supercritical fluid has low cost, is a nonflammable compound and devoid of oxygen, thus protecting lipid samples against any oxidative degradation.

PRINCIPLES FOR THE ANALYTICAL SFE OF LIPIDS

The first guiding principle is the optimization of the solubility of lipids in supercritical CO2 and the improvement of the fractionation with respect to a particular lipid species.

Important data on the solubility of vegetal oils and other lipids may be found in the detailed study of Stahl et al. (Dense gases for extraction and refining, Springer Verlag, Heidelberg, 1987). These data have led to perform oil and fat extractions above 600 bar and temperatures from 80 to 100°C.

It should be emphasized that many lipid solutes have similar solubility parameters, making their separation by SFE difficult. An improvement in the separation of complex lipid mixture may be found by the integration of adsorbent compound into the extraction cell with the sample. Several compounds such as alumina, silica, Celite, Florisil or synthetic resins were proposed for the optimization of lipid differential extraction.

The improvement of lipid SFE needs also the study of the kinetics of the lipid removal from the sample matrix. It must be noticed that the fast back-diffusion of analytes in the supercritical fluid reduces the extraction time since the complete extraction step is performed in about 20 min instead of several hours.

A common practice in SFE, which must be mentioned in connection with the physicochemical properties of supercritical fluids, is the use of modifiers (co-solvents). These are compounds that are added to the primary fluid to enhance extraction efficiency. Thus, the addition of 1 to 10% of methanol or ethanol to CO2 expands its extraction range to include more polar lipids. When the extraction was performed with supercritical carbon dioxide and 20% of ethanol, more than 80% of the phospholipids were recovered from salmon roe (Tanaka Y et al., J Oleo Sci 2004, 53, 417).

INSTRUMENTATION

Those wishing to build their own experimental equipment should read t he d et a i le d st ud y of H a w th or ne e t a l . (i n P r a c ti ca l su pe rc ri ti ca l chromatography and extraction, Caude M., Thiebaut D, Eds, Harwood Academic, 1999).

ISCO Inc was one of the first companies to address the off-line SFE market. Extraction cells of 0.5 up to 15 ml are offered.

An automatic version permits automated valve operation for extraction of one or two samples and another model permits 24 samples to be automatically and sequentially extracted. ISCO has also offered a extraction system (FastFat HT) specifically made for the rapid determination of fat content in foods and agriculture products ("The Isco FastFat HT provides rapid, accurate % fat determination in a wide range of foods- a critical parameter in quality control, product labeling, and calibrating on-line process control equipment. With FastFat HT, you get reliable results in minutes, and eliminate costly delays in production decisions").

Applied Separation offers several extraction units offering great flexibility with respect to sample size and experimental design. Extractor cell sizes can range from several ml to one liter. Off-line and in-line trapping of solutes may be realized.

IECO Corporation is offering a total fat analyzer designed with a triple parallel channel system ("LECO's new TFE2000 Fat/Oil Determinator is specifically designed to determine fat/oil content and eliminate the need for hazardous chemicals used in Soxhlet, Mojonnier/Roese-Gottlieb, acid hydrolysis, and other solvent extraction methods.

Using inexpensive compressed CO_2 as the solvent, the analyte is extracted from the sample and transferred to the removable ultra efficient solid phase collection traps. Precise calculations are determined by the integrated balance based on sample weight, and the before and after weights of the collection vials"). Application notes may be found on the LECO site.

The use of high purity SFE-grade CO_2 is not required but impurity and moisture in industrial grade CO_2 can accumulate and may interfere with further analytical operations (gas or liquid chromatography).

Thus, an on-line fluid cleanup system may be used to remove trace contaminants.

Extractions can be performed in static, dynamic or recirculating mode. During static extraction, the cell is filled with the supercritical fluid, pressurized and allowed to equilibrate. In the dynalic mode, the fluid is run continuously through the cell, and in the recirculating mode, the same fluid is repeatedly pumped in the cell before being pumped out to the collection vial.

IMPORTANT PARAMETERS

A. *Sample Matrix:* The levels of lipid content and moisture are important for the analytical process. Lipid levels may be from 1 up to 50% (w/w).

B. *Sample Preparation:* Moisture may inhibit contact between extraction fluid and sample. Thus, removal of water by freeze drying is recommended prior to SFE.
It may be also efficient to disperse the sample matrix, to grind the sample to increase the mass transfer of lipids. The choice of drying agent can be made by consulting the study of Bulford (Bulford MD et al., J chromatogr A 1993, 657, 413).

C. *Collection of the Lipid Extract:* The collection method for the resultant extract must be optimized to avoid incomplete extraction. The open vials are most frequently used, a sub-ambient cooling being useful for volatile species. It is best to use a collection vial packed with a surface area material, i.e. glass beads, glass wool (Snyder J. M. et al., JAOCS 1994, 71, 261) or containing some volume of a chosen solvent. The supercritical CO2 can be separated from the collected analytes without trouble or disposal problems.

APPLICATION OF SFE TO LIPIDS

Several reviews were devoted to the application of SFE for the extraction of lipids in various sample types. Those of Clifford A et al. (in Supercritical fluid technology in oil and lipid chemistry, AOCS Press, chap. 19, 1996), Eller FJ et al. (Sem Food Technol 1996, 1, 145) and King J.W. (Grasas y Aceites 2002, 53, 8) should be consulted for specific applications.

Food and various agricultural products were successfully analyzed for their fat and levels by SFE. Progressively, SFE may be regarded as an alternative to organic solvent extraction methods. The extraction efficiencies of SFE and organic solvent methods (Soxhlet or liquid-liquid extractions) were frequently compared and shown to be in good agreement (Eller FJ et al., J Agric Food Chem 1998, 46, 3657). It must be noticed that gravimetric-based results can be influenced by the sample matrix, the moisture and non-lipid moieties and the extraction solvent.

Total fat determinations were done in meat products with two different extractors and compared with a standard method (Berg H et al., J AOAC Int 2002, 85, 1064). The amount and the composition agreed well with results from the standard procedure. To obtain quantitative recoveries by SFE, 1 ml ethanol was added to 1 g sample in the extraction cells before extraction.

Extracting conditions largely affected the composition of dissolved lipids in freeze-dried animal samples (Tanaka Y et al., J Oleo Sci 2003, 52, 295). Thus, one group of triglycerides was extracted from salmon roe while another group remained in the matrix together with phospholipids and a large part of astaxanthin. It is now well known that the extraction yield and composition of triglycrides depend on the extracting conditions. This was verified for the extraction of oil from seaweed (Cheung PCK et al., J Agric Food Chem 1998, 46, 4228), tomato seeds (Bhupesh CR et al., J Food Sci Technol 1996, 31, 137) or soyabean oil (Snyder JM et al., JAOCS 1984, 61, 1851).

The extraction and separation of phospholipids from tuna fish have been described using various concentrations of methanol in supercritical CO_2 (Tanaka Y et al., J Oleo Sci 2005, 54, 569). Good recovery of DHA-rich phospholipids were claimed in a series of industrial processes.

A detailed description of a relia ble procedure a dapted for the determination of total fat in milk- and soy-based infant formula powder has been published by LaCroix DE et al. (J AOAC Int 2003, 86, 86).

The extraction of a specific lipid moiety is generally influenced by substances which are co-extracted, all having a high solubility in supercritical CO_2.

One technique to overcome this problem is to use a sorbent to retard the analyte of interest, the interfering substances being removed first. Then, a higher CO_2 extraction density or a co-solvent is used to removed the analyte of interest from the sorbent. Thus, it was shown that NH2-bonded silica is able to retard sterols.

Analytical SFE has also been used for lipid-derived volatiles such as aroma in various food samples. For the application of SFE to the study of total fat and lipid classes in meats, the studies of Berg H et al. (J Chromatogr A 1997, 785, 345) and Chandrasekar R. (JAOAC int 2001, 84, 466) should be consulted.

FIELD OF THE INVENTION

The extraction of the principal significant components of herb and spice plants containing pigment, flavor, and aroma and, when present in the starting material, antioxidant, using edible, food-grade solvent.

Of especial interest is the extraction of the principal significant components of spices and herbs represented by plants of the family Solanaceae, representatively Capsicums such as paprika, red pepper, and chili, and Lycopersicon, representatively tomato, all containing carotenoid pigments; Umbelliferae, representatively celery, lovage, dill, carrot, cilantro, fennel, cumin, caraway, parsley, angelica, and anise; Compositae, representatively marigold, artemisia, and tarragon; Leguminosae, representatively fenugreek; Labiatae, representatively rosemary, thyme, sage, oregano, marjoram, mint, savoury, and basil; Zingerberacae representatively ginger, cardamom, and turmeric, Lauraceae, representatively laurel, cinnamon, cassia, and bay; Myrtaceae, representatively allspice and clove; of the genus Myristica, representatively mace and nutmeg; of the genus Piper, representatively black and white pepper; of the genus Vanilla, representatively vanilla; of the genus Allium, representatively onion and garlic; of the genus Sesamum, representatively sesame seed; Cruciferae, representatively mustard and horseradish; the defining characteristic being that it is of a spice or herb plant material from which flavor, aroma, colour, and/or antioxidant can be extracted and used to flavor and/or colour foods and beverages or otherwise employed to enhance the palatability of foods and beverages.

BACKGROUND OF THE INVENTION AND PRIOR ART

The present invention relates to a method of increasing the stability and reducing the microbial counts of both spice or herb oleoresin and the residual cake from which the oleoresin has been extracted. The process simultaneously extracts and concentrates the principal flavor, aroma, colour, and other active components, produces a concentrated and standardized food-grade extract of active components, and a standardized food-grade residual solid, with both the extract and residual solids having significantly reduced microbial counts and frequently also improved stability.

Concentrated extracts of spices and herbs are universally used for flavoring and coloring of food, beverages, and pharmaceuticals. These extracts are traditionally used where a standardized, sterile, and uniform concentrate offers the benefits of control which are inherently difficult to obtain from raw spice or herb, or where the bulk of the raw material is not needed or undesirable.

Ground spice and herb solids are universally used for flavoring, coloring, and imparting otherwise favourable characteristics to food and beverages where the bulk, functional characteristics, and appearance of the food or beverage is important.

Dried spices and herbs, most often in their ground form, are used in the preparation of food and beverages to add flavor, aroma, colour, and preservative properties that make the food more palatable and appealing. The dried spices, ground or unground, are usually added to the food or beverage during preparation at such a point in the preparation that time is allowed for the principal components of interest to be extracted into the food or beverage to impart the desired combination of attributes to the food or beverage. Further, as spices and herbs are notoriously known to have inconsistent levels of the flavor, aroma, colour, or antioxidants, it is commonly required that spices of varying levels of the principal components of interest be blended to make a final product that is consistent with regard to the principal components of interest to achieve predictable and repeatable performance with respect to the flavor, aroma, colour, or antioxidant release into the food or beverage system in which they are used. This is a costly and time consuming process.

As suggested in prior art, much of the flavor, aroma, and/or colour often is not effectively transferred to the food or beverage. U.S. Pat. No. 2,507,084 overcomes this obstacle of under-utilization of the principal components of interest by first extracting the principal components of interest and subsequently coating the spent spice from the extraction process with a portion of the extract originally removed, thereby extending the useful amount of flavor and aroma that can be derived from a given quantity of spice. It is also disclosed that this process derives value from the exhausted spice solids, from which the flavor, aroma, colour, or antioxidants have been removed, which would otherwise be a waste product. This is a complicated and costly process for recovery of the maximum value of the spice and its principal components of interest.

Traditional extraction processes for the manufacture of concentrated extracts (concentrated several fold as compared with the raw material) involve not only the use of various non-edible solvent systems, but also a large proportion of solvent in relation to the compounds of interest. Many require the use of petroleum distillates, chlorinated solvents, or highly flammable solvents which must be eliminated almost completely from the finished products to make them safe for consumption. These systems require expensive distillation equipment and special precautions must be taken to ensure worker safety and to limit environmental impact.

The intensive processing required often destroys, modifies, or loses some of the more unstable compounds, delicate aromas, flavours, or pigments. More significantly, the last traces of undesirable non-edible solvents are very difficult to separate from the concentrated extract. The residual solid must necessarily contain the same residual non-edible solvents, which are removed only with difficulty. Such residual solvents limit the potential use of the residual solid for human consumption, and are potential environmental contaminants.

Other concentration techniques rely on high pressure equipment to obtain good solvating properties from gases, e.g., liquid or supercritical CO2 (U.S. Pat. No. 4,490,398). High pressure liquefied or supercritical gas extraction requires expensive equipment and has limited solvating abilities for some compounds requiring the addition of cosolvents, or solvents such as propane and butane, which are also difficult to control and may be environmentally sensitive or undesirable in a finished product.

Following extraction and desolventization, the concentrated extract is often standardized with edible solvents and emulsifiers to provide a concentrate with reproducible levels of the active or principal compounds of interest to the user. In an effort to overcome the shortcomings and risks associated with the above-mentioned processes, extraction has been carried out using edible solvents such as vegetable oils or lard. Typical extraction procedures are disclosed in U.S. Pat. Nos. 3,732,111; 2,571,867; and 2,571,948. These methods require a relatively large volume of solvent in relation to the compounds of interest and result in a dilute extract which is limited in its application and which has few of the advantages of the concentrates which can be produced using volatile solvents.

U.S. Pat. No. 4,681,769 discloses a method for simultaneously extracting and concentrating in a series of high pressure countercurrent mechanical presses using relatively small amounts of vegetable oil as the solvent in an attempt to overcome the problem of dilution inherent in earlier processes. This method suffers from severe limitations in temperature and pressure ranges in an attempt to avoid unacceptable oxidative damage, colour loss, yield losses, and flavor changes with the final result being that contact times must be unduly extended for up to 16-24 hours, adding greatly to the cost of the process. Extraction cycle times are unduly long for a given size pressing operation, and the process does not provide for a controlled degree of browning or for sterilization of the extract or of the residual solid. It is also limited to temperatures of less than 100° F. to avoid alleged undue oxidation and thus it does not allow for the use of edible solvents which have a melting point of more than 100° F. or which are highly viscous at temperatures of less than 100° F. Maximum pressures of up to about 500 PSI (cone pressure) are claimed and this severely limits the efficiency and throughput rate for a given size pressing operation, as shown by the disclosure of this patent.

Traditional methods for the sterilization of ground spices and herbs involve the use of extremely toxic substances such as ethylene oxide or methyl bromide, irradiation, or steam and moisture treatment to reduce plate counts to less than 100,000. Chemical sterilization and irradiation of spices and herbs are disagreeable to the consumer because of the perceived risk of residual chemicals and/or radiation remaining in the plant matter and, as a result, several processes using added moisture, such as water or steam, at elevated pressures have been developed as alternatives. Typical sterilization procedures are disclosed in U.S. Pat. Nos. 4,210,678, 4,790,995, and 4,910,027. All sterilization processes are inherently costly in that they require a separate processing step or steps to accomplish the sterilization, and also present the possibility of further degrading the more unstable components. Addition of moisture or water vapour, as disclosed in U.S. Pat. Nos. 4,210,678 and 4,910,027, prior to or during the heating and sterilization process results in a cooked aroma not typical of the fresh, dehydrated spice or herb and also results in steam distillation and loss of some of the volatile flavor and aroma constituents.

U.S. Pat. Nos. 4,790,995 and 4,910,027 require the addition of a coating of animal protein to protect the spice from the loss of volatile aroma compounds during the sterilization process with water vapour. U.S. Pat. No. 4,210,678 requires bringing the moisture of the spice to above 8-14%, in some cases up to 16-20%, and holding the spice for an extended period of time prior to sterilization to equilibrate the moisture. This additional step is costly and time consuming. In the case of Capsicums, severe browning and off aromas and flavours are developed in the presence of moistures in excess of 10% at elevated temperatures above 180° F.

Traditional methods for controlling the brownness or degree of caramelization of Capsicum solid to enhance its visual appearance involve the use of elevated temperatures and the addition of vegetable or animal fats or oils to bring up the surface colour and luster of the ground spice. This requires a separate and costly processing operation.

Above all, there is the unsolved problem of obtaining satisfactory yields, quality, and throughput rates of acceptable extract having an acceptable content of active principle in the edible solvent without undesirable oxidative damage to, and reduced stability of, the principal compounds of interest, while at the same time providing for simultaneous sterilization of both the herb or spice solid and extract.

Obviously, existing prior art procedures leave much to be desired, and it is a primary objective of the present invention to provide a procedure for the production of sterilized spice and herb products having enhanced stability and which otherwise obviates the shortcomings of the prior art.

AROMATHERAPY VS. "NORMAL" MEDICINE

Many people take Aspirin for headaches although many tests have proven that Aspirin can cause stomach upsets, thin the blood, cause liver damage and contribute to anaemia. Yet people take many of these a day to relieve headaches, and think they are safe.

Antibiotics are used for infections because they kill bacteria. However there are good bacteria living in our bodies, without which our bodies can not work efficiently. Antibiotics kill off all bacteria, and many people suffer from thrush and other illnesses as a result. The other concern with antibiotics is that each time they are used, the body builds up a resistance to them, much the same way our bodies build up a resistance to the Smallpox or Measles virus when we are vaccinated. Stronger doses of antibiotics are then needed to fight the infections, and the circle continues.

Aromatherapy works on the wholistic approach. It treats the whole body at the one time. Aromatherapy has no negative side effects when used properly, and is non- addictive.

AROMATHERAPY EXPLAINED (SIMPLY)

People think of Aromatherapy as being smell therapy, but this isn't the case. The essential oils can used in many different methods, I will be explaining those later... but the reason people think of them as being smell therapy, is that the blood vessels in your nose are very close the surface of your skin.... so the molecules of "healing goodness" can be absorbed into the body quickly (and they do smell nice...well....some of them!) the healing effects can also pass through the skin anywhere on your body, and enter the blood stream, where they work on the troubled areas of the body.

Essential oils, unlike prescription drugs, work only on those areas that are "broken" i.e. they do not go into healthy tissues, and start working there... they travel around your body, and look for the illnesses, and target them, leaving the rest of your body alone. It is because of this, that if you run lavender oil into your fingertip, it will help your infected toe...even though the oil never touches the actual toe. (and your headache, and cut finger!!!).

USING ESSENTIAL OILS

There are 8 main ways to use the Essential oils, they are as follows:

Inhalation:

(1) Straight from the bottle—Headache, memory booster, nausea etc.

(2) Oil burner—Kill airborne bacteria (prevents colds spreading to others), insomnia, stress etc. Put 3-5 drops in a water filled well of the oil burner, and replace as needed. NEVER burn Essential oils without water... it damages them

(3) Drops on a tissue (carry with you or place under pillow etc.)—colds, coughs, migraine etc. 1-2 drops on a tissue will be ample

(4) Drops in sink/bowl of hot water—colds, respiratory infection, catarrh (runny nose) etc. stick your head over the sink/bowl, with eyes closed and inhale the vapour. No more than 5 drops to half a sink full of water (which is all you need)

Bat:

(1) Hot/warm bath—colds, muscle cramp, stiffness etc. 10 drops Maximum

(2) Cold bath—Fever. 10 drops Maximum

(3) Foot bath—Athlete's foot, blisters, aching feet etc. Use a bucket or bowl big enough to comfortably put your feet in. 5 drops Maximum

(4) Shallow bath—Thrush, Piles etc. a bath deep enough to cover the problem area. 5 drops maximum

If using peppermint oil, you may want to use only half the recommend drops.... as my Aromatherapy teacher said "It runs amok amongst your genitals" it has a cooling effect that you may not wish to have touching sensitive areas.

You will need to swish the water around. There is a product called Solubalizer that may be useful. It makes the oil dissolve in water, although the same effect can be to mix the oil with isopropyl alcohol (rubbing alcohol) or vodka, which will make it water soluble. 5 drops to 1tsp alcohol. I have also heard that the same effect can be achieved with milk, but I am not sure.

Massage:

(1) Massage diluted oil onto effected area - varicose veins, strains, constipation Muscle aches etc.

(2) Massage diluted oil all over body - Stress, insomnia, anxiety etc.

Both, use a 3% dilution for normal skin, 1% for face or sensitive skin (explained further below).

Internally: Most Essential oils are toxic and should NEVER be taken internally. It is safest to assume that ALL Essential oils are toxic and therefore none should be taken internally.

Many Aromatherapy books suggest a mouth wash or a gargle for gum problems or throat infections, however it is dangerous and other methods ork just as well. There are many different species of the same oil, for example

Birch has 2 varieties, white and sweet.

White birch is non-toxic, but sweet birch is fatally toxic. I would not use ANY Essential oils internally, especially in their pure state, as there are many other methods of application which are much safer. {as I was saying in a previous section, even rubbing an oil on your toe will help a sore throat, so it isn't worth ingesting something that is potentially harmful, although I have gargled with 2 drops Bergamot oil mixed with a cup of warm water}

Directly To The Skin: There are only four Essential oils which may safely be applied directly onto the skin an all should have a patch test done first. All essential oils are acidic, have you ever seen what they do to plastic?

Place a drop of the oil onto the back of your wrist, cover with a Band- Aid and leave for 1 hour. If no irritation has occurred you may use it. If irritation does occur, bathe the area in cool water and dilute the oil with a carrier oil. Only the four Essential oils listed below may be applied to skin directly, and only onto an effected area i.e. a cut or burn. Do not use as a massage oil, or slather it all over your skin:

Lavender, Sandalwood, Tea tree and some say Lemon, ylang ylang or Chamomile.

There is no need to apply any essential oil directly onto the skin, an essential oil blended 3% into a carrier oil will have exactly the same healing properties as a full strength oil... so not only do you run the risk of burning the skin by applying them neat, you are also wasting oil:)—Scrooge McObsidian here:)

(1) Drops of oil in cold water for cold compress - fever, swelling etc. (2). Drops of oil in hot water for hot compress - Headache, period pain etc.

To make a compress, half fill a bowl or sink of either hot or cold water, and add 3-5 drops of essential oil.... soak the cloth in this water for a few moments, wring out, and apply to the effected area.

Perfume:

(1) Use same dilution as massage oil, use a carrier oil of Apricot kernel or other light oil. Dab behind ears, wrists etc.

Skin/Hair Tonic:

(1) Use this when an oil is not suitable, for example on an oily scalp, or to dry out a cut. use 5 drops essential oil into a teaspoon of Isopropyl alcohol (rubbing alcohol) or vodka Dilutions:

Babies 0-12 months—1 drop of Rose or Lavender or chamomile in 1 teaspoon of carrier oil, or in a bath.

Infants 1-5 years - 2-3 drops of Rose, Lavender, Chamomile, Sandalwood, Tangerine, Ylang Ylang or Neroli in 1 teaspoon of carrier oil or in a bath.

Children 6-12 years -Use as for adults, but half the concentration.

3% dilution:

For 100 mls of carrier oil use 60 drops of Essential oil. For 25 mls of carrier oil use 15 drops of Essential oil.

For 5 mls of carrier oil (1 teaspoon) use 3 drops of Essential oil. 1% dilution:

For 100 mls of carrier oil use 20 drops of Essential oil. For 25 mls of carrier oil use 5 drops of Essential oil.

For 5 mls of carrier oil (1 tsp) use 1 drop of Essential oil. For normal use do not exceed 3% Essential oil dilution.

For use on face or other sensitive skin use a 1% Essential oil dilution.

Pregnancy - use half the dilution and none of the contraindicated oils.

Contraindications

Aromatherapy oils are concentrated and should not be applied to the skin or taken internally.

There are also other times when Essential oils should be treated with caution or not be used at all, these are called Contraindications. The following is a list of the contraindications for the various Essential oils.

Oils not to be Used at All: These oils are dangerous for anyone except a qualified Aromatherapist to use. They are either extremely toxic or cause severe skin irritation even in a diluted state. These oils are:

Bitter Almond, Arnica, Boldo, Broom, Buchu, Calamus, Camphor (brown & Yellow), Cassia, Chervil, Cinnamon (bark), Costus, Deertongue, Elecampane,

Fennel (bitter), Horseradish, Jaborandi, Melilotus, Mugwort, Mustard, Oregano,

Pennyroyal, Pine (dwarf), Rue, Sage (common), Santolina, Sassafras, Savine,

Savoury, Tansy, Thuja, Thyme (red), Tonka, Wintergreen, Wormseed and Wormwood.

Oils that should be Used in Small Doses for no Longer Than 2 Weeks: These oils are fairly toxic or may have side effects such as nausea, vomiting and headaches and should be used with extreme caution:

Ajowan, Anise star, Aniseed, Basil (exotic), Bay laurel, Bay (west indian) Calamintha, Camphor (white), Cascarrilla bark, Cassie, Cedarwood (virginian), Cinnamon (leaf & bark), Clove (bud), Coriander, Eucalyptus, Fennel (sweet), Hops, Hyssop, Juniper, Nutmeg, Parsley, Pepper (black), Pine, Sage (spanish), Tagetes, Tarragon, Thyme (white), Tuberose, Tumeric, Turpentine and Valerian.

Oils that Irritate the Skin if Used in High Concentration: These oils should be used in half the recommended dilution, and no more than 3 drops.

Borneol, Cajeput, Caraway, Cedarwood (Virginian), Cinnamon (leaf), Clove (bud), Cornmint, Eucalyptus, Garlic, Ginger, Lemon, Parsley, peppermint, Pine (needle, Scotch & Longleaf), Thyme (white) and Tumeric.

Oils that Cause Irritation on Sensitive Skin: These oils may cause eczema or dermatitis with people who have very sensitive skin. (For people with senstive skin always test the oil on the back of your wrist, and leave for an hour. If irritation occurs bathe area with cold water and try a weaker concentration.) These oils are:

Aniseed, Basil (french), Bay laurel, Benzoin, Bergamot, Cade, Cajeput, Cananga, cedarwood (virginian), Chamomile (Roman and German), Citronella, Garlic, Geranium, Ginger, Hops, Jasmine, Lemon, Lemongrass, Lemon balm (Melissa), Litsea cubeba, Loveage, Mastic, Mint (pepper & spear), Orange, Peru balsam, Pine (scotch & longleaf), Styrax, Tea tree, Thyme (white), Tolu balsam, Tumeric, Turpentine, Valerian, Vanilla, Verbena, Violet, Yarrow and Ylang Ylang.

Oils that are Phototoxic: These are oils which can cause the skin to darken if exposed to direct sunlight. Do not use these oils at all if the area will be exposed to sunlight. These oils are:

Angelica root, Bergamot, Cumin, Ginger, Lemon, Lime, Loveage, Mandarin, Orange and Verbena.

Oils that should be Avoided during Pregnancy: Due to the effects of these oils on the reproductive organs, and the sensitivity of the foetus, certain oils should not be used at all during pregnancy. These oils are:

Ajowan, Anjelica, Anise star, Aniseed, Basil, Bay laurel, Calamintha, Cedarwood (all types), Celery seed, Cinnamon (leaf), Citronella, Clary sage, Clove, Cumin, Cypress, Fennel (sweet), Hyssop, Jasmine, Juniper, Labdanum, lovage, Marjoram, Myrrh, Nutmeg, Parsley, Penyroyal, Peppermint, Rose, Rosemary, Snakeroot, sage, Tarragon and Thyme (white).

Oils that should be Avoided with High Blood Pressure: These oils should not be used:

Black pepper, Hyssop, Lemon, Lemongrass, Nutmeg, Rosemary, Sage (spanish & Common) and Thyme.

Oils that should be avoided with low blood pressure. - These oils should not be used:

Chamomile (Roman & German), Lemon balm, Lavender (true), Marjoram (sweet) and Ylang ylang.

The oil that should be avoided for diabetes. Anjelica.

The oil that should be avoided for kidney problems. Juniper.

Oils that should be not be Used with Homeopathic Treatments: These oils are not to be used by anyone receiving homeopathic treatment:

Black pepper, camphor, eucalyptus and peppermint.

Oils that should be Avoided with Alcohol Consumption: These oils will increase the effects of alcohol:

Aniseed, clary sage and fennel.

The oil that should be avoided with depression. Basil.

Oils that should be Avoided with Epilepsy: These oils should not be used: Fennel, Hyssop, Sage and Rosemary.

THE COMMON ESSENTIAL OILS

The following information has been gathered from many books over many years. Some oils work by promoting balance, which is why they are listed as working well with things such as oily skin and dry skin. What this means is that if your skin is oily, it will help dry it out, if it is dry it will help add moisture. In other words, it will balance.

Different sources will give different properties to the Essential oils - some may even contradict others. It is for this reason that it is best to leave Aromatherapy to trained professionals. The following information is not intended to prescribe or diagnose in any way.

It is not meant to be a substitute for professional medical advice/ assistance. The intention of this list is to give information on the historical usage of Aromatherapy.

Please consult your doctor or other health professional if you have any medical complaints. Do not attempt to self diagnose or self prescribe herbal treatments for yourself or others. The Author (Obsidian) shall not be responsible for any misuse or abuse of this information.

Aniseed

Botanical Name: Pimpinella Anisum

Note - Top to middle

Type - Spice

Family - Umbelliferae

Part - Herbs/seeds

Extraction - Steam Distillation

Aroma: Sweet and spicy, pungent, Licorice like, very warming.

Blends well With: Amyris, Bay, Cardamon, Caraway, Cedarwood, Coriander, Dill, Fennel, Galbanum, Mandarin, Petitgrain, Rose wood.

Contraindications: Sensitive skin, Pregnancy, Over use can cause sluggishness, drowsiness and dizziness. In extreme cases can cause cerebral congestion and circulatory problems.

Parasiticide, Antiemetic, Aphrodisiac, Cardiac, Digestive aid, Diuretic, Expectorant, Galactagogue, Insecticide, Laxative, Parturient, Pectoral stimulant, Stomachic.

Uses: Respiratory problems, Digestive problems, Flatulence, Indigestion, Period pains, Stimulate lactation, Lice, Scabies, Muscular aches and pains, Rheumatism, Bronchitis, Coughs, Colic, Cramp, Colds, Stimulate the mind, Dyspepsia, Nausea, Vomiting, Stimulating peristalsis, Oliguria (low quantity of urine), Stimulates cardiac fatigue, Lice, Scabies, Infectious skin diseases.

Cautions: Not generally recommended for use in the home as prolonged or over use may be harmful.

Basil (Sweet)

Botanical Name: Omicum Basilicum

Note - top Type - Herb Family - Labiatae

Part - Flowering top

Extraction - Steam Distillation

Aroma: Very clear, sweet and slightly spicy.

Blends well With: Bergamot, Black pepper, Citronella, Chamomile, Clary Sage, Geranium, Hyssop, Lavender, Lemongrass, Lime, Marjoram, Melissa, Neroli, Peppermint, Rose, Sandalwood, Verbena.

Contraindications: Pregnancy, Sensitive skin, Do not use to excess.

Properties: Soothing, Uplifting, Antiseptic, Insect repellent, Digestive aid, Antispasmodic, Emmenagogue, Analgesic, Antidepressant, Antispasmodic, Antivenomous, Aphrodisiac, Bactericide, Carminative, Cephallic, Expectorant, Febrifuge, Galactagogue, Insecticide, Nervine, Stomachic, Sudorific, Tonic, Restorative, Stimulant, Vermifuge, Effects adrenal cortex, Imitates oestrogen, Minimise uric acid in muscles, stimulates blood flow, Helps expel afterbirth, Cleanse intestines and kidneys.

Uses: Fatigue, Depression, Respiratory infections, Colds, Cough, Bronchitis, Asthma, Sinusitis, Fever, Gout, Indigestion, Insect bites and stings, Breast engorgement, Fainting, Flatulence, Insomnia, Muscular aches and pains, Rheumatism, Anxiety, Migraine, Nervous tension, Sharpening senses, Nerve tonic, Concentration, Hysteria, Headaches, Temporary paralysis, Nasal polyps, Earache, Allergies, Bronchitis, Emphysema, Flu, Whooping cough, Catarrh, Vomiting, Gastric spasm, Nausea, Dyspepsia, Hiccups, Menstrual problems, Scanty periods, Fertility problems, Fatigue, Stress, Poor circulation.

Bay

Botanical Name: Laurus Nobilis

Note - top

Type - Spice

Family - Lauraceae

Part Leaves and twigs

Extraction - Steam Distillation

Aroma: Sweet and spicy, similar to Cinnamon

Blends well With: Citrus Oils, Cedarwood, Clary Sage, Coriander, Cypress,

Eucalyptus, Ginger, Hyssop, Juniper, Lavender, Lemon, Marjoram, Myrtle, Orange, Rose, Rosemary, Thyme, Ylang Ylang.

Contraindications: Sensitive skin, Pregnancy, Irritate mucous membranes. Properties: Analgesic, Antineuralgic, Antiseptic, antispasmodic, Aperitif, Astringent, Cholagogue, Diuretic, Emmenagogue, Febrifuge, Hepatic, Insecticides, Parturient, Stimulant, Stomachic, Sudorific, Tonic, Mildly narcotic,

Warms emotions, Reproductive tonic, Uplifting.

Uses: Colds, Flu, Bronchitis, Digestive aid, Dyspepsia, Flatulence, Appetite stimulant, Settles stomach, Liver and Kidney tonic, Rheumatism, Aches and pains, Sprains, Fever, Infectious disease, Scanty periods, Speeds up childbirth, Ear infections, Dizziness, Restores balance, Minor respiratory problems, Indigestion.

Cautions: People prone to sensitive or allergy prone skin should not use Bay oil. Use in moderation and never undiluted.

Bergamot

Botanical Name: Citrus Bergamia

Note - top Type - Citrus Family - Rutacaea Part - Peel

Extraction - Expression

Aroma: Light, delicate, refreshing, something like Orange and lemon with slight floral undertones.

Blends well With: Basil, Cardamon, Chamomile, Coriander, Cypress, Eucalyptus, Geranium, Juniper, Jasmine, Lavender, Lemon, Marjoram, Mimosa, Myrtle, Neroli, Palmarosa, Patchouli, Petitgrain, Sandalwood, Ylang ylang.

Contraindications: Phototoxic, sensitive skin.

Pro pertie s: An tise ptic , Pa r a sit icid e, An tide pres sa nt, Ana lges ic, Antispasmodic, Carminative, Cicatrisant, Cordial, Deodorant, Digestive, Expectorant, Febrifuge, Insecticide, Sedative, Stomachic, Tonic, Vermifuge, Vulnerary, Keeps pets away from plants, Uplifting, Vitalising, Anti-inflammatory,

Uses: Dandruff, Urinary and Respiratory infections, Skin infections, Throat and mouth infections, Scalp and skin, Psoriasis, Acne, Ulcers, Stress related conditions, Depression, Coldsores, Shingles, Insomnia, Anxiety, Stress, Bad breath, Deodorant, Worms, Intestinal parasites, Colic, Appetite stimulant, Vaginal infections, Flatulence, Boils, Eczema, Varicose Ulcers, Wounds, Tonsillitis, Colds, Fever, Flu, Abscesses, Cystitis, Digestive aid, Eczema, Insect repellent, Oily skin, Infectious diseases, PMS, Dyspepsia, Flatulence, Colic, Indigestion, Gallstones, Anorexia, Breathing difficulties, TB, Chickenpox, Uterine Tonic, STDs, Gastro-intestinal spasm, Cellulite, Sore throat, Bronchitis.

Black Pepper

Note - Middle

Type - Spice

Family - Piperaceae

Part - fruit

Extraction -Distillation

Aroma: Sharp and Spicy.

Blends well With: Basil, Bergamot, Cedarwood, Cypress, Frankincense, Geranium, Grapefruit, Juniper, Lemon, Marjoram, Palmarosa, Rosemary, Sandalwood, Ylang Ylang.

Contraindications: Kidney Problems, Sensitive Skin.

Properties: Analgesic, Antiemetic, Antiseptic, Antispasmodic, Aphrodisiac, Cardiac, Carminative, Detoxicant, Digestive, Diuretic, Febrifuge, Laxative, Rubefacient, Stimulant, Stomachic, Tonic, Helps frustration, Warms the heart with there is indifference, Dilates local blood vessels, Stimulates peristalsis, Stimulates circulation, Helps form new blood cells, Antidote for fish and mushroom poisoning, Reduces fat, Increases flow of Saliva, Stimulates appetite, Expels wind, Fortifying stomach, Expels toxins.

Uses: Muscle aches and pains, Tired and aching limbs, Muscle stiffness, Rheumatoid Arthritis, Temporary Paralysis, Vomiting, Bowel problems, Anaemia, Respiratory illnesses, Fever (Small amounts).

Cajuput

Note - top

Type - Herb

Family - Myrtacaea Part - leaves and twigs Extraction - Distillation

Aroma: Sweet, herbaceous and rather penetrating.

Blends well With: Angelica, Bergamot, Birch, Cardamon, Cedarwood,

Clove, Eucalyptus, Geranium, Immortelle, Lavender, Myrtle, Niaouli, Nutmeg,

Pine, Rose, Rose wood, Thyme.

Contraindications: Use with caution, sensitive skin, irritate mucous membranes

Properties:Analgesic, Antidontalgic, Antineuralgic, Antirheumatic, Antiseptic, Antispasmodic, Balsamic, Cicatrisant, Decongestant, Expectorant, Febrifuge, Insecticide, Pectoral, Stimulant, Sudorific, Vermifuge, Clears the mind, Balances mind and body, Imitates Oestrogen.

Uses: Respiratory tract infections, Fever, Colds, Pharyngitis, Laryngitis, Bronchitis, Asthma, Ease Chronic Pulmonary Disease, Colic, Inflammation of the intestines, Enteritis, Dysentery, Gastric spasm, Nervous vomiting, Intestinal Parasites, Urinary infections, Cystitis, Urethritis, Neuralgia, Headaches, Toothache, Earache, Gout, Chronic rheumatism, Muscle Stiffness, Muscle aches and pains, Menopausal problems.

Cedarwood

Note - Base

Type - Wood

Family - Cupressacae/Pinaceae

Part - Wood

Extraction - Distillation

Aroma: Woody, reminiscent of sandalwood but slightly "drier" and almost pine tones.

Blends well With: Benzoin, Bergamot, Black pepper, Cajuput, Cinnamon, Cypress, Frankincense, Ginger, Jasmine, Juniper, Lavender, Lemon, Linden, Myrrh, Neroli, Patchouli, Pine, Rose, Rosemary, Sandalwood, Vetiver, Ylang Ylang.

Contraindications: Sensitive Skin, Pregnancy.

Properties: Calming, Soothing, Antiseptic, Astringent, Diuretic, Emollient,

Expectorant, Fungicide, Insecticide, Sedative, Tonic, Better for chronic (long standing) problems than acute (recent) ones, Balances body and mind, Insect repellent, Aphrodisiac.

Uses: Nervous Tension, Anxiety, Meditation, Bronchitis, Coughs, Catarrh, Excess phlegm, Cystitis, Genito-Urinary tract problems, Kidney problems, Rheumatism, Arthritis, Oily skin, Acne, Clearing scabs, Dermatitis, Psoriasis, Hair tonic, Seborrhoea, Dandruff, Alopecia, Softening skin (especially when mixed with Cypress and Frankincense), Respiratory infections, Glandular problems, Stress, Insect bites and stings, Dermatitis, Eczema, Itching, Coughs, Fungal infections, Hair loss, Ulcers, Bronchitis, Catarrh, PMT, Tiredness, Vaginal infections, Urinary tract infections, Congestion, Sinusitis.

Chamomile

Note -Middle

Type - Flower

Family - Compositae Part - Flowers Extraction - Distillation

Aroma: Fruity, apple-like.

Blends well With: Angelica, Basil, Benzoin, Bergamot, Clary sage, Geranium, Jasmine, Lavender, Lemon, Marjoram, Neroli, Palmarosa, Patchouli, Rose, Star Anise, Ylang Ylang.

Contraindications: Pregnancy (early Months)

Properties: Emmenagogue, Analgesic, Antiallergenic, Anticonvulsive, Antidepressant, Antibacterial, Antiemetic, Antiphlogistic, Antipruritic, Antirheumatic, Antiseptic, antispasmodic, Carminative, Cholagogue, Cicatrisant, Digestive, Diuretic, Emollient, Febrifuge, Hepatic, Nervine, Sedative, Splenetic, Stomachic, Sudorific, Tonic, Vermifuge, Vulnerary, Soothing, Calms the mind, Regulates menstruation, Stimulates growth of white corpuscles.

Uses: Anxiety, Tension, Anger, Fear, Promotes relaxation, Gives patience and peace, Allay worry, Insomnia, Muscular pain, Lower back pain, Headache, Neuralgia, Toothache, Earache, Menstrual problems, Period pain, PMT, Menopause, Soothes stomach, Gastritis, Diarrhoea, Colitis, Peptic Ulcers, Vomiting, Flatulence, Irritated bowels, Liver problems, Jaundice, Genito-urinary problems, Anaemia, Burns, Blisters, Inflamed wounds, Ulcers, Boils, Dermatitis, Acne, Herpes, Psoriasis, Broken Capillaries, Improves skin elasticity, Itching, Puffiness, Strengthen tissues, Skin cleanser, Hair tonic, Cramps, Nappy Rash, Nervous Tension, Neuralgia, Bleaching hair, Cracked nipples, Children's tantrums, Fevers, Insomnia, Mastitis.

Cinnamon

Note - Base

Type - Spice

Family - Lauracaea Part - Bud/Bark/leaf Extraction - Distillation

Aroma: Spicy, Sharp, Sweet and Musky

Blends well With:Benzoin, Cardamon, Clove, Coriander, Eucalyptus, Frankincense, Galbanum, Ginger, Grapefruit, Lavender, Lemon, Mandarin, Orange, Pie, Rosemary, Thyme.

Contraindications: (Leaf is safer as Bud and Bark can irritate skin more)

Use with care in small doses, Pregnancy, High doses could cause convulsions

Properties: Anaesthetic, Antidontalgic, Antiseptic, Antiputrefative, Antispasmodic, Aphridesiac, Astringent, Cardiac, Carminative, Emmenagogue, Escharotic, Haemostatic, Insecticide, parasiticide, Sialogue, Stimulant, Stomachic, Vermifuge, Stimulates tears, Stimulates saliva and mucous, Stimulates secretion of gastric juices, Stimulates Circulatory system.

Uses: Respiratory infections, Colds, Flu, Breathing difficulty, Fainting, Infectious diseases, Viral infections, Intestinal infections, Digestive spasm, Asthenia, Dyspepsia, Colitis, Flatulence, Gastralgia, Diarrhoea, Nausea, Vomiting, Cholera, Typhoid, Period pain, Scanty menstruation, Leucorrhoea, Impotence, Muscle spasm, Rheumatism, Insect bites, Respiratory and digestive problems, Lice, Scabies, Tooth and Gum care, Warts, Wasp stings, Poor circulation, Rheumatism, Anorexia, Colitis, Aids childbirth, Frigidity, Cough, Depression, Flu.

Citronella

Note - Top Type - Citrus Family - Graminae Part - Grass

Extraction - Distillation

Aroma: Sweet and Lemony

Blends well With: Bergamot, Cajuput, Cedarwood, Eucalyptus, Geranium, Lavender, Lemon, Mandarin, Neroli, Orange, Peppermint, Petitgrain, Pine, Sage, Ylang Ylang.

Contraindications: May irritate Sensitive Skin, Pregnancy.

Properties: Antidepressant, Antiseptic, Deodorant, Insecticide, Parasiticide, Tonic for heart and nervous system, Stimulant, Clearing mind, uplifting.

Uses: Insect repellent, Excessive perspiration, Oily skin, Cold, flu, Minor infections, Fatigue, Headache, Migraine, Neuralgia, Tired feet, Rheumatic aches and pains, Softens skin.

Clary Sage

Note - Top to Middle

Type - Herb

Family - Labiatae

Part - Herb/Flowering tops and leaves

Extraction - Distillation

Aroma: Heavy herby and nutty.

Citronella, Coriander, Cypress, Frankincense, Geranium, Grapefruit, Jasmine, Juniper, Lavender, Lemon, Lime, Myrtle, Petitgrain, Rose,

Sandalwood, Ylang Ylang.

Contraindications: Not before driving or operating heavy machinery, Not with Alcohol consumption, Large doses can cause headaches, Pregnancy, Epilepsy

Properties: Anticonvulsive, Antidepressant, Antiphlogistic, Antiseptic, Antispasmodic, Antisudorific, Aphrodisiac, Balsamic, Carminative, Deodorant, Digestive, Emmenagogue, Hypotensive, Nervine, Parturient, Sedative, Stomachic, Tonic, Uterine, hormone balancing, Kidney tonic, Soothing, Uplifting, Balance, Encourages hair growth, Astringent, Anti-inflammatory, Antibacterial, Powerful muscle relaxant.

Uses: Nervous tension, Anxiety, Uterine problems, Scanty periods, PMT, Menstrual cramps, Stress, Fertility, Digestive problems, Flatulence, Gastric spams, Headaches, Migraine, Tension, cramp, Excessive perspiration, TB, Asthma, Sore throats, Throat infections, Brings vigour after illness, Convalescence, Overcoming drug addictions, Depression and hopelessness, Cell regenerate, Scalp problems, Dandruff, Oily hair, Inflamed and puffy skin, Hypertension, Colds, Menstrual problems, Dry skin, Digestive problems.

Clove

Note -Base

Type - Spice

Family - Myrtaceae

Part - (Tree) Bud or Leaf Extraction - Distillation Aroma: Spicy, strong.

Blends well With: Basil, Benzoin, Black pepper, Cinnamon, Citronella, Grapefruit, Lemon, Nutmeg, Orange, Peppermint, Rosemary.

Contraindications: (Highly irritant), Sensitive skin, Pregnancy, Not for use with children

Properties: Analgesic, Anaesthetic, Antidontalgic, Antiemetic, Antineuralgic, Antiseptic, Antispasmodic, Aperitif, Aphrodisiac, Carminative, Caustic, Cicatrisant, Disinfectant, Insecticide, Parturient, Splenetic, Stimulant, Stomachic, Uterine, Vermifuge, Expectorant, Antihistamine, Aids digestion, Antidepressant, Parasiticide, Tonic for the Kidneys; spleen and stomach, Antibacterial.

Uses: Dyspepsia, Gum infections, Toothache, Bronchitis, Catarrh, Scabies, Athletes foot, Cold, Flu, Tinea, Acne, Bruises, Burns, Cuts, Ulcers, Wounds,

Arthritis, Rheumatism, Sprains, Asthma, Colic, Nausea, Minor infection,

Diarrhoea, Flatulence, General weakness, Muscular aches and pains, Tension,

Scar tissue, Memory, Lethargy, Vomiting, Intestinal spasm, Halitosis, Headache,

Respiratory problems, TB, Impotence, Frigidity, Helps child birth pains, Lupus.

Cypress

Note - Middle to base

Type - Wood

Family - Cupressaceae

Part - (Tree) Leaves and cones

Extraction - Distillation

Aroma: Woody and spicy, but refreshing and clear

Blends well With: Benzoin, Bergamot, Clary Sage, Juniper, Lavender, Lemon, Linden, Orange, Pine, Rosemary, Sandalwood.

Contraindications: High Blood pressure, Pregnancy,

Properties: Antiseptic, Astringent, Aids healing, Insecticide, Vaso-constricting, Tonic for circulatory system and liver, Cicatrisant.

Uses: Urinary problems, Fluid retention, Excessive perspiration, Diarrhoea, Menorrhagia, Tired aching legs, Oily skin, Rheumatism, Back ache, Haemorrhage, Swelling, Nasal congestion, Cold, Flu, Scars, Wounds, Haemorrhoids, Varicose veins, Asthma, Cellulitis, Menstrual cramp, Poor circulation, Spasmodic coughs, Dysmenorrhoea, Stress, Nervous tension, Acne, Eczema, Gum disorders, Incontinence, Menopausal problems, Nose bleeds, Whooping cough.

Eucalyptus

Note - Top

Type - Wood

Family - Eucalyptus globulus

Part - (Tree) leaves

Extraction - Distillation

Aroma: Clear, sharp and piercing

Blends well With: Benzoin, Cajeput, Cedarwood, Coriander, Cypress, Juniper, Lavender, Lemon, Lemongrass, Marjoram, Melissa, Peppermint, Pine, Rosemary, Star Anise, Teatree, Thyme.

Contraindications: Sensitive skin, Kidney problems, Toxic if taken internally, Heart problems, Not for children, High Blood pressure, Pregnancy, Epilepsy, Do not use if you are on any Homoeopathic medication.

Properties: Analgesic, Antirheumatic, Antipholgistic, Antiseptic, Antispasmodic, Antiviral, Antibacterial, Balsamic, Cicatrisant, Decongestant, Insecticide, Rubefacient, Stimulant, Vermifuge, Vulnerary, Parasiticide, Cools and soothes, Strengthens nervous system,

Uses: Respiratory complaints, Croup, Bronchitis, Ringworm, Insect bites, Shingles, Chicken pox, Herpes, Muscle aches and pains, Dysentery, Hay fever, Burns, Throat infections, Colds, Chest infections, Acne, Asthma, Boils, Cold sores, Cuts, Fever, Flu, Lice, Laryngitis, Rheumatism, Skin infections, Sore throat, Urinary infections, Aids concentration, Catarrh, TB, Sinusitis, Migraine, Typhoid, Diphtheria, Malaria, Cystitis, Diarrhoea, Gall stones, Nephritis, Gonorrhoea, Diabetes, Haemorrhage, Neuralgia, Pyorrhoea.

Fennel

Note - Top to middle

Type - Herb

Family - Umbelliferae Part - (Herb) seed Extraction - Distillation

Aroma: Floral, herbal and spicy

Blends well With: Basil, Geranium, Lavender, Lemon, Rose, Rosemary, Sandalwood.

Contraindications : Pregnancy, Epilepsy, Toxic if used in large doses, not for babies.

Properties : Antiphlogistic, Antiseptic, Antispasmodic, Aperitif, Carminative, Detoxicant, Diuretic, Emmenagogue, Expectorant, Galactagogue, Insecticide, Laxative, Resolvent, Splenetic, Stimulant, Stomachic, Sudorific, Tonic, Vermifuge, Reduces lactobacillus, Has an action similar to Oestrogen, Stimulates lactation, Reduces the toxic effect of alcohol, Body cleansing and detoxifying.

Uses : Kidney Stones, Menstrual problems, PMT, Respiratory problems, Urinary tract infections, Flatulence, colic, Menopausal problems, Diuretic, Gout, Liver problems, Children's complaints, Intestinal parasites, Nausea, Vomiting, Indigestion, Cellulitis, Obesity, Odema, Rheumatism, Asthma, Bronchitis, Anorexia, Bruises, Dull skin, Oily skin, Alcohol poisoning, Appetite reduction, Arthritis, Colitis, Constipation, Fluid retention, Mouth and gum problems, Hangovers, Stomach ailments, Eases digestion, Hiccups, Whooping cough, Scanty periods.

Frankincense

Note - Middle to base

Type - Resin

Family - Burseraceae

Part - (Tree) Bark

Extraction - Distillation

Aroma: Woody, spicy, and a hint of lemon

Blends well With: Basil, Black Pepper, Cedarwood, Cinnamon, Citrus oils, Galbanum, Geranium, Ginger, Grapefruit, Lavender, Orange, Melissa, Myrrh, Neroli, Patchouli, Pine, Sandalwood, Vetiver.

Contraindications: Pregnancy.

Properties: Uterine tonic, Astringent, Blood coagulant, Calming, Deepens breathing, Induces sweating, Pulmonary antiseptic, Calming, Clears the lungs, Anti-inflammatory.

Uses: Bronchitis, Laryngitis, Asthma, anxiety, Stress, Emotional upsets, Urinary tract infections, Cystitis, Uterine tonic, Wounds, Mature skin, Blemishes, Dry skin, Scars, Catarrh, Dysmenorrhoea, Cold, Flu, Nervous tension, Acne, Coughs, Laryngitis, Meditation, Menstrual problems, PMS, Menorrhagia, Respiratory conditions, Scar tissue, Improves skin tone, genito-urinary infections, Catarrh, Nephritis, Genital infections, Uterine haemorrhage,

Post natal depression, Calms during labour, Breast inflammation, Dyspepsia, Belching, Wrinkles, Oily skin, Ulcers, Carbuncles.

Geranium

Note - Middle

Type - Floral

Family - Geraniacea

Part - (plant) Flowers and leaves

Extraction - Distillation

Aroma: Sweet and heavy, a little like rose with a hint of mint.

Blends well With: Angelica, Basil, Bay, Bergamot, Carrot Seed, Cedarwood, Citronella, Clary Sage, Grapefruit, Hyssop, Jasmine, Lavender, Lemon, Lime, Mandarin, Marjoram, Neroli, Orange, Patchouli, Petitgrain, Rose, Rosemary, Sandalwood, Tea Tree.

Contraindications: Sensitive skin, Pregnancy.

Properties: Analgesic, Anticoagulant, Antidepressant, Aphrodisiac, Antiseptic, Anti-funga l, Anti-infla mma tory, Astringent, Cica trisa nt, Cytophylactic, Diuretic, Deodorant, Haemostatic, Hypoglycemiant, Insecticide, Styptic, Tonic, Vasoconstrictor, Vulnerary, Cleanses the body of toxins, Stimulates lymphatic system, Clears digestive mucous, Balances Sebum, Skin cleanser, Improves flow of blood.

Uses: Anxiety, Depression, Balances mind, Stress, PMT, Menorrhagia, Lack of vaginal secretions, Inflammation, Breast Congestion, Congested system, Jaundice, Kidney stones, Gallstones, Diabetes, Urinary infections, Fluid retention, Swollen ankles, Throat infections, Mouth Infections, Neuralgia, Gastritis, Colitis, Insect Repellent, Eczema, Shingles, Herpes, Ringworm, Chilblains, Oily skin, Sluggish skin, Congested skin, Cuts, Menopausal conditions, Cellulitis, Mastitis, Emotional problems, tonsillitis, Burns, Muscular aches and pains, Respiratory conditions, Rheumatism, Swelling, Ulcers, Apathy, Acne, Bruises, Broken capillaries, Dermatitis, Haemorrhoids, Lice, Mature skin, Mosquito repellent, Wounds, Engorgement of breasts, Poor circulation, Sore Throat, Nervous tension, Abscesses, Boils, Bronchitis, Indigestion, Insect bites.

Jasmine

Note - Middle to Base

Type - Floral

Family - Jasminacaea

Part - Flowers

Extraction - Enfleurage/Solvent Extraction

Aroma: Sweet and flowery.

Blends well With: Bergamot, Citrus oils, Chamomile, Clary Sage, Coriander, Frankincense, Geranium, Guaiacwood, Immortelle, Lavender, Mandarin, Melissa, Mimosa, Myrtle, Neroli, Orange, Palmarosa, Patchouli,

Peppermint, Petitgrain, Rose, Rose wood, Sandalwood, Vetiver, Ylang Ylang.

Contraindications: Sensitive skin, Pregnancy, Not for Babies, Excessive use can cause problems with bodily fluids such as phlegm, May have a narcotic effect and cause lack of concentration.

Properties: Menstrual regulator, Sedative, Antidepressant, Stimulates lactation, Boosts confidence, Analgesic, Balances hormones, Increases male fertility.

Uses: Stress, Skin Care, Throat infections, Coughs, Catarrh, Listlessness, Apathy, Melancholy, Hopelessness, Menstrual cramps, Back pain, Labour Pain, Impotence, Frigidity, Dry Skin, Itchy skin, Muscle aches and pains, Child Birth, Lethargy, Nervous tension, PMS, Post natal depression, Vaginal infections, Premature ejaculation, Hoarseness.

Juniper

Note - Middle

Type - Herb

Family - Cupressacea

Part - Berries

Extraction - Distillation

Aroma: Slightly woody

Blends well With: Benzoin, Bergamot, Cedarwood, Citrus oils, Cypress,

Frankincense, Geranium, Ginger, Grapefruit, Orange, Lavender, Lemongrass,

Lime, Melissa, Pine, Rosemary, Sandalwood, Vetiver.

Contraindications: Pregnancy, Kidney problems, not for use with babies. Properties: Antiseptic, Anti-rheumatic, Antispasmodic, Aphrodisiac, Astringent, Carminative, Cicatrisant, Clears Mucous from intestines, Depurative, Detoxicant, Digestive aid, Disinfectant, Diuretic, Emmenagogue, Nervine, Insecticide, Parturient, Regulating appetite, Regulating periods,

Rubefacient, Stimulating, Stomachic, Sudorific, Tonic, Vulnerary.

Uses: Genito-Urinary infections, Cystitis, Strangury (Inability to pass urine), Kidney stones, Cellulitis, Dropsy, Fluid retention, releasing toxins, Piles, Obesity, Cirrhosis, Arthritis, Rheumatism, Gout, Sciatica, Stiff joints, Menstrual cramps, Childbirth, Problem skin, Oily skin, Congested skin, Seborrhoea, Acne, Blocked pores, Dermatitis, Eczema, Psoriasis, Swelling, Haemorrhoids, Ulcers, Stress, Oily Hair, Indigestion, Insomnia, Menstrual problems, Loss of appetite, Muscular aches and pains, PMS, Intestinal parasites, Colds, Flu, Anxiety, Purifying the blood, Circulation problems, Cough, Diarrhoea, Fatigue,

Lavender

Note - Middle Type - Flower Family - Labiatae Part - Flowers

Extraction - Distillation

Aroma: Floral and slightly woody

Blends well With: Basil, Bay, Bergamot, Cedarwood, Chamomile, Citronella, Clary Sage, Cypress, Eucalyptus, Geranium, Grapefruit, Hyssop, Jasmine, Lemon, Lemongrass, Lime, Mandarin, Marjoram, Myrtle, Neroli, Nutmeg, Orange, Patchouli, Peppermint, Petitgrain, Pine, Thyme, Rosemary, Tea Tree.

Contraindications: Low Blood pressure, Early Pregnancy.

Properties: Analgesic, Anticonvulsive, Antidepressant, Antiphlogistic, Antirheumatic, Antiseptic, Antispasmodic, Antiviral, Bactericide, Balances central nervous system, Carminative, Cholagogue, Cicatrisant, Cordial, Cytophylactic, Decongestant, Deodorant, Detoxicant, Diuretic, Emmenagogue, Fungicide, Hypotensive, Increases gastric secretions, Nervine, Promotes growth of new skin cells, Restorative, Sedative, Splenetic, Stimulates bile production, Sudorific, Vulnerary.

Uses: Anger, Exhaustion, High blood pressure, Heart palpitations, Insomnia, Muscular spasm, Sprains, Strains, Rheumatic pains, Bronchitis,

Asthma, Catarrh, Colds, Laryngitis, Throat infections, TB, Infections, Period pain, Scanty periods, Leucorrhoea, Childbirth, Cleanse spleen and liver, Nausea, Vomiting, Colic, Flatulence, Insect repellent, Burns, Sunburn, Acne, Eczema, Psoriasis, Abscesses, Boils, Carbuncles, Fungal growths, Swelling, Scars, Gangrene, Alopecia, Headaches, Lice, fleas, Appetite stimulating, Whooping cough, Flu, Nervous Tension, Stress, Vertigo, Shock, Athlete's foot, Genito- urinary problems, Cystitis, Scalds, Wounds, Sores, Varicose veins, PMT, Ulcers, Spider bites, Ringworm.

Lemon

Note - Top

Type - Citrus

Family - Rutaceae

Part - Peel

Extraction - Expression/Distillation

Aroma: Citrus, Sharp and fresh

Blends well With: Bay, Benzoin, Black pepper, Cardamon, Chamomile, Citronella, Citrus oils, Eucalyptus, Fennel, Frankincense, Geranium, Ginger, Jasmine, Juniper, Lavender, Linden, Neroli, Peppermint, Rose, Sandalwood, Ylang-Ylang.

Contraindications: Sensitive skin, Phototoxic, High Blood pressure.

Properties: Antacid, Antisclerotic, Antiscorbutic, Antineura lgic, Antirheumatic, Antipruritic, Antiseptic, Astringent, Bactericide, Carminative, Cicatrisant, Decongestant, Depurative, Diuretic, Emollient, Escharotic, Febrifuge, Haemostatic, Hepatic, Hypoglycemiant, Hypotensive, Insecticide, Laxative, Stomachic, Tonic, Vermifuge.

Uses: Varicose veins, Easing blood flow, High Blood pressure, Anaemia, Restoring vitality to Red blood cells, Stimulating white corpuscles, Infectious diseases, Nosebleeds, Sore throat, Coughs, Colds, Flu, Fever, Cold sores,

Herpes, Digestive complaints, Counteracting acidity in stomach, Diabetes, Cleanses body, Constipation, Cellulite, Headaches, Migraine, Neuralgia, Rheumatism, Arthritis, Insect bites and stings, Removes dead skin cells, broken capillaries, Cleansing greasy skin, Corns, Warts, Verrucae, Scars, Strengthens nails, Cuts, Circulation problems, Boosts immune system, Asthma, Bronchitis, Catarrh, Dyspepsia, Sinusitis, Tonsillitis, Chilblains, Mouth sores, Middle ear infections, Depression, Indigestion, Boils, Debility, Fluid retention, Mouth Ulcers, Oily skin, Wounds.

Lemongrass

Note - Top
Type - Citrus
Family - Graminaea
Part - Leaves
Extraction - Distillation
Aroma: Strong, sweet and lemony

Blends well With: Basil, Cedarwood, Coriander, Eucalyptus, Geranium, Jasmine, Lavender, Neroli, Niaouli, Palmarosa, Peppermint, Rosemary, Tea Tree, Thyme, Vetiver, Yarrow.

Contraindications: Sensitive skin, use in low dose, High Blood pressure. Properties: Antidepressant, Antiseptic, Bactericide, Carminative, Deodorant, Digestive, Diuretic, Fungicide, Galactagogue, Insecticide,

Prophylactic, Stimulant, Tonic, Tones the skin, Sedative, Relaxing.

Uses: Exhaustion, Boosting parasympathetic nerves, Digestive complaints, Illness, Loss of appetite, Colitis, Indigestion, Gastro-enteritis, Infectious disease, Respiratory infections, Sore throat, Laryngitis, Fever, Aching muscles, Muscular aches and pains, Tired legs, Jet Lag, Headaches, Fatigue, Insect repellent, Fleas, Aids flow of breast milk, Open pores, Acne, Oily skin, Athlete's foot, Thrush, Digestive disturbances, Stress, Anxiety, Fluid retention, Gastric infections, Gout, Lice, Mental fatigue, Poor Circulation, Rheumatism, Scabies.

Lime

Note - Top Type - Citrus Family - Rutaceae Part - Peel
Extraction - Expression/Distillation
Aroma: Sharp and Tangy

Blends well With: Angelica, Basil, Bergamot, Citronella, Citrus oils, Clary Sage, Geranium, Linden Blossom, Lavender, Neroli, Nutmeg, Palmarosa, Rose, Rosemary, Violet, Ylang Ylang.

Contraindications: Phototoxic, Sensitive skin.

Properties: Antiscorbic, Antiseptic, Antiviral, Apertif, Astringent, Bactericide, Disinfectant, Febrifuge, Haemostatic, Insecticide, Restorative, Tonic, Stimulating, Activating, Refreshing, Uplifting, Digestive stimulant, Stimulates appetite, Stimulates digestive secretions.

Uses: Apathy, Anxiety, Depression, Fever, Colds, Sore Throat, Flu,

Coughs, Chest congestion, Catarrh, Sinusitis, Immune system tonic, Infections, Anorexia, Alcoholism, Rheumatic pain, Greasy skin, Acne, Cuts, Wounds, Anaemia, Brittle nails, Boils, Chilblains, Corns, Herpes, Insect bites, Mouth Ulcers, Spots, Varicose veins, Warts, Arthritis, Cellulitis, High Blood Pressure, Nose bleeds, Obesity, Poor circulation, Rheumatism, Asthma, Throat infections, Bronchitis, Dyspepsia, Headaches, Stress.

Mandarin

Note - Top to Middle

Type - Citrus Family - Rutacaea Part - Peel

Extraction - Expression

Aroma: Sweet and tangy

Blends well With: Basil, Bergamot, Black Pepper, Chamomile, Cinnamon, Citrus oils, Clary Sage, Coriander, Cumin, Geranium, Grapefruit, Juniper, Lavender, Lemon, Lime, Marjoram, Nutmeg, Palmarosa, Petitgrain, Rose.

Contraindications: Phototoxic.

Properties: Antispasmodic, Cholagogue, Cytophylactic, Digestive tonic, Emollient, Sedative, Tonic, Uplifting, Stimulates appetite, Stimulates liver, Regulate Metabolic processes, Aids secretion of Bile, Aids breaking down of fats, Calms the Intestines, Revitalising, Skin tonic.

Uses: Depression, Anxiety, Flatulence, Morning sickness, PMT, Stretch Marks and scarring, Digestive weakness, Good for children/pregnant women and the elderly, Insomnia, Nervousness, Acne, Oily skin, Fluid retention, Obesity, Hiccups, Restlessness, Constipation, Digestive problems.

Marjoram

Note - Middle Type - Herb Family - Labiatae Part - Leaves

Extraction - Distillation

Aroma: Slightly Spicy

Blends well With: Basil, Bergamot, Cedarwood, Chamomile, Cypress, Eucalyptus, Geranium, Lavender, Mandarin, Melissa, Orange, Nutmeg, Peppermint, Rosemary, Rose wood, Tea Tree, Thyme, Ylang Ylang.

Contraindications: May cause drowsiness with prolonged use, Pregnancy. Properties: Analgesic, Anaphrodisiac, Antiseptic, Antispasmodic, Carminative, Cephalic, Cordial, Digestive, Emmenagogue, Expectorant, Hypotensive, Laxative, Nervine, Restorative, Sedative, Tonic, Vulnerary, Calming, Dilates the arteries and capillaries, Cleanses toxins, Regulates

Menstrual cycle, Hypnotic,

Uses: Stress, Anxiety, Psychological trauma, Confronting "issues", Grief, Loneliness, Hyperactivity, Muscular aches and pains, Lower back pain, Rheumatic aches and pains, Swollen joints, Stiff joints, After-sports rub, High Blood pressure, Headache, Migraine, Insomnia, Digestive problems, Stomach cramps, Indigestion, Constipation, Flatulence, Sea Sickness, Chest infections, Colds, Sinusitis, Bronchitis, Asthma, Congestion, Painful periods, Bruises,

Sprains, Arthritis, Menstrual problems, Coughs, Colic, Chilblains, Ticks, Lumbago, Strains, Dyspepsia, Leucorrhoea, PMS, Nervous tension, Cramps, Emotional comfort, Flu, Circulation.

Orange

Note - Top

Type - Citrus

Family - Citrus Vulgaris/Aurantium/ Sinesis

Part - Peel

Extraction - Expression

Aroma: Zesty and refreshing citrus

Blends well With: Angelica, Black Pepper, Cedarwood, Cinnamon, Citrus oils, Coriander, Clary Sage, Clove, Cumin, Cypress, Frankincense, Geranium, Ginger, Hyssop, Jasmine, Juniper, Lavender, Myrrh, Neroli, Nutmeg, Petitgrain, Rose, Rose wood.

Contraindications: Sensitive skin, Phototoxic.

Properties: Antidepressant, Antiseptic, Antispasmodic, Carminative, Digestive, Febrifuge, Sedative, Stomachic, Tonic, Stimulates bile, Helps digestion of fats, Stimulates Appetite, Aids digestion of Vitamin C, Aids formation of collagen, Lowers cholesterol, Uplifting, Calming.

Uses: Depression, Tension, Stress, Boredom, Lethargy, "Butterflies" in the stomach, Diarrhoea, Constipation, Viral infections, Colds, Bronchitis, Fever, Repairing body tissues, Sore muscles, Rickety bones, Insomnia, Anxiety, Congested skin, Wrinkles, Dermatitis, Skin complaints, Flu, Oily skin, Coughs, Heartburn, Indigestion, Dull complexion, Dyspepsia, Mouth ulcers, Obesity, Palpitations, Water retention, Nervous tension.

Patchouli

Note - Base

Type - Herb

Family - Pogostemon patchouli

Part - Leaves

Extraction - Distillation

Aroma: Earthy and woody, a bit spicy (sort of mouldy)

Blends well With: Angelica, Bergamot, Black pepper, Cedarwood, Clary Sage, Elemi, Frankincense, Galbanum, Geranium, Ginger, Lavender, Lemongrass, Myrrh, Neroli, Orange Pine, Rose, Rose wood, Sandalwood, Ylang Ylang.

Contraindications: Sedative in low doses but Stimulating in high doses, May cause loss of appetite, May cause a headache in some people.

Properties: Grounding, Balancing, Antidepressant, Antipholgistic, Antiseptic, Anti-infla mmatory, Aphrodisia c, Astringent, Cicatrisa nt, Cytophylactic, Deodorant, Diuretic, Febrifuge, Fungicide, Insecticide, Sedative, Tonic, Soothing, Calming, Opens pores, Cell regeneration.

Uses: Lethargy, Clarifying problems, Loose skin, Weight loss, Diarrhoea, Water Retention, Cellulite, Sweating, Insect bites and stings, Snake bites, Scars, Cracked skin, Sores, Wounds, Acne, Eczema, Fungal infections, Scalp disorders, Skin disorders, Athlete's foot, Dry Skin, Oily Skin, Tinea, Excessive Menstrual flow, Dandruff, Dermatitis, Hair care, Impetigo, Wrinkles, Frigidity, Nervous exhaustion, Stress, Anxiety, Bed sores, Depression.

Peppermint

Note - Top

Type - Herb

Family - Labiatae

Part - Leaves and flowering tops

Extraction - Distillation

Aroma: Minty

Blends well With: Basil, Benzoin, Cedarwood, Cypress, Eucalyptus, Jasmine, Lavender, Lemon, lemongrass, Mandarin, Marjoram, Niaouli, Pine, Rosemary.

Contraindications: (Very cooling on the skin - so best used in very small concentration on the skin), Sensitive skin, Pregnancy, Nursing Mothers (can discourage flow of milk), Should not be used with Homoeopathic remedies.

Properties: Analgesic, Antidontalgic, Anaesthetic, Antigalactagogue, Antiphlogistic, Antiseptic, Antispasmodic, Astringent, Carminative, Cephalic, Cholagogue, Cordial, Decongestant, Emmenagogue, Expectorant, Febrifuge, Hepatic, Nervine, Stimulant, Stomachic, Sudorific, Vasoconstrictor, Vermifuge, Encourages sweating, Insecticide, Softens skin, Improves thinking, Uplifting.

Uses: Anger, Hysteria, Nervous trembling, Mental fatigue, Depression, Colds, Mucous, Fever, Respiratory disorders, Dry coughs, Sinus congestion, Asthma, Bronchitis, Cholera, Pneumonia, Tuberculosis, Food poisoning, Vomiting, Diarrhoea, Constipation, Flatulence, Halitosis, Colic, Gall stones, Nausea, Travel sickness, Kidney disorders, Liver disorders, Numbness in the limbs, Shock, Vertigo, Anaemia, Dizziness, Fainting, Headaches, Migraines, Toothache, Aching feet, Rheumatism, Neuralgia, Muscular aches, Scanty menstruation, Painful periods, Mastitis, Dermatitis, Ringworm, Scabies, Pruritus, Itching, Inflammation, Sunburn, Blackheads, Oily hair and skin,

Abdominal cramps, Digestive upsets, Flu, Morning Sickness, Shingles, Insect bites, Nervous stress, Indigestion, Acne, Palpitations.

Rosemary

Note - Middle Type - Herb Family - Labiatae

Part - Flowering tops and leaves

Extraction - Distillation

Aroma: A strong refreshing herbal scent

Blends well With: Basil, Black Pepper, Cedarwood, Frankincense, Geranium, Ginger, Grapefruit, Hyssop, Lavender, Lemongrass, Lime,

Mandarin, Melissa, Myrtle, Orange, Peppermint, Petitgrain, Pine, Tea Tree, Tangerine.

Contraindications: Pregnancy, High Blood pressure, Epilepsy, Not to be taken with Homoeopathic remedies.

Properties: Analgesic, Antidepressant, Antirheumatic, Antiseptic, Antispasmodic, Astringent, Carminative, Cephalic, Cholagogue, Cicatrisant, Cordial, Decongestant, Digestive, Diuretic, Emmenagogue, Hepatic, Hypertensive, Nervine, Resolvent, Stimulant, Stomachic, Sudorific, Tonic, Vulnerary, Invigorating, Strengthens the mind, May help restore speech; hearing and sight, Heart tonic, Cardiac stimulant, Encourages hair growth.

Uses: Memory, Mental Strain, Dullness, Lethargy, Weakness, Mental exhaustion, Headaches, Migraines, Gastric problems, Vertigo, Paralysed limbs, Gout, Rheumatic pains, Tired and overworked muscles, Low blood pressure, Anaemia, Colds, Asthma, Chronic bronchitis, Flu, Hepatitis, Cirrhosis, Gallstones, Jaundice, Blocked bile ducts, Colitis, Dyspepsia, Flatulence, Stomach pains, Menstrual cramps, Scanty periods, Water retention, Cellulite, Obesity, Sagging skin, Skin congestion, Puffy skin, Swelling, Scalp disorders, Dandruff, Infections, Halitosis, Stress, Eyesight, Apathy, Muscle fatigue, Poor circulation, Aches and pains, Acne, Dermatitis, Eczema, Oily hair, Insect repellent, Lice, Seborrhoea, Scabies, Varicose veins, Rheumatism, Whooping cough.

Sandalwood

Note - Base

Type - Wood

Family - Santalaceae Part - Inner wood Extraction - Distillation

Aroma: Woody and Exotic

Blends well With: Basil, Benzoin, Bergamot, Black Pepper, Cedarwood,

Cypress, Frankincense, Geranium, Jasmine, Lavender, Lemon, Mimosa, Myrrh,

Neroli, Palmarosa, Patchouli, Rose, Rose wood, Vetiver, Ylang Ylang.

Contraindications: Depression? (May cause mood to drop lower, may act as an antidepressant)

Properties: Antiphlogistic, Antiseptic, Anti-inflammatory, Antispasmodic, Aphrodisiac, Astringent, Bechic, Carminative, Diuretic, Emollient, Expectorant, Sedative, Tonic, brings peace and acceptance, Stimulates immune system.

Uses: Nervous tension, Anxiety, Obsessional attitudes, Cutting ties with the past, Meditation, Genito-urinary problems, Cystitis, Frigidity, Impotence, Chest infections, Sore throat, Dry coughs, Bronchitis, Lung infections, Insomnia, Catarrh, Heartburn, Diarrhoea, Dry skin, Oily skin, Aging skin, Dehydrated skin, Itching, Acne, Boils, Infected wounds, Cracked skin, Chapped skin, Shaving rash, PMS, Upset stomach, Stress, Urinary tract infections, Laryngitis, Nausea, Depression, Eczema, Fatigue, Respiratory problems, Skin problems, Sunstroke, Venereal infections.

Tea Tree

Note - Top

Type - Wood

Family - Myrtaceae

Part - Leaf

Extraction - Distillation

Aroma: Pungent and Sterile

Blends well With: Black Pepper, Cinnamon, Clary Sage, Clove, Coriander, Cumin, Cypress, Eucalyptus, Geranium, Ginger, Lavender, Lemon, Mandarin, Marjoram, Nutmeg, Orange, Pine, Rosemary, Thyme.

Contraindications: Sensitive skin, Pregnancy

Properties: Antibiotic, Antipuritic, Antiseptic, Antiviral, Antibacterial, Balsamic, Cicatrisant, Cordial, Disinfectant, Expectorant, Fungicide, Insecticide, Stimulant, Sudorific, Boosts immune system.

Uses: Shock, Infectious diseases, Eliminating toxins, Flu, Colds, Cold sores, Catarrh, Glandular fever, Gingivitis, AIDS (not a cure, but may boost immune system to be of benefit), Post-operative shock, Convalescence, Vaginal thrush, Genital infections, Urinary tract infections, Cystitis, Genital and anal pruritus, Chickenpox, Itching, Rashes, Insect bites and stings, Ear infections, Tonsillitis, Enteritis, Intestinal parasites, Infected wounds, Boils, Carbuncles, Spots, Acne, Shingles, Burns, Sores, Sunburn, Ringworm, Warts, Tinea, Herpes, Athlete's foot, Dry scalp, Dandruff,. Bronchitis, Verrucae, Asthma, Hysteria, Abscesses, Calluses, Blisters, Respiratory problems.

OBJECTS OF THE INVENTION

Accordingly, it is an object of the present invention to provide a process for simultaneously and rapidly extracting and concentrating the principal components of herb and spice solids, at temperatures of at least 130° F., preferably 130 to about 450° F., in a process which is completely free of petroleum, chlorinated or highly flammable solvent, does not require high pressure gas handling equipment, does not require distillation for solvent removal, uses only food-grade edible solvents which are typically used in the trade to standardize the resulting extract to a desired concentration, and provides a product of reduced bacterial count which is free of adulterants and impurities.

Another object of this invention is to prepare such a concentrated extract by a process which is simple, environmentally friendly, and economical.

A further object of this invention is to prepare a residual solid or press cake which is edible, free of residual petroleum distillates, chlorinated solvent, or other adulterants, which is standardized with respect to the principal components of commercial interest, which has a predictable and controlled degree of brownness or caramelization, and which has a controlled level of water activity with its attendant increased resistance to oxidative deterioration of carotenoid pigments and colour loss where this is otherwise a problem.

Still another object of this invention is to prepare a residual solid or press cake that is standardized with respect to the principal components of interest, that when reground rapidly and efficiently imparts flavor, aroma, colour, and/ or other principal components of interest to a food or beverage in which it is used, and all without the use of undesirable non-edible solvents that are inherently difficult to remove from spice solids remaining after extraction prior to standardization with respect to the principal components of interest, are environmentally unfriendly, and are perceived by the consumer as being undesirable in the preparation of a food ingredient. A still further object of this invention is to provide such a process wherein antioxidants can be added to the edible solvent system so as to protect the concentrated extract and the residual solids against oxidative degradation of the principal components of interest, i.e., flavor, aroma, and colour, which are extracted from the raw plant material or left in the residual solids.

Still a further object of this invention is to prepare an edible extract and an edible residual solid with reduced microbial activity by a process wherein the moisture of the herb or spice is kept below 10%, preferably below 8%, thereby avoiding the loss of volatile flavor and aroma constituents and avoiding the development of uncontrolled browning and off flavor development at temperatures in excess of 130° F. which are necessary to effect high extraction efficiencies, reduction in microbial activity, and improved stability of the carotenoid pigments in both the extract and in the residual solids.

Yet a further object of this invention is to prepare an extract with increased resistance to oxidative degradation of pigments and consequent colour loss. Still an additional object is to provide a process wherein and whereby the residual spice or herb plant solids have their tissue ruptured so as to produce quick release of the flavor, aroma, colour, or antioxidant component therein and thereof when in use in a food or beverage thereby greatly enhancing its use effectiveness, and whereby all products of the process may be conveniently standardized with respect to the principal flavor, aroma, colour, or antioxidant component of interest.

Other objects will be apparent to one skilled in the art to which this invention pertains and still others will become apparent hereinafter as the description proceeds.

BRIEF DESCRIPTION OF THE DRAWINGS

The process of the present invention, including the several process steps involved in the simultaneous extraction and concentration of herb or spice solids, e.g., Capsicum solids, to produce the desired extract and sterilized residual solid, both of which have increased resistance to oxidative degradation, and which can be readily standardized to desired levels of the principal components of interest. Although the process illustrated comprises three extraction stages, the number of stages can be decreased to two or increased to more than three to effect the desired relative principal component concentration in the extract and in the residual solid.

SUMMARY OF THE INVENTION

The invention, then, inter alia, comprises the following, alone or in combination:

A continuous multistage mixing, high pressure pressing, and countercurrent extraction process for the production of a concentrated edible extract and quick-release edible residual solids, both of reduced bacterial content, and both of which contain herb or spice pigment, flavor, and aroma and, when present in the starting material, antioxidant, from herb or spice plant solids, comprising the following steps: subjecting said herb or spice solids to a countercurrent extraction process involving a plurality of mixing and pressing stages, including first and last mixing stages and first and last pressing stages, together with up to about fifty percent by weight of an edible solvent, to produce an extract and residual solids, continuously returning the extract from each pressing stage to the previous mixing stage, and finally separating the extract from the first pressing stage and separating the residual solids from the last pressing stage, all pressing stages being carried out at a temperature of at least 130° F.; such a process wherein the temperature is 130 to about 450° F.; such a process wherein the solids are subjected to internal pressures in the press stages of at least 6,000 pounds per square inch; such a process wherein the weight of the edible solvent is 5% to about 20% by weight of the solids; such a process wherein the moisture content of the starting solids is less than 10% by weight, and wherein bacterial count reduction is effected at this low moisture content, thereby avoiding undesirable loss of volatile flavor and aroma constituents and avoiding the development of cooked, off flavours and aromas which occur at higher moisture contents; such a process wherein the solids extracted in the process are selected from the group consisting of chipotle, turmeric, black pepper, onion, rosemary, and oregano; such a process wherein the edible solvent is selected from the group consisting of soybean oil, corn oil, cottonseed oil, rapeseed oil, peanut oil, mono-, di-, or triglycerides, lecithin, edible essential oils, sesame oil, edible alcohols, hydrogenated or partially hydrogenated fats or oils, polyoxyethylene sorbitan esters, limonene, edible animal fats or oils, mixtures thereof, and edible derivatives thereof; such a process wherein fine particulate solids are filtered or centrifuged from the extract and alternatively discarded, returned to a mixing or pressing stage of the process, or incorporated in the final residual solids; such a process which includes the steps of hydrating the final extract to add water to the extent of 5% to 200% by weight of the gums and fine particulate solids therein and filtering or centrifuging to remove said gums and solids; such a process including the step of returning the separated hydrated gums and solids to the final residual solids; such a process including the step of rehydrating the final residual solids with water to a water activity greater than 0.3 AW for stabilization thereof; such a process wherein the solids are rehydrated to a water activity of about

0.4 to 0.6 AW; such a process wherein an effective stabilizing amount of an edible antioxidant or chelator is included in the edible solvent; such a process wherein the antioxidant comprises an antioxidant selected from the group consisting of lecithin, ascorbic acid, citric acid, tocopherol, ethoxyquin, BHA, BHT, TBHQ, tea catechins, sesame, and the antioxidant activity from an herb of the Labiatae family; such a process wherein the antioxidant comprises a naturally-occurring antioxidant from an herb of the family Labiatae or powdered ascorbic acid; such a process wherein the antioxidant comprises the antioxidant activity from an herb selected from the group consisting of rosemary, thyme, and sage; such a process wherein the temperature is greater than 180° F.; and such a process wherein the temperature is between about 180° F. and 235° F. having a high level of principal flavor, aroma, colour, or antioxidant components of interest and a low bacterial count due to the high temperature employed in its production and due to the low water content not greater than 10% in the starting solids; and an extract of herb or spice plant solids having a low bacterial count due to the high temperature employed in its production and having improved stability produced according to the process due to edible antioxidant therein; and residual spice or herb plant solid having a low bacterial count due to the high temperature employed in its production and having its tissue ruptured so as to produce quick release of the principal flavor, aroma, colour, or antioxidant component therein, and which is standardized with respect to the principal flavor, aroma, colour, or antioxidant component of interest, produced by the process of the present invention.

THE PRESENT INVENTION

In General

Raw Capsicum or other spice or herb solids, either ground (usually to pass US 40 mesh, and preferably to pass at least US 20 mesh) or unground if coarse particles are desired in the residual solid or cake, e.g., spice solids having a moisture range of about 0.5% to 16% by weight, preferably 0.5 to 12%, and most preferably 1.5% to 10% by weight (ASTA method 2.0), are subjected to a mixing stage, preferably high shear, and in at least one stage an edible solvent is thoroughly dispersed throughout the raw plant material solids.

Typical spice starting plant materials include, for example but without limitation, those of the genus Capsicum including the dried ripe fruits of Capsicum frutescens L. (chilies), Capsicum annum L. (Spanish peppers), Capsicum annum L. var. longum Sendt, its hybrid Louisiana Sport Pepper, and Capsicum chinense (Scotch Bonnet or habenero), all by way of example and not by way of limitation.

Other spices and herbs of interest include those of the family Solanaceae, as stated representatively Capsicums such as paprika, red pepper, and chili, and Lycopersicon, representatively tomato, all containing carotenoid pigments;

Umbelliferae, representatively celery, lovage, dill, carrot, cilantro, fennel, cumin, caraway, parsley, angelica, and anise; Compositae, representatively marigold, artemisia, and tarragon; Leguminosae, representatively fenugreek; Labiatae, representatively rosemary, thyme, sage, oregano, marjoram, mint, savoury, and basil; Zingerberacae, representatively ginger, cardamom, and turmeric, Lauraceae, representatively laurel, cinnamon, cassia, and bay; Myrtaceae, representatively allspice and clove; of the genus Myristica, representatively mace and nutmeg; of the genus Piper, representatively black and white pepper; of the genus Vanilla, representatively vanilla; of the genus Allium, representatively onion and garlic; of the genus Sesamum, representatively sesame seed; Cruciferae, representatively mustard and horseradish; the defining characteristic being that it is a spice or herb plant material from which flavor, aroma, colour, and/or antioxidant can be extracted and used to flavor and/or colour foods and beverages or otherwise employed to enhance the palatability of foods and beverages.

The comminuted or uncomminuted plant material is subjected to a plurality of mechanical pressing stages, whereby a concentrated extract of principal components is obtained and a final utilizable and preferably standardized residual solid is produced. The selected edible solvent is introduced into the residual solid at a mixing stage at some point prior to the last pressing stage. The edible solvent, now containing extract, is cycled back to the previous stage, thus always supplying a solvent extract with increasing principal component concentration to the previous mixing and pressing stages. As the extract/edible solvent is passed through each stage countercurrent to the solids flow, a portion of the edible solvent is squeezed or pressed out, thereby extracting a portion of the principal components of interest. As the edible solvent/extract passes countercurrent to the solids, the extracted principal components are progressively concentrated in the extract in a continuous process and the residual principal components end up in the final residual solids known as the cake.

By varying the pressure, temperature, spice solids feed rate, solvent addition rate, and the number of mixing and pressing stages, the concentration of the principal components can be controlled in both the extract and the residual solid.

As will be apparent to one skilled in the art, variations in the process of the present invention can be employed to produce variations in result, the most advantageous of which are the production of both plant material extract of standardized marketable potency and edible residual solid plant material also characterized by standardized marketable potency, and with the edible residual solids also characterized by rapid release of the principal components of interest. Moreover, in the process of the present invention, the spice or herb plant solids have their tissue ruptured so as to provide quick release of the flavor, aroma, colour, or antioxidant component therein when in actual use, i.e., when incorporated into foods or beverages.

For example, using 200 ASTA paprika starting material of about 5% moisture, a 20% soy oil addition, and leaving a residual cake extractable yield of 9.8% by weight of the starting plant solids material, gives an extract with a colour value of 850 ASTA and a residual cake colour value of approximately a cake having about 65 ASTA colour value and, by increasing the residual cake extractable yield to 12.5% by weight of starting plant solids material, the colour value of the residual cake rises to about 100 ASTA and that of the extract to about 1400 ASTA. The lowest colour extract for paprika normally traded is 1,000 ASTA.

Although less than 20% edible oil addition is highly desirable and can be used in many cases, with some edible solvent systems wherein the principal compounds of interest have a limited solubility, or when a more dilute extract and/or lower concentration of principal compounds is desired in the residual solids, more than 20% by weight of edible solvent addition will be required inasmuch as a suitable concentration of principal compounds in the finished extract and in residual solid can in some cases be produced only by the employment of the higher dilution.

Due to the successive treatments of high pressure and pressure relief, with pressures ranging from 6,000 to 30,000 PSI in the pressing stages of the operation, in the presence of added edible solvent, e.g., vegetable oil, and due to frictional heat generated in these high pressure zones, both the residual solid and the extract exiting the process surprisingly have a significantly reduced microbial load over that of the starting material even at moisture levels significantly lower than those indicated by the prior art and, also surprisingly, exhibit increased resistance to oxidative degradation of the carotenoid pigments which are responsible for the characteristic red-yellow colour of various spices, e.g., Capsicums.

The extract from the first or any selected pressing stage may be centrifuged or filtered to provide the finished extract free of particulate solids. Preferably, the fine particulate solids and gums in the extract may be hydrated to about 5% to 200% by weight of the gums and solids prior to centrifugation or filtration to give a crystal clear extract. If water is not used to hydrate the solids and gums, the fine particulate solids from the extract may conveniently be combined with the final residual solids, recycled back into mixing and pressing stages of the process, or alternatively discarded. If water is used to hydrate the solids and gums, it is preferred that the solids and gums be added back to the final residual press solids or discarded.

The edible solvent employed according to the process of the present invention, as illustrated by the following Examples, may be any edible solvent and especially those selected from the group consisting of soybean oil, corn oil, cottonseed oil, rapeseed oil, sesame oil, peanut oil, mon-, di-, and triglycerides, lecithin, essential oils of spices, herbs, or other plants, edible alcohols, propylene glycol, glycerine, hydrogenated or partially hydrogenated fats or oils, limonene, polyoxyethylene sorbitan esters, or any other edible vegetable or animal fat or oil, or mixture thereof, or edible derivatives thereof, the essential aspects of the solvent being that it serves as an extraction aid in which the principal components of the material being extracted are soluble and that it be edible.

The edible solvent, according to the present invention, is combined with the raw material solids to be processed in a proportion of about 5% to about 50% by weight, and frequently amounts as low as 5 to 20% by weight are possible, based on the weight of the starting raw material solids to be extracted. The lower percentages frequently produce a more acceptable and marketable concentration of principal components of interest in both the extract and the residual solids.

The temperature to be employed during the processing and especially in the pressing stages of the process of the invention may be varied widely, but the process is generally carried out at a temperature below about 450° F., and between about 130° F. and 325° F., most preferably above 180° F. and especially between about 180° F. and 235° F.

Temperatures in excess of 130° F. are advantageously employed to achieve acceptable yields and increased throughput rates as compared to the prior art. Higher temperatures are employed to control an increased degree of browning and, most importantly, to reduce the microbial load of both the solids and the extract while at the same time imparting increased resistance to oxidative degradation of the carotenoid pigments of Capsicums in both the extract and the residual solids. Thus, when it is desired that the residual solids from the process have a desirable darkened, caramelized appearance and/or flavor, a reduced microbial load, and increased resistance to oxidation, this is readily attained by increasing the temperature of the solids and the extract during the process, especially during the pressing stages thereof.

When an antioxidant or chelator is introduced into the process for protection of the spice or herb being processed, this is preferably another plant material or an extract thereof, preferably of the Labiatae family, such as rosemary, thyme, or sage, which is known for its protective antioxidant activity (U.S. Pat. No. 5,209,870), or sesame, or tea catechins, but may alternatively be a suitable edible and preferably an approved food grade additive such as ethoxyquin, BHA, BHT, TBHQ, tocopherol, Vitamin C (e.g., as in U.S. Pat. Nos. 5,290,481, 5,296,249, or 5,314,686), citric acid, EDTA, or the like. The process of the present invention is particularly adaptable to the extraction of any spice or herb plant material solids containing carotenoid pigments or other components which provide colour and/or flavor, pungency, aroma, or antioxidant activity, such as present in rosemary, thyme, sage of the Labiatae genus, to a food with which combined.

VARIOUS NON-CAPSICUM SPICE OR HERB PLANT SOLIDS

In addition to the foregoing, the following examples show the applicability of the process of the present invention in the production of herb or spice plant extracts and solids having greatly reduced bacterial counts and without the deterioration alleged by the prior art to occur at temperatures above about 100° F., especially at low water contents which are also contraindicated by the prior art, and with the production in each case of residual spice or herb plant solids having its tissue ruptured so as to produce quick release of the flavor, aroma, colour, or antioxidant component therein when in actual use in a food or beverage, thereby greatly increasing the use effectiveness thereof, and both extract and solids produced by the process being readily standardized with respect to the principal flavor, aroma, colour, or antioxidant component of interest.

Example 3: Paprika Extraction and Flavor/Aroma Activation : Paprika is processed in the same manner as given in Examples 1, 1a, 1b, or 2 using a multiple stage, counter-current process with temperatures being in excess of 130° F. with the residual solids being rehydrated to a water activity of 0.6. By adjusting the amount of edible, food grade solvent, and the pressures and temperatures in the pressing stages, the residual cake solids are standardized with respect to ASTA colour value to produce paprika solids with ASTA colour values equivalent to ground paprika commonly used commercially as described in the above examples.

A sample of the residual cake solids at 120 ASTA was reground to pass US 40 mesh and was compared to the starting, unextracted spice, also ground to pass US 40 mesh and rehydrated to a water activity of 0.6, with respect to flavor and aroma intensity. Ten grams each of the residual cake solids and the unextracted spice were thoroughly mixed with 50 grams of flour salt to make a dispersion that would typify a coating for snack foods used to impart a paprika flavor and aroma. Triangle tests were done on the samples.

The samples were coded with random three digit numbers and twelve expert panelists were asked to identify the sample that had the highest paprika flavor and aroma. Twelve of twelve panelists picked the reground residual cake solids as having a more intense paprika aroma. Eight of twelve picked the reground residual cake solids as having a more intense paprika flavor. By statistical analysis (according to methods described in Sensory Evaluation Techniques, Vol II, by Morten Meilgaard, 1987, page 133) this clearly demonstrates that the residual cake solids have more intense paprika aroma and flavor available in a food system as a result of the high pressure, high shear forces and the attendant disruption of the flavor and aroma containing tissue of the spice.

Example 3a: Colour Activation : A sample of 120 ASTA ground residual cake solids was prepared as in Example 3 above. This was compared to a sample of commercially available 120 ASTA paprika with regard to effective colour release into water to model colour release under conditions typical of those used to prepare a marinade or sauce. One (1) gram each of the ground residual cake solids and commercial ground paprika were added to 100 ml of distilled water and stirred for two minutes at ambient temperature.

The slurries were then filtered to remove all particulate solids and the absorbance of each of the solutions was measured spectrophotometrically at 460 nm. The absorbance of the water solution prepared using the residual press solids was 0.566. The absorbance of water solution prepared with the commercial ground paprika was 0.294. This clearly demonstrates that the effective utilization of the colour, and the colour intensity of the model sauce system, were significantly enhanced by the high pressure, high shear, and high temperature of the pressing and extraction process, which ruptures the tissues of the plant solids.

Example 4: Chipotle Extraction and Flavor/Aroma Activation : Chipotle (smoked and dehydrated Jalapeno capsicum pepper) at 4% moisture is ground to pass US 40 mesh and extracted in a two-stage countercurrent pressing operation with the addition of 6% of an edible solvent mixture consisting of 95% soybean oil and 5% decaglycerol tetraoleate (Mazol PGO 104K) by weight of the starting spice in the same manner as described in the above Examples. The principal components of interest in this spice are the flavor (including capsaicinoids which impart the pungent flavor typical of chili peppers) and aroma compounds (including the smokey aroma).

The pungency of the starting ground Chipotle is 35,000 Scoville (ASTA method 21.0). The pungency of the extract is 200,000 Scoville and the pungency of the residual cake solids is 20,000. Both the extract and the residual cake solids have the characteristic smokey aroma of the starting spice. By varying the addition rate of the soybean oil, the concentration of pungent principles is varied in both the extract and the residual solids. For example, using a 12.5% soy oil addition results in an extract with a Scoville pungency of 165,000 and a residual cake solid of 15,000 Scoville. Increasing the soy oil addition to 15% results in an extract of 150,000 Scoville and a residual solid of 7,500 Scoville. This clearly demonstrates that the spice solids can be predictably standardized effectively and efficiently with respect to the principal flavor compounds without the requirement of traditional blending and replating of solvent-extracted oleoresins as described in prior art (U.S. Pat. No. 2,507,084).

The aroma of the residual cake solids is compared to that of the starting unextracted spice using the Triangle method described in Example 3 by dispersing 10 grams of each in 50 grams of flour salt. Six of the twelve panelists unextracted starting spice, clearly demonstrating that the high pressure, high shear process provides for a ruptured spice residual solid with equivalent aroma intensity even though a portion of the principal components of interest have been removed with the extract.

The starting raw spice has an aerobic plate count of 80,000,000. The plate count of the final extract and residual cake solids are 15,000 and 1,100,000 respectively, again demonstrating that significant reduction in microbial activity can be achieved at such low water contents.

Example 5: Onion Ex traction—Flavor and Aroma Activation : Dehydrated, toasted onion powder (Gilroy Foods, Inc. 92700 Toasted Special Onion Powder) was processed in a high pressure extraction system comprising two pressing stages, using Egon Keller Model KEK-100 Screw Presses. Glycerol monooleate containing 10% propylene glycol (Mazol DF300K) was added to the high shear mixing stage prior to the second pressing stage at 25% by weight of the starting spice. The raw material onion was continuously fed at a rate of about 150 lbs per hour with a total contact time in the pressing stages of about 120 seconds. The pressing stage was operated at about 6,000 psi internal pressure and about 190° F., which was maintained by cooling with water through the bore of the press shaft as needed.

The principal components of interest in both the extract and the residual solids are flavor and aroma constituents typical of toasted onion powder. The resulting final extract from the pressing process has the characteristic aroma and flavor profile at a level approximately 4 times the strength of the starting spice as determined by plating the extract on flour salt at varying concentrations and subjecting the resulting dispersions to triangle tests as described in previous examples compared to the unextracted spice. This clearly demonstrates that the flavor and aroma components of the raw spice can be effectively extracted using high pressure, high temperature mechanical pressing.

The residual cake solids are compared to the unextracted spice by dispersing 20 grams of each in 200 ml of salad oil as in Example 3a above, stirring for 5 minutes, and filtering to remove all particulate solids to compare the effectiveness of flavor release into a model salad dressing system. Twelve trained panelists are asked to pick which salad oil has a more intense toasted onion flavor. Twelve of twelve pick the salad oil prepared with the residual cake solids as having superior and more intense toasted onion flavor and aroma. This is a very surprising and unexpected result as a significant portion of the flavor and aroma of the starting spice was removed with the extract.

Without in anyway being limited by theoretical considerations, it is hypothesized that the nature of the edible solvent system used, in combination with the high temperature, high pressure, and high shear forces generated during the processing of the spice, result in a ruptured spice tissue matrix with the flavor and aroma compounds remaining in the residual cake solids being readily soluble in salad oil which otherwise does not readily dissolve the principal components of interest. It is clear that this process provides very significant economic and functional value over prior art.

Example 6: Black Pepper Extraction, Standardization, and Flavor Activation : Black Pepper, ground to pass US 30 mesh, was subjected to a two- stage, countercurrent extraction process as demonstrated in the previous Examples using Triacetin (glycerol triacetate) as the edible solvent at 7% by weight of the starting spice. The temperature of the residual cake solids exiting the pressing stages was maintained at about 215° F.

The piperine content of the starting spice was 11% by ASTA method 12.1. Piperine is responsible for the characteristic pungent flavor of black pepper. The final extract, after filtering to remove the fine particulate solids, had a piperine content of 41.6% and the residual cake solids had a piperine content of 4.1%, typical of commercially-traded grades of black pepper commonly used in food preparation.

An expert panel compared the ground residual cake solids to commercial ground black pepper at 4% piperine. The panelists unanimously picked the residual cake solids as being more pungent, demonstrating that the high pressure, high shear treatment in combination with an edible food solvent provide a surprisingly improved residual spice solid, as compared to an untreated spice having equivalent levels of the principal compound of interest. This presents a clear advantage over prior art.

Example 7: Rosemary Extraction and Standardization of Antioxidants : Ground, dried Rosemary at 6% moisture was processed in accordance with the procedures described in Example 6 but using a medium chain triglyceride based on caprylic/capric fatty acids (Neobee M-5, produced by the Stepan Company) at a level of 40% by weight of the starting spice, with temperatures of the residual cake solids maintained at about 250° F. with cooling water or steam as needed through the bore of the press shafts. The starting raw material had levels of Carnosol and Carnosic acid, two of the primary antioxidant compounds present in rosemary, of 0.46% and 2.47% respectively, for a total of 2.93% by weight of active compounds. Carnosic acid and Carnosol levels were determined by extracting a sample with a methanolic solution of Bisphenol A (internal standard).

The extract therefrom was analyzed by reverse phase HPLC on a C-18 column using a gradient mobile phase of methanol and methanol: aqueous citric acid buffer and UV detection at 280 nm. The method can be calibrated using a pure sample of Carnosic acid and Carnosol had 0.49% Carnosol and 5.80% Carnosic acid for a total of 6.2% by weight of active compounds or a two-fold increase in concentration from that of the starting spice. The residual cake solids contained 0.21% Carnosol and 0.23% Carnosic Acid for a total of 0.44% by weight active compounds. This represents about 15% of the active compounds found in the starting spice.

This surprisingly demonstrates that, contrary to prior art, the antioxidant compounds can be efficiently extracted in a continuous, high speed, high pressure process with levels of edible solvent considerably below those disclosed by prior art, providing an extract produced by such a process that is clearly superior in levels of antioxidants. Prior art, in particular U.S. Pat. No. 3,732,111, discloses a method for extraction of Labiatae herbs using prohibitively high ratios of edible solvent in relation to the weight of the starting spice. This necessarily, by simple dilution, results in an extract of low antioxidant concentration that make the extract so weak with respect to the active compounds that it cannot be used in many food systems where the volume of edible solvent in relationship to the compounds of interest is simply too high.

By varying the ratio of edible solvent to ground spice, and the number of countercurrent pressing stages, the levels of active compounds in the extract and residual solids can be controlled in the same manner as described in previous examples.

The starting ground rosemary had an aerobic plate count of 7,000,000. The final extract and residual cake solids had plate counts of 600 and 35,000 respectively. Again, contrary to prior art which suggests that elevated moisture contents and lengthy holding time are necessary, the present process dramatically and rapidly sterilized both the extract and residual solids at such low moisture contents due to the high temperatures, pressures, and shear forces employed.

Example 8: Turmeric Extraction, Standardization, and Sterilization : Using the general procedures as described in the previous Examples, turmeric at 3% moisture and containing 6% curcumin (ASTA method 18.0) was extracted using 10% by weight of Polysorbate 80.RTM., a polyoxyethylene sorbitan ester, in a countercurrent, two-stage pressing operation with the temperature of the residual cake solids being maintained at about 220° F. Curcumin is the pigment responsible for the intense yellow colour of turmeric. The final filtered extract and the residual cake solids are 20% and 3.5% curcumin respectively.

The plate count of the starting spice is about 50,000,000, the final extract 25,000, and the final residual cake solids 1,500,000. Again, contrary to the teachings of prior art, at such low moisture contents.

By varying the amount of edible solvent added prior to the second pressing stage, the levels of curcumin can be accurately and predictably controlled in both the extract and residual cake solids as described in previous examples.

Example 9: Oregano Extraction, Standardization, Activation, and Sterilization : In the same manner as given in previous Examples, ground oregano at 5% moisture is processed in a two-stage, countercurrent extraction process using 10% by weight of soy bean oil. The presses are operated at about

230° F. as measured by the temperature of the cake exiting the pressing stages. The presses are operated at about 20,000 PSI. The plate count of the starting herb is 5,000,000. The plate counts of the final extract and residual cake solids are 800 and 50,000 respectively demonstrating again, contrary to prior art, that the plate counts of spice and herb solids can be significantly reduced at such low moisture contents.

The residual cake solids are compared for flavor strength to the starting ground herb using the method as described in Example 5. Only six of twelve panelists are able to pick the residual cake solids as being less flavourful than the starting ground herb.

Example 10: Other Families and Species of Herb and Spice Plant Materials In the same general manner as given in previous Examples, other spices and herbs at moisture contents of less than 10% that contain colour, flavor, aroma, or antioxidant principles, are processed and extracted in accord with the method of the present invention.

Such plant materials include, but without limitation, oregano, basil, mint, marjoram, anise, mace, caraway, carrot, garlic, cinnamon, allspice, clove, ginger, cilantro, parsley seed, sesame, cumin, lovage, tarragon, cardamom, fenugreek, mustard, and vanilla, the primary characteristic of such plant materials being that they impart flavor, aroma, colour, or preservative qualities to the food or beverage system in which they are used, and by way of illustration but not by way of limitation, in each case to produce a concentrated extract from the first pressing stage and residual cake solids from the last pressing stage, both standardized with respect to the principal components of interest, both with significantly reduced microbial load, and the residual cake solids having "activated" or quick-releasing principal components of interest in the food or beverage system in which they are used, and for those containing carotenoid pigment, increased stability of the pigment in both the extract and residual cake solids.

All this being accomplished under conditions contrary to prior art: without the use of non-edible solvents, low temperatures, and high moisture contents which develop off flavours, aromas, and colours; and without excessive volumes of edible solvents resulting in extracts and residual solids of limited application that an improved countercurrent process for the extraction of spice and herb plant solids using an edible solvent, whereby improved yields of both extract and residual solids are obtained, whereby both the extract and the residual solids have improved stability and freedom from bacterial contamination due to the higher temperatures employed, whereby due to optional advantageous rehydration of residual solids and level of water activity employed an improved stability in the residual solids is attained, whereby an extract in the form of a clear solution can be obtained by removal of gums and particulate solids in the form of their insoluble hydrates, whereby even greater stability can be effected by the employment of edible antioxidants in the solvent utilized, whereby controlled browning of the residual solids may be conveniently effected, and whereby the residual spice or herb plant solids have their tissue ruptured so as to produce quick release of the flavor, aroma, colour, or antioxidant component therein thereby to provide greatly improved use effectiveness, and whereby all products of the process can be conveniently standardized with respect to the principal flavor, aroma, colour, or antioxidant component of interest, all without the expected disadvantages from employing higher temperatures and lower water content as clearly indicated by the prior art, and whereby all of the stated objects of the invention have been accomplished, has been provided.

It is to be understood that the invention is not to be limited to the exact details of operation, or to the exact compositions, methods, procedures, or embodiments shown and described, as obvious modifications and equivalents will be apparent to one skilled in the art, and the invention is therefore to be limited only by the full scope which can be legally accorded to the appended claims.

❐

Sustainable Use of Medicinal Plants

Wild plants have been an important component of healthcare throughout human history. Medicinal plants continue to make important contributions to healthcare and livelihoods, and were recently identified by FAO as being among the most valuable non-wood forest products (FAO, 1999). Unfortunately, harvests to meet the demand for a growing number of medicinal species are in many cases exceeding sustainable levels. Wild medicinal plant populations and the benefits derived therefrom are coming under threat as a result.

More effective co-operation among the variety of institutions concerned with the use and trade of medicinal plants, including those from the healthcare, conservation, development and commercial sectors, is required to ensure the conservation of biodiversity and continued availability of medicinal resources.

MEDICINAL PLANTS AND HEALTH

Medicinal plants underpin healthcare practices across the globe. Much of the world's population depends on traditional medicine to meet daily health requirements, especially within developing countries. Traditional medicine in turn relies heavily on medicinal plants. Reliance on natural medicinal resources can be attributed to cultural preferences as well as to the high cost and inaccessibility of western medicine.

Use of plant-based remedies is also widespread in many industrialised countries. Herbal remedies are made directly from plant materials, and numerous pharmaceutical products are based on or derived from plant compounds. Similarly, cosmetics and other household products may contain plants of medicinal or therapeutic value. The use of medicinal plants for healthcare is believed to be increasing throughout much of the world, e.g. in Africa (Cunningham, 1993; Marshall, 1998), China (He and Sheng, 1997), Europe (Lange, 1998) and North America (Brevoort, 1998).

Commercial Trade in Medicinal Plants

The large and growing demand for plant-based medicines and changing population patterns have prompted a growing domestic and international trade in medicinal plants. The following information from Lange (1997, 1998) gives an indication of the scale of the trade.

According to Customs data, approximately 440 000 t of medicinal and aromatic plants were traded internationally in 1996, with a reported value of USD1.3 billion. Hong Kong, Japan and Germany were the largest importers during 1994 and 1995, the United States being the third largest importer overall during the period 1992 to 1996. Approximately 60% of imports into Germany in 1996 originated from non-European countries, with exports from Asia dominating the trade, followed by exports from Africa. China was also by far the largest exporter of medicinal and aromatic plants to world markets during the mid-1990s, with average exports topping 140 000 t from 1992 to 1996. The second largest exporter was India, with export volumes averaging approximately 36 000 t during this period.

A wide diversity of medicinal plant species are used and traded for medicinal purposes. A recent TRAFFIC 1 study of the European medicinal plant trade (Lange, 1998) estimates that over 2000 medicinal and aromatic plant species are used commercially in Europe, of which 1200 to 1300 are native. Approximately 90% of the European species are collected from the wild, with eastern Europe and the Mediterranean regions being the main suppliers (Lange, 1998). In India it has been estimated that approximately 7500 species are used for medicinal and veterinary purposes (Uniyal et al., 2000). Over 10,000 species are used medicinally in China (He and Cheng, 1991), with 1,000 species commonly used in medicinal preparations, of which 80% are wild-collected (He and Sheng, 1997).

Harvest of medicinal plants to supply domestic and foreign markets provides an important source of cash income in many countries. In Nepal, for example, Olsen (1998, cited in Olsen, 1999) has estimated that 470 000 households are engaged in commercial collection of medicinal plants. Several publications in the FAO Non-Wood Forest Product Series have drawn attention to the current and potential role of medicinal plants in economic development.

Declines in Medicinal Plant Populations

There is growing evidence that the populations of many medicinal plant species are declining in the wild. These declines are the result of several factors, key among them being habitat degradation and expanding harvests. TRAFFIC's study of the European medicinal plant trade identified approximately 150 European species reported to be threatened in at least one. European country (Lange, 1998); a TRAFFIC study in East/Southern Africa identified approximately 100 species of conservation concern in one or more countries (Marshall, 1998). Reviews of the status of medicinal plant species according to the 'Red List' (threat) criteria of IUCN-The World Conservation

Union in three regions of India identified approximately 70 species considered at risk (Anon., 1998).

Fourteen species have been included in the Appendices of the Convention on International Trade in Endangered Species of Wild Fauna and Flora (CITES) owing to concern that they might be threatened unless international trade is subject to specific controls.

A MULTI-SECTORAL CHALLENGE

A variety of individuals and institutions have an interest in securing the future of medicinal plant species both because of the direct benefits they provide and in the wider context of biodiversity conservation. These range from local collectors, healers and communities to national governments, multi- national corporations, non-governmental organisations and international treaty bodies. Areas of concern include the role of medicinal plants in healthcare (both local and national) and development, biodiversity conservation, the use of traditional knowledge, intellectual property rights and benefit sharing, marketing and trade.

Individuals acting within different sectors are frequently unaware of the shared and/or conflicting interests and motivations of other sectors. In some cases, this can lead to different sectors unnecessarily working at cross-purposes. For example, government agencies charged with species conservation may be unaware of the importance accorded medicinal plants by health agencies. Similarly, health agencies may be unaware of the status of certain species in the wild. The former may seek to restrict use and trade of specific species, while the latter seeks to expand it.

In many cases, the long-term interests sought by different sectors might be better served through increased information sharing, dialogue and cooperation. For example, efforts to promote commercial trade of medicinal plants as a basis for economic development would benefit from greater knowledge of species biology and market dynamics. Efforts to ensure the conservation of medicinal plant species and their availability for healthcare would similarly benefit from such knowledge. Policies intended to support these and/or other objectives similarly seem more likely to succeed if the full range of stake-holder perspectives and interests are understood and taken into account.

The need for more effective cross-sector collaboration to address medicinal plant conservation issues was first brought to world attention by the International Consultation on the Conservation of Medicinal Plants, convened by the World Wide Fund for Nature (WWF), IUCN and the World Health Organisation in Chiang Mai, Thailand, in 1988. This message was reiterated a decade later during the international conference Medicinal Plants for Survival, hosted by the Foundation for Revitalization of Local Health Traditions in Bangalore, India in 1998. More recently, 20 participants at the symposium Medicinal Utilisation of Wild Species signed a 'Joint Declaration for the Health of People and Nature', which emphasises the need to address conservation concerns in a multi-disciplinary and collaborative manner. Signatories include representatives of the phytopharmaceutical industry, practitioners' associations and conservation organisations. The depository for the Joint Declaration is WWF Germany, who organised the symposium with TRAFFIC Europe—

Germany, and, who, with TRAFFIC, is working to encourage and monitor the Declaration's transformation from words into actions.

These and other initiatives indicate the potential for more and more effective cooperation among individuals and institutions concerned with the use, trade and conservation of medicinal plants. Additional effort needs to be invested in putting these good intentions into practice in order to secure the future of medicinal plant populations and the benefits they provide.

DEVELOPING THE MEDICINAL PLANTS

The medicinal properties of plant species have made an outstanding contribution in the origin and evolution of many traditional herbal therapies. These traditional knowledge systems have started to disappear with the passage of time due to scarcity of written documents and relatively low income in these traditions.

Over the past few years, however, the medicinal plants have regained a wide recognition due to an escalating faith in herbal medicine in view of its lesser side effects compared to allopathic medicine in addition the necessity of meeting the requirements of medicine for an increasing human population. Through the realization of the continuous erosion of traditional knowledge of plants used for medicine in the past and the renewed interest at the present time, a need existed to review this valuable knowledge of medicinal plants with the purpose of developing medicinal plants sectors across the different states in India. Our major objectives therefore were to explore the potential in medicinal plants resources, to understand the challenges and opportunities with the medicinal plants sector, and also to suggest recommendations based upon the present state of knowledge for the establishment and smooth functioning of the medicinal plants sector along with improving the living standards of the underprivileged communities.

Medicinal plants, and attempts are being made at different levels for sustainable utilization of this resource in order to develop the medicinal plants sector.

Background

Forests have played key roles in the lives of people living in both mountains and lowland areas by supplying fresh water and oxygen as well as providing a diversity of valuable forest products for food and medicine. The age-old traditional values attached with the various forest types and the varieties of forest products (i.e., medicinal plants) have gained tremendous importance in the present century.

Furthermore, the cosmetic industries are increasingly using natural ingredients in their products, and these natural ingredients include extracts of several medicinal plants. India and China are two of the largest countries in Asia, which have the richest arrays of registered and relatively well-known medicinal plants. Since the Indian subcontinent is well known for its diversity of forest products and the age-old healthcare traditions, there is an urgent need to establish these traditional values in both the national and international perspectives realizing the ongoing developmental trends in traditional knowledge.

Apart from health care, medicinal plants are mainly the alternate income-generating source of underprivileged communities; therefore, strengthening this sector may benefit and improve the living standard of poor people. A great deal of traditional knowledge of the use of various plant species is still intact with the indigenous people, and this fact is especially relevant with the mountainous areas such as the Himalaya due to less accessibility of terrain and comparatively slow rate of development.

The ongoing growing recognition of medicinal plants is due to several reasons, including escalating faith in herbal medicine. Allopathic medicine may cure a wide range of diseases; however, its high prices and side-effects are causing many people to return to herbal medicines which have fewer side effects.

The instant rising demand of plant-based drugs is unfortunately creating heavy pressure on some selected high-value medicinal plant populations in the wild due to over-harvesting. Several of these medicinal plant species have slow growth rates, low population densities, and narrow geographic ranges; therefore they are more prone to extinction. Conversely, because information on the use of plant species for therapeutic purpose has been passed from one generation to the next through oral tradition, this knowledge of therapeutic plants has started to decline and become obsolete through the lack of recognition by younger generations as a result of a shift in attitude and ongoing socio-economic changes.

Furthermore, the indigenous knowledge on the use of lesser-known medicinal plants is also rapidly declining. Through the realization of the continuous erosion in the traditional knowledge of many valuable plants for medicine in the past and the renewal interest currently, the need existed to review the valuable knowledge with the expectation of developing the medicinal plants sector.

The present paper is therefore concerned with the following major objectives: (1) discovering the role, value, diversity and potential in medicinal plants resources, (2) assessing various aspects of medicinal plant sector, which includes challenges and opportunities, and (3) suggesting recommendations based on existing information for the benefit and development of medicinal plants sector in northern India.

Use and Diversity in Medicinal Plants

In India, of the 17,000 species of higher plants, 7500 are known for medicinal uses. This proportion of medicinal plants is the highest proportion of plants known for their medical purposes in any country of the world for the existing flora of that respective country. Ayurveda, the oldest medical system in Indian sub-continent, has alone reported approximately 2000 medicinal plant species, followed by Siddha and Unani. The Charak Samhita, an age-old written document on herbal therapy, reports on the production of 340 herbal drugs and their indigenous uses. Currently, approximately 25% of drugs are derived from plants, and many others are synthetic analogues built on proto type compounds isolated from plant species in modern pharmacopoeia.

The northern part of India harbours a great diversity of medicinal plants because of the majestic Himalayan range. So far about 8000 species of angiosperms, 44 species of gymnosperms and 600 species of pteridophytes have been reported in the Indian Himalaya, of these 1748 species are known as medicinal plants. The maximum medicinal plants (1717 species) have been reported around the 1800 m elevation range. On the regional scale, the maximum species of medicinal plants have been reported from Uttaranchal, followed by Sikkim and North Bengal. The trans-Himalaya sustains about 337 species of medicinal plants, which is low compared to other areas of the Himalaya due to the distinct geography and ecological marginal conditions.

Several plant species are endemic to the Himalayan region. Out of total known number of higher plants from India, approximately 46% are endemic to the Himalaya. Of the total medicinal plant species, sixty-two species of to the adjacent areas, and are therefore classified as near endemic. Over 200 species of Himalayan medicinal plants are consumed raw, roasted, boiled, fried, cooked, or they are used in the form of oil, spices, jams or pickles.

The indigenous communities use some medicinal plant species as a source of food, fodder, timber as well as various other ethnobotanical purposes. For example, apart from the use of Myrica esculenta and Terminalia bellirica as medicines, the fruits of these species are edible, the leaves are used for fodder and the wood is used for fuel. Approximately 81 species of Himalayan medicinal plants are known to be used for the extraction of oil. Of the total 675 species of Himalayan wild edibles, 171 are used for the treatment of diseases. The crop plants diversity is also a source of traditional medicine .

Apart from the human use, animal husbandry uses many plant species as its primary source of healthcare in northern India. The reliance on medicinal plants is also due to cultural preferences. Medicinal plants have strong acceptance in religious activities of north Indian native communities, who worship the plants in the form of various gods, goddesses and minor deities. Origanum vulgare, Saussurea obvallata, Ocimum sanctum, Cedrus deodara, Cynodon dactylon, Aegle marmelos, Juniperus communis, Musa paradissica, Nardostachys grandiflora, Zanthoxylum armatum, Ficus benghalensis, and

Ficus religiosa are examples of the medicinal plants highly used for medicinal as well as a religious purposes by the Hindus in northern India.

The Buddhist community in northern India regards Terminalia chebula as an important medicine as well as sacred fruit. It has been stated long ago that the therapeutic potency of medicinal plants is more effective and better suited to a person of a particular region or culture in which the plant is naturally growing. This idea has given a way to the development of a new drug for heart patients of specific ethnic groups in African countries .

INDUSTRY ROLES IN MEDICINAL PLANT CONSERVATION

This is the story of one company's efforts to source its herbal ingredients from sustainable sources, according to its own account. Pukka Herbs, founded in the UK in 1999, imports plant materials from India and Sri Lanka for the manufacture of ayurvedic preparations. In an interview with Alan Hamilton of Plantlife International, Sebastian Pole, co-founder of Pukka Herbs, emphasised his company's interest in providing high quality health-giving products. Sebastian believes that organic production can be a key to such quality assurance. As with ecological sustainability, verification of organic status requires traceability back to the source areas of the plants, so that Pukka Herbs has a prima-facie motivation to establish traceability.

Pukka Herbs does not buy raw plant materials directly from individual farmers or collectors (which would be a hard task for all but the smallest manufacturers), but does have close relationships with producer companies that work closely with farmers. Pukka does try to restrain the length of its supply chains (which tend to be extensive in the herbal business). Long supply chains, with many intermediate traders between producers and manufacturers, compound the difficulties of tracing the movements of plant materials. They make it difficult for manufacturers to verify that adequate 'production quality' has been achieved for any of the quality categories in which they might be interested - ecological sustainability, product quality (such as organic) and fair trade.

A maximum of three trade links separates Pukka Herbs from the producers of the medicinal plants and usually only two. Pukka purchases plant materials from exporting companies in India and Sri Lanka, that either buy these materials directly from the producers or else buy them from intermediate companies that themselves are directly connected.

EXPORTING COMPANY—PUKKA HERBS

Pukka's ability to achieve traceability for its raw materials, as well as required standards of organic production, has been recognised by the Soil Association, with Pukka's products certified as organic to EU and US standards (the latter under the National Organic Programme). Field certification was by the certifiers SKAL and ECOCERT, their certification being passed on to the Soil Association through recognition of standards' equivalence. Certification was to the normal organic standard of the Soil Association (used mainly for cultivated plants) and not to according to its Organic Wild Crafting Standard, which has more stringent sustainability requirements relating specifically to wild plants.

Principles of 'Production Quality' and their Sharing

Pukka's relationships with a few exporting companies in India and Sri Lanka are central to its business. These exporters are reported by Pukka Herbs to be ecologically and ethically minded agricultural companies that purchase crops from farmers, as well as providing them with training, advice, seeds and fair-trade relationships. Pukka's trading partners were not involved in some of the more specialised Ayurvedic medicinal plants prior to their relationships with Pukka.

Pukka Herbs is committed through its business principles to high quality in three aspects of production: high quality ingredients from the medicinal perspective, ecological sustainability and fair trade. As regards sustainability, Pukka Herbs has its own working document on standards and guidelines to guide its efforts to achieving sustainable harvest. This document is based closely on the standards of the Soil Association, covering both cultivated and wild plants. Special emphasis is placed on the need for management systems for wild plants to be adaptive, allowing rapid and appropriate response to changing circumstances.

The social agenda of Pukka Herbs aims to enhance the livelihoods of the producers of the medicinal plants through enhancing their autonomy. Specific objectives are to develop long-term relationships with the producers (including for the promotion of sustainable production practices and long-term planning), the payment of premium prices that include the cost of sustainable production, the provision of technical assistance and advice, the encouragement or strengthening of community groups for self-empowerment, and the promotion of local markets for organic production (to spread the risks to the producers, so that they are not uniquely bound to Pukka Herbs for market access).

Pukka's business principles must be shared by its business partners in India and Sri Lanka, if they are to be carried into effect. It is these business partners that can give field reality to Pukka's own objectives, which, in the sustainability arena, include the establishment of systems of sustainable harvesting for wild plants, the training of farmers in organic agriculture and assistance for the establishment of nurseries (whether to produce seedlings for field crops or for enrichment planting in the wild).

Pukka Herbs has developed memoranda of understanding (MOU) with its business partners regarding intentions, aspirations and operating standards, covering:

- Organic farming standards
- Commitment to fair trade

- Medicinal plant quality
- Processing standards
- Attainment of Good Agricultural Practice (GAP) and Good Manufacturing Practice (GMP).

Pukka Herbs undertakes an annual exercise in relationship building, technical auditing and quality inspection at randomly selected growing and processing areas to ensure that the terms of the MOU are being met. Relationships are being built 'inclusively', recognising that current practices are not perfect, but rather 'work-in-progress'. The company reports that, with a willingness to learn and a spirit of co-operation, steady progress is proving possible, year-by-year.

The Forest Gardens

Most of the plant materials purchased by Pukka Herbs are actually derived from field crops, rather than wild plants. Of course, there are benefits for plant conservation from organic agriculture, but the parts of Pukka's business most strongly relevant to wider plant conservation are two cases of harvesting wild or semi-wild plants in Sri Lanka. One of these involves the production of medicinal plants in 'forest gardens' and the other the collection of medicinal plants from natural habitats. The exceptional plant conservation interests here are the possibilities of conserving natural populations of plants with their genetic diversity and ecological connections, and opportunities to provide incentives for the conservation of natural or semi-natural habitats containing a diversity of plants.

The forest (or home) gardens of Sri Lanka are famous for their plant diversity, with a total of more than 400, mostly indigenous, species of woody plants recorded. These gardens are tended patches of vegetation of intermediate status between fully wild and fully domesticated. Found in all climatic parts of the island - from the wet rainforest regions of the southwest and centre to the drier wooded savannas of the north and east- the forest gardens of Sri Lanka are economically important to the nation, being the source of 41 per cent of its saw-logs and 26 per cent of its biofuel (Ariyadasa 2002; FSMP 1995). They contain a large number of medicinal plants, including the scrambler Asparagus racemosus, the small shrub Munronia pinnata, the large climbers Coscinum fenestratum and Tinospora cordifolia, and the trees Strychnos nux-vomica and Syzygium cumini.

For the purposes of judging ecological sustainability, a choice must be made for the forest gardens as whether to regard them as cultivated or wild. Sustainability can be judged very differently in the two cases. As typically defined, sustainable agriculture refers to a quite different set of required criteria to sustainability for a wild plant resource. Sustainable agriculture primarily requires maintenance of the basic quality of the land, particularly as regards the quality of the soil, and there is no special need for continuing production of any particular crop in a particular field. In contrast, sustainability with reference to a wild plant resource typically requires that the resource re-grows - most stringently defined as reforming at a rate at least as fast as its rate of extraction. For the purposes of resource management (as opposed to certification requirements), Pukka Herbs decided to regard the forest gardens as wild rather than cultivated (an excellent decision from the wider plant conservation perspective). There then ensued questions about how to ensure that the management and harvesting of medicinal plants in these gardens conformed to standards required for sustainability.

Developing Management Systems for the Forest Gardens

Garden ownership, allowable off-take and enrichment planting were among matters that required addressing to establish satisfactory systems of garden management for sustainability. On ownership, it is widely recognised that a key requirement for proper management of a natural resource is security of rights over its use. For example, the Organic Wild Crafting Standard of the Soil Association requires the designation of a responsible manager for each production area. When Pukka Herbs turned its attention to the forest gardens, it discovered that many were not legally registered, creating an obstacle for certification and possibly also for good management.

A lack of legal title for land or plant resources is a common condition in many developing countries and does not necessarily imply a lack of proper management. Customary rules that are publicly respected can also convey the necessary degree of recognised authority. However, in this case, Pukka Herbs, in association with a producing partner (Lanka Organics), considered it necessary to devote considerable effort to getting the land registered, so that the farmers then legally owned the land and their produce could be certified as organic.

The approach taken to setting levels of off-take for the forest gardens was to request officers from the Forest Department to set annual quotas for each species to be harvested, based on discussions with the producer companies and the farmers, and judgements of the levels at which they could be sustainably harvested in particular gardens. These estimates were rule-of-thumb assessments, based on fairly casual observations of the abundance of the species and general knowledge of their ecologies.

No precise measurements were made of the amounts of the species present or of their rates of regeneration or re-growth. In view of the many uncertainties, the levels of allowable off-take were set conservatively, following the precautionary principle. The Forest Department undertakes annual inspections to verify adherence to the set harvesting levels.

The owners of the forest gardens were encouraged to establish small nurseries of some valuable medicinal plants to produce seedlings for enrichment planting. Criteria for species selection included appropriateness for growing in particular climatic regions, saleability and price. Only local and indigenous species were used, examples including Phyllanthus emblica, Piper longum and Tinospora cordifolia.

Harvesting Medicinal Plants from Natural Habitats

The other example of special relevance for wider plant conservation is also in Sri Lanka and concerns the harvesting of medicinal plants in an area of natural forest. The site, near the town of Bibile in the 'intermediate' climatic zone of Sri Lanka, had earlier been chosen as one of five representative Medicinal Plant Conservation Areas (MPCA) in Sri Lanka by a project of the World Conservation Union (IUCN).

The MPCA at Bibile consists of a core forested area and a surrounding zone with farms. During its period of involvement, the IUCN project started to develop systems of sustainable harvesting for medicinal plants in buffer zones of the forest, as well as inaugurating a medicinal plant demonstration garden and involving around 50 local farmers in medicinal plant production.

However, linkages to the market were poor and, as its project came to an end, IUCN requested Lanka Organics in partnership with Pukka Herbs to see whether it could assist the initiatives that it had started to continue and be developed. As a consequence, Lanka Organics, a local business associate of Pukka, has helped some local farmers to achieve certified organic production of medicinal plants and assisted in the development of sustainable harvesting systems for a few species of wild medicinal trees.

The species selected for sustainable wild production are all plants in which it is the fruits that are required by the medicinal trade, making over-harvesting less of a worry than it would be, for example, if it was roots that were needed. They include Phyllanthus emblica, Terminalia cheluba and T. bellirica.

Possible Future Steps

This case study raises questions about how best to develop practical management and harvest guidelines for each species of medicinal plant harvested from natural vegetation at a particular location. Detailed information on the abundance, regeneration and re-growth rates of harvested species has either been unavailable or not of practical use, either in the case of the forest gardens or at Bibile.

Rather, the approach used has been to set conservative limits to the types or amounts of products allowed for harvest, based on rule-of-thumb estimates of species abundance and recovery rates, and the likely damage likely to be incurred to the plants through collection. Species- and site-specific collection guidelines may be further developed.

A related issue is about how far quantitative rigour is required or possible for the certification of wild-collected medicinal plants as sustainable. In the present case, organic certification was achieved without the need for a high degree of quantitative rigour in resource assessment or monitoring. Conservation organisations have recently been giving increased thought to certifica tion schemes for susta ina bility, sometimes requiring ma ny measurements and observations on the status of medicinal species and their habitats to achieve certification.

On the other hand, the herbal and botanical sectors are beset with increasing amounts of regulations, compliance with which can be especially difficult for smaller companies, and there are also the challenges of finding finance and expertise required for sophisticated schemes. The challenge of developing workable systems for certifying sustainable wild collection remains.

MEDICINAL PLANTS

Traditional medicines are used by about 60 per cent of the world's population. These are not only used for primary health care not just in rural areas in developing countries, but also in developed countries as well where modern medicines are predominantly used. While the traditional medicines are derived from medicinal plants, minerals, and organic matter, the herbal drugs are prepared from medicinal plants only.

Use of plants as a source of medicine has been inherited and is an important component of the health care system in India. In the Indian systems of medicine, most practitioners formulate and dispense their own recipes, hence this requires proper documentation and research.

In western world also, the use of herbal medicines is steadily growing with approximately 40 per cent of population reporting use of herb to treat medical illnesses within the past year. Public, academic and government interest in traditional medicines is growing exponentially due to the increased incidence of the adverse drug reactions and economic burden of the modern system of medicine.

There are about 45,000 plant species in India, with concentrated hotspots in the region of Eastern Himalayas, Western Ghats and Andaman & Nicobar Island. The officially documented plants with medicinal potential are 3000 but traditional practitioners use more than 6000. India is the largest producer of medicinal herbs and is appropriately called the botanical garden of the world.

There are currently about 250 000 registered medical practitioners of the Ayurvedic system (total for all traditional systems: approximately 291 000), as compared to about 700,000 of the modern medicine system. In rural India, 70 per cent of the population is dependent on the traditional system of medicine, the Ayurveda.

MEDICINAL PLANTS—INDUSTRIAL PROFILES

Which well known plant never touches the ground, does not follow a 12- month vegetation cycle, stays green year round, blooms in the winter, and sells predominately in December? The answer, of course, is mistletoe. Current research questions the efficacy of this highly controversial plant. "Rejected by clinical oncologists but used by practitioners and cancer patients, it is applied as a remedy to treat a broad spectrum of different diseases, such as epilepsy, diabetes, hypertension, arthrosis, hepatitis, HIV infection, labour pains, and cancer."

Now a new book on the therapeutic uses and industrial applications of Viscum has been published. Rarely mentioned in traditional books on herbal medicine mistletoe research remains questionable. Because the "extracts may exert different effects than purified substances" individual immune responses vary greatly. There is a great need for further investigation. Currently no clinical data are available documenting long-term therapy treatment.

Whether the extracts of Viscum become a major player in the fight against cancer, this book makes for provocative reading. Researchers in pharmacognosy and phystochemistry will find this book documented with references to hundreds of research articles invaluable. While most articles feature the European point of view, there is one article from Japan and another from South Africa. Although none of the articles originate from the United States, American research is well represented in the bibliographies, as are traditional Chinese uses for this herb.

Responding to the increased demand for information on medicinal and aromatic plants this fascinating look at this highly controversial plant is the 16th volume in the series Medicinal and Aromatic Plants Industrial Profiles. This series brings together articles scattered through a variety of sources, is international in scope, and includes many little known sources. Each article is well documented and is introduced by the editor Arndt Bussing, head of the Department of Applied Immunology at the foundation Krebsforschung Herdecke, University of Witten/Herdecke. Mistletoe: the Genus Viscum is illustrated with colour photographs of the plant, line drawings, and chemical structures. With few exceptions most references are current, dating from 1990 to 2000.

While this book would be of interest to scientists in botany, agriculture, and phytochemistry, those working in alternative medicine, pharmaceutical, and health sciences should find it of greater interest. Recommended for academic and research libraries.

NEW SUPPORT FOR MEDICINAL PLANTS

Aspirin, ginseng tea, Aloe lotions and gels are simple healthcare remedies used in many parts of the world to treat a variety of illnesses. They all also have a common beginning: wild plants. Aspirin, for instance, owes its origins to the willow tree.

Hippocrates used powder extracted from willow bark to treat pain and reduce fever in the fifth century BC. Over 2000 years later, the chemical compound salicin was isolated from willow bark, the precursor to the active compound found in modern aspirin. Today, it is estimated that more than 80 billion aspirin tablets are used each year in the USA alone. Unlike aspirin, ginseng tea, used to improve vital energy and slow aging, is still produced from the raw product: ginseng roots. However, much of the ginseng in trade is cultivated, as is all of the aloe vera gel found in skin-care products and health drinks.

Less well known are the tens and perhaps hundreds of thousands of other medicinal plant species used around the world, some of which, like willow trees, have been recognised for their healing properties for thousands of years.

These plants form the basis of health care systems throughout much of the developing world, a source of new compounds on which to base new pharmaceutical products, and a major component of the burgeoning markets for herbal health care remedies and natural products. They also provide a source of income for growers, traders, collectors and manufacturers of plant-based medicines.

In this dual role as a source of healthcare and income, medicinal plants make an important contribution to the larger development process. Unfortunately, however, some plant species of medicinal value are already in short supply, which poses a threat to human welfare and the wild species themselves. Immediate actions are therefore required to ensure harvest and trade of medicinal plant species are conducted sustainably.

TRAFFIC has been working on the medicinal plant trade for many years, including collaboration with important partners such as the IUCN/SSC Medicinal Plant Specialist Group.

Germany's Federal Ministry for Economic Cooperation and Development (Bundesministerium fur wirtschaftliche Zusammenarbeit, more commonly known as BMZ) is supporting a suite of new actions by TRAFFIC. Through a Funds in Trust Agreement with WWF International, BMZ has pledged DM1 million (US$560 000) to the TRAFFIC Network's medicinal plant work during 1998-2000. Much of the funding is directed toward regionally focused work in East Asia, the Indian subcontinent and South America.

In addition, BMZ is supporting efforts to build and/or strengthen links with others working on medicinal plant trade issues. It aims to enhance the communication of TRAFFIC's research results to those who need it, from traditional medicine communities to policy makers.

The regional work to be undertaken through BMZ support is as diverse as the medicinal plant trade itself, with each region home to different, but in the case of India and East Asia, overlapping, medicinal traditions.

East Asia

The major traditional medicine systems in this region are derived from traditional Chinese medicine (TCM), which has a history of several thousand years and is well-documented. These species such as rhinoceros and Tiger in TCM, animal ingredients actually make up less than 20% of those used in TCM. TCM is largely a plant-based medicinal system. It is believed that as many as 1000 plant species are in use for TCM in China and that about 80 per cent of them are taken from the wild. An initial TRAFFIC East Asia study in Hong Kong in 1995/96 revealed a massive trade involving a number of threatened plant species: of the 388 plant species listed in the China Plant Red Data Book, 69 were found to be used in TCM, and 22 of these were in common use.

Through work supported by BMZ, TRAFFIC East Asia seeks to promote the security and conservation of wild plant resources used in traditional medicine in East Asia to support basic health care needs. TRAFFIC East Asia will convene a series of meetings to promote dialogue and understanding of the links between conservation and medicinal security issues among producers, regulators and medicinal communities.

Other activities planned include the compilation of an overview of the nature of and trends in medicinal plant harvest, propagation and trade in East Asia; identifying species at risk; and reviewing national legislation and policies relevant to production, supply and conservation of medicinal plants. Work will also be undertaken to help build capacity within governments and TCM communities to implement any needed trade controls.

The Indian subcontinent

The Himalayas provide more than a meeting point for China and the Indian subcontinent. They also provide a huge variety and volume of medicinal plants used in TCM, Tibetan medicine, and Ayurved. Like TCM, Ayurved has a long history (over 3000 years), is well-documented, and is widely used both locally and in Asian communities established in other parts of the world. There are also a large number of localised traditional medicine systems.

Harvest of native plants to supply India's own healthcare needs and a growing export market provides an important source of income for local communities. However, demand for plant materials is huge and growing, while many of the region's medicinal plant resources are dwindling.

Recent reviews applying IUCN threat criteria found that a significant number of medicinal plant species are threatened or endangered within India. Large quantities of raw medicinal plant materials are also imported into India from neighbouring countries and exported to overseas markets.

A number of organizations within India are concerned with maintaining India's traditional medicine systems. In addition, there is a widespread development network, an established pharmaceutical industry and a wealth of botanical experts in the country. Until now, however, there has been little effort to document the volume and impact of national or international trade in India's medicinal plants.

TRAFFIC India is already well on its way toward establishing working relationships with key stake-holders such as those above and government personnel and toward collecting information required if plants in trade are to be managed on a sustainable basis.

A key challenge within India will be to inform these and other stake-holders of the nature and impact of the medicinal plant trade, and to facilitate their co-operation in developing and implementing measures that will secure the conservation of medicinal plants. Original research will be combined with meetings and workshops to discuss findings and develop workable solutions to any problems identified.

South America

In contrast to East Asia and India, South America's traditional medicine practices are far more localised, with neither the geographic extent or the written texts that characterise TCM and Ayurved. As a result, an important first step is to study and describe the medicinal plant trade in the region, to identify commonly used species, and to begin the process of identifying whether any species are at risk.

Preliminary research in 1996 and 1997 by TRAFFIC International's South America Plants Officer confirmed that, as in Asia, medicinal plants are important components of local health care, are in some cases used unsustainably, and are exported as well as used locally.

BMZ funding is supporting the completion of a regional overview of the medicinal plant trade as well as more detailed studies of individual species in trade, existing trade controls, and the potential role of regional and international treaties in this region. Two species already identified for further research are Cat's Claw Uncaria tomentosa and Dragon's Blood Croton lechleri.

The results of this research will be shared with governments, traditional healthcare associations and relevant agencies to further raise the profile of medicinal plant trade issues and stimulate discussion and actions necessary to ensure more effective management.

MEDICINAL PLANTS AND CITES

The Challenge of Sustainable Harvest

Plants of medicinal value originate from all over the world. Harvest occurs for both local and international use. A growing problem, which is compounded by global population growth and increased demand for raw of medicinal plants used in traditional medical systems and natural products industries are collected from the wild. While propagation occurs for a few species such as American Ginseng Panax quinquefolius and Kuth Saussurea costus, propagation is generally limited due to the expense and time periods required for plants to reach salable size. Harvest and trade can be an important source of income for rural peoples. Regrettably, unsustainable harvest is an increasingly common occurrence that threatens not only the future of these species, but also the livelihoods and health status of people throughout the world.

The Current Situation

At present an estimated 230 plant species included in CITES are traded for medicinal purposes, or are likely to be traded in the future. Fourteen of these were specifically included in the Appendices expressly because of the need to regulate trade in medicinal material. A further six species, Adonis vernalis, Camptotheca acuminata, Cistanche deserticola, Harpagophytum procumbens, Harpagophytum zeyheri and Panax ginseng, are proposed for inclusion in Appendix II at COP11. The Parties' implementation of the

Convention for the species currently included in the Appendices is poor, and is in many cases non-existent. This is surprising, given the importance of these species to the health care of the peoples of these nations, to the livelihoods of the millions who derive income from medicinal plant harvest and trade, and to the industries and consumers who benefit from these resources. Indeed, some Parties have made notable efforts to implement CITES for medicinal plants, such as Germany with the publication of the Checklist of Medicinal and Aromatic Plants and their Trade Names covered by CITES and EU Regulation 2307/97 and Identification Training for Medicinal and Aromatic Plants covered by CITES and EU Regulation 2307/97, and USA with the establishment of a ginseng management programme to monitor wild populations and regulate harvest and commerce.

The Plants Committee has examined the trade through the Medicinal Plant Significant Trade Study, and additional significant plant trade surveys have been undertaken by TRAFFIC. However, these efforts are few in number and although Parties may have taken domestic measures to conserve native plant populations, in general, implementation of the Convention for medicinal plants is unsatisfactory.

Over-exploitation of medicinal plants, and lack of attention to illegal and unsustainable trade, is having serious repercussions around the world. As the global population expands, the demand for medicine increases correspondingly. International trade in medicinal and aromatic plants is already massive, for example, annual global market imports totalling 440,000 metric tonnes in 1996, at a value of USD 1.3 billion. The medicinal plant trade can make a considerable contribution to the economies of producer countries.

Searching for Solutions

As medicinal plant populations decline, governments, natural resource managers, local communities and a variety of other stake-holders have attempted to address the problem in order to conserve medicinal resources. Efforts have been varied.

For example, these initiatives include: promotion of sustainable harvesting techniques; improvement of marketing and trade opportunities to ensure better management; training in quality control and packaging to reduce wastage and derive higher earnings; increased regulation and control at local, national and international levels; and propagation of medicinal plant species. Increasingly, these efforts are designed taking into consideration the complexity of the medicinal plant issue and the realization that demand will not decrease, hence solutions must factor in the aspect of a continuously increasing trade.

The market for medicinal plants is dynamic and complex. Demand for new natural products, and growing interest in traditional medical systems around the world, means that greater volumes of plant material are required to satisfy the market. Medicinal plants are traded in a variety of forms, for example: raw material such as leaves, bark, and roots, unprocessed broken material such as chips or slices, derivatives and semi-processed or manufactured material such as powders, extracts, tonics, pills, teas and other products, as well as finished pharmaceutical products.

Trade occurs far from the area of production, and processing often takes place in countries other than those where the plants originate. For example, approximately 120,000 metric tonnes of medicinal and aromatic plants were imported into Europe in 1996, and this material came from over 120 countries, 60% of which were African and Asian nations. During this same year, Europe exported about 70,000 metric tonnes of plant material. Understanding the dynamics of the trade in medicinals can be difficult, and although overall volumes and values may be known, species-specific information is not at all comprehensive. The dearth of such data is one reason for the lack of attention countries have directed toward the medicinal plant resource.

Insufficient knowledge about the scope of the trade, in particular at the range state level, has resulted in ineffective implementation of existing regulations and initiatives in producing countries, to the detriment of the resource and those who will depend on it in the years to come. Perhaps most important is that there is little appreciation for the increasingly critical imbalance between supply and demand.

Can CITES Help?

CITES addresses only a small portion of the medicinal plant issue, but it has the potential to help achieve sustainable and legal trade in medicinal resources. Specifically, CITES can do the following:

- identify trends at the species level and on the global level, to highlight critical issues and address them;
- help to make the trade more transparent, by documenting the species and parts in trade, and volumes traded, because this information is necessary for designing and implementing sustainable management plans;
- stimulate cooperation between importing and exporting countries to ensure that trade is conducted in a legal and sustainable manner;

So What is the Problem?

When the trade is so large, and the implications of unsustainable harvest and trade so serious, why is implementation of CITES for medicinal plants unsatisfactory? Some possible explanations include the following:

- Parties are unaware that CITES-listed medicinal plants are in international trade, because of insufficient knowledge about the parts and derivatives that aretraded.
- Regulatory officials responsible for inspection of plant material are unfamiliar with CITES and do not know that certain traded plant species require CITES documentation.
- Plants are frequently afforded less attention than animal species.

- The variety of parts and derivatives in trade is numerous, and the annotations for CITES- listed medicinal plants vary from species to species, therefore it may be difficult for inspectors to keep track of what should be regulated.
- The majority of trade in medicinal and aromatic plants is not regulated by CITES, and therefore CITES-listed species may be accorded a low priority.

Will these Efforts help Medicinal Plants?

At present the sustainability of the medicinal plant trade is on precarious ground. Through CITES, there is an opportunity to promote sustainable harvest and trade. While regulation is only part of the solution, it is an integral part of a strategy that must entail efforts from many sectors and many directions.

Because of the importance of a sustainable trade in medicinal plants, it is entirely appropriate for CITES to collaborate and indeed advise other global bodies that deal directly with human health issues, on the conservation aspect of this problem. With regard to medicinal plants, the objectives of CITES and the CBD are complementary.

Demand for Medicinal Plants in KwaZulu-Natal

Medicinal plants are used extensively by the black population throughout KwaZulu-Natal (KZN), and indeed South Africa. An active trade and market in medicinal plant material occurs in KwaZulu-Natal as a result of:

- a fragmented distribution of medicinal plant species due to the varied land use, topography and climate in the region,
- large spatial concentrations of consumer demand as more than half the province's population is concentrated in two urban centres,
- local extinctions of plants and the need to access more remote plant populations due to intensive harvesting, and
- various socio-economic factors (including culture and accessible health care) which maintain and stimulate demand.

In KwaZulu-Natal over 400 plants are actively traded [Cunningham 1988; McKean 1996] with an estimated trade volume of some 4 300 tonnes per year. As the market is large and dynamic, several market segments have developed in response to the users' demands and the supply of plants. The extent of trade and the market segments are discussed in the following sections.

Quantity and Trends in Consumer Demand

A survey of several Durban City medical clinics indicated that 53% of the black clinic patients made use of indigenous healers at least once during the previous year, with an average of 3.34 visits in the previous year. The term indigenous healers or medicine is preferred by the author to the more conventional term traditional healers or medicine. The healing practices used, while originating in African culture, are not purely traditional. The practice is dynamic, addressing new illnesses like AIDS, and adopts new technologies and new medicines.

The healers also deal with all manner of urban social problems, which are not traditional. The term indigenous medicine may therefore be more appropriate as it relates to the practices of healing and divination within an indigenous but modem African culture which may not necessarily be traditional.

While respondents asked whether they visited a indigenous healer in the previous year, the survey omitted to ask respondents whether they purchased indigenous medicine without a healer's prescription. As a consequence, the above estimate of indigenous medicine use may be an underestimate. An indication of the extent of self-medication can be obtained from the expressed preference for hygienically packed medicines.

Eighty-four percent of the black clinic patients indicated that they would prefer more hygienically packed indigenous medicines, indicating that 31% of the sample may not have visited an indigenous healer in 1995 but probably make use of indigenous medicine.

Assuming that the clinic sample is representative of the black population in Durban, the total number of users is estimated to be around 2 million people [that is 84% of 2.442 million blacks resident in Durban (Durban Metropolitan Government 19.96)]. This estimate can be considered a conservative minimum level, as 6% of the indigenous healers patients indicated that they did not make use of western clinics, and therefore using the clinic patients as a proxy for the Durban black population may be a slight underestimate.

The Quantity of Plant Material Reported to be Consumed

Basing the quantity demanded on the reported number of times which the population sample visits indigenous healers (3.34 times per annum), it is estimated that between 900 tonnes and 1 500 tonnes of plant material were consumed in Durban in 1995 .

As most of the estimates are based on relatively imprecise data regarding the numbers of market participants, the broad estimates will generally be rounded off to make for easier reading. However, detailed measurements made within the survey will be retained for descriptive accuracy and where calculations are made.

This estimate assumes that the indigenous medicine users not visiting indigenous healers, that is the remaining 31% of users, would use indigenous medicine at the same rate at which healers are visited (3.34 times a year). The estimate of 900 tonnes is derived if 53% of the population is assumed to use medicine at an average mass of 83.3g per use (the average mass of plant material prescribed by healers and shop traders) and the remaining consumers use the medicine at 216.5g per use (the average mass of plant material traded in the street markets). The estimate of 1 500 tonnes is obtained if all 84% of the black population uses medicine at 216.5g per use. This last estimate is likely to be more realistic given the extent of wastage associated with the poor storage of plant material.

The Quantity of Plant Material Reported to be Traded

The shop traders are estimated to trade 340 tonnes per year, with approximately 50% reported to be purchased directly from plant gatherers (170 tonnes) and the remaining 50% purchased from street traders (170 tonnes).

The quantities traded by the healers was problematic to estimate due to the unknown number of healers in the survey area. Various reports [Holdstock of indigenous healers to the population but these have not been used for a number of reasons.

Firstly, the mode of operation differs considerably between healers, with some healers being extremely busy whilst others may only practise part-time. Secondly, the various healers' organizations have provided a rough indications of the number of healers which are registered with them, but it has not been possible to obtain membership lists from these groups (in addition, the membership makes no differentiation regarding the nature of the practitioners operation, that is, whether it is either full-time or part-time).

Due to the above problems, estimates are based on the visitation frequency reported by the clinic patients and the average number of patients, which the indigenous healers indicate they may treat per day. Following this approach an estimated 936 tonnes of medicinal plants are traded per year by indigenous healers in Durban.

The indigenous healers reported that they purchase plant material from two sources, approximately 50% from the street markets and 50% directly from plant gatherers. This suggests that approximately 468 tonnes are bought from each group.

This estimate uses an average mass of 216.5 g for a prescribed medicine dosage. This mass is the average mass of street traded products and is believed to be a more appropriate mass than the mass dispensed in traders shops and by healers (an average 83.3 g) for estimating the quantity used by healers. The traded products are generally unprocessed and poorly packaged, with a significant proportion (not quantifiable at present) of the plant material spoiled in the transportation and storage process. The author therefore considers the larger street traded mass to be a more accurate reflection of the quantities which healers will utilise but not necessarily dispense.

Of the plant mass traded in the street markets, an estimated 20% of the trade or 220 tonnes, is reported to be traded between the street traders themselves and not to consumers, healers or shop traders. This implies that of the 1 100 tonnes traded in the market as a whole, only 880 tonnes of plant material is the physical stock of plants entering the street markets in a year. By summing the quantities sold by the various market players to end consumers, it is estimated that some 1 500 tonnes of plant material were sold in the Durban markets in 1996.

This estimate of 1 500 tonnes traded in the market approximates the estimate derived in 4.1.1 regarding the maximum quantity of plant material which may be consumed in Durban given the consumption rates of the clinic patients interviewed. While the two approaches are not entirely independent as both models use a common number in estimating the use associated with healers, there is sufficiently different information in the other sectors which gives confidence to the similarity of estimates.

Potential Provincial and National Consumption Levels

Several studies in different geographic localities throughout South Africa and in different cultural groups have shown that between 58 and 100% of the black population uses indigenous medicine. Holdstock [1978] estimated that between 80 and 85% of the black population in Soweto (a black township in Johannesburg) consumed indigenous medicine. Ellis [1986] found that 100% of a random sample of hospital patients in the Estcourt area (a typical rural population) used indigenous medicine. More recently, a study in peri-urban Bushbuckridge [Mander 1997a] estimated that 58% of the clinic patients used indigenous medicine. However, this estimate is known to be conservative due to the persecution of people suspected of witchcraft in the area, and consequently an unwillingness to admit to the use of indigenous medicine. Assuming that the characteristics of the Durban consumers are representative of the rest of the population in KwaZulu-Natal and South Africa, it is possible to provide a preliminary indication of provincial and national consumption patterns. In KwaZulu-Natal the current population is estimated to be 8.7 million, with the black population comprising 83% of the total population or 7.2 million people [Central Statistical Services 1996]. Assuming that 84% of the black population use indigenous medicine in KwaZulu-Natal, the number of potential users of indigenous medicine could therefore be 6 million people. Based on an average frequency of uses of 3.34 visits/uses per year (this translates to 20 million uses a year), and assuming an average mass of 216.5g per use, then total quantity of medicinal plants used in KwaZulu-Natal could amount to 4 339 tonnes per year.

Similarly, at a national level there are 33 million blacks in South Africa [Central Statistical Services 1996] with an estimated 28 million (84%) users. Using the same visitation rate per year and the mass per use as above, the total national consumption could amount some 90 million uses per year with a mass of 19 500 tonnes of plant material.

Trends in the Use of Indigenous Medicine

The survey of consumer trends at western clinics and at indigenous healers indicated that a large section of the population has not changed their use patterns, with similar percentages indicating both an increase and a decrease in use. There is, however, an overall increase in the use of indigenous medicine. The following figures (4.3 to 4.8) and discussion outline the changes and reasons for change in use frequency cited by healers and clinic patients indigenous medicine would remain high. The shop traders shared the same perspective that trade would remain at high levels.

Discussions with market players and observations of the markets in southern Africa (South Africa, Mozambique, Swaziland, Lesotho and Namibia) have pointed to an increase in the demand for medicines [Scott pers. comm. 1996; Maseko pers. comm. 1997]. While the individual consumers surveyed may not have indicated a trend of increasing use, there is common consensus among traders and researchers that there has been an increase in the number of individuals consuming indigenous medicine. This may be the result of the following factors.

The population growth throughout the region is around 2.4% per year [Central Statistics 1996], leading to an increase in the potential number of people who may make use of indigenous medicine. Coupled with this increase, are the accelerated urbanization rates, which increase the competition for resources and services, especially where economic growth lags behind population growth. Indigenous medicines are actively used to reduce competition for employment, housing, and other social resources that are associated with increasing urban competition. Competition in urban areas may also contribute to psychological stress, and indigenous healing and healers are used extensively to treat stress-related illness.

The existence of poverty also fuels the demand for medicinal plants as households are forced to make use of affordable medicine. While consulting a healer may be more expensive than visiting a clinic, medicines bought directly from the street traders are much cheaper than any other forms of health care, and consequently are an important health care option.

Past government policies in South Africa discriminated against indigenous healing, giving it no positive recognition, and generally labelling the activities as primitive and even legislating against witchcraft practices (Suppression of Witchcraft Act). Perceptions are now changing from several quarters, with increasing official and societal recognition. For example, medical aids in South Africa are increasingly accepting claims, by their members, for visits to indigenous healers [Daily News, 14 January 1997], and black people themselves are developing increasing pride in the culture of indigenous healing.

One of the greatest drivers of the demand for indigenous medicine are the widely held views by the black community that certain illnesses are cultural' sicknesses which can only be treated by indigenous medicine. In addition, AIDS is rapidly increasing within the South African community, and with little relief from western medicine, healers report that people with AIDS consult them. There are many healers who now advertise that they have a cure for AIDS, promoting the increased use of indigenous medicine.

Apart from the above, the remote geographical location of many large rural populations also promotes the use of indigenous medicine as it is usually the most accessible source of health care, and the most available health care, as western clinics are either far away or visit rural communities only periodically.

In view of the above factors, the local demand for indigenous medicine is unlikely to decline and will probably increase as the population increases.

Apart from growing local demand, there are also indications of a growing international demand. Neighbouring countries (particularly Namibia and Botswana) are increasing their demand for South African medicinal plants due to the greater diversity, reliability of supply and quantities available. The dry environments have relatively low diversities of high value medicinal plants and in addition, the frequent and regular movement of people between southern African states results in considerable exchange in ideas and information, with foreign healers learning to use South African products. In addition, the declining ability of many countries to maintain the importation of synthetic drugs promotes the continued use of indigenous medicines8. International demand for local plant products is also likely to increase with the growing popularity of alternative medicines and natural products in developed countries [Lange 1997].

For example, discussions in 1996 with women from a remote area in western Mali, reported to the author that they did not bother travelling to the local clinic, in this case only a few kilometres away, as the only medicine which the clinic could provide was quinine and aspirin, and good alternatives for these drugs were more easily accessible in the bush close to where they lived.

❐

Traditional Systems of Medicinal Plants

ACTIVE HYPOGLYCEMIC CONSTITUENTS FROM PLANTS

Many active compounds have been isolated from the plant and herb species of India. These active principles are dietary fibres, alkaloids, flavonoids, saponins, amino acids, steroids, peptides and others. These have produced potent hypoglycemic, anti-hyperglycemic and glucose suppressive activities.

The above effects achieved by either insulin release from pancreatic â-cells, inhibited glucose absorption in gut, stimulated glycogenesis in liver or increased glucose utilization by the body. These compounds also exhibited their antioxidant, hypolipidemic, anticataract activities, restored enzymatic functions, repair and regeneration of pancreatic islets and the alleviation of liver and renal damage. Some active constituents have been obtained from plants possess insulin like activity and could be provide alternate for insulin therapy. Chemical structures of few active compounds having anti-diabetic potentials from above mentioned plants are provided.

Metabolic imbalance causing diabetes mellitus is a characteristic of materialistic world. Differences in social structure, psychic stress, obesity, hormonal imbalance and heredity are optimizing the growth of pandemic. Increasing population with diabetes has a huge requirement of effective remediation.

The Indian flora has a vast variety of medicinal plants, which are used traditionally for their anti-diabetic property. However, careful assessment including sustainability of such herbs, ecological and seasonal variation in activity of phyto-constituents, metal contents of crude herbal anti-diabetic drugs, thorough toxicity study and cost effectiveness is required for their popularity.

These efforts may provide treatment for all and justify the role of novel traditional medicinal plants having anti-diabetic potentials.

BIO-INFORMATICS ON MEDICINAL PLANTS AND TRADITIONAL KNOWLEDGE

Medicinal Plants Master Database

A comprehensive master database on medicinal plants of India has been systematically built up at FRLHT over the last 8 years. Currently, this database incorporates more than 7, 500 botanical names which are linked to more than 1,40,500 vernacular names in 13 different languages like Tamil, Kannada, Malayalam, Hindi, Sanskrit, etc. Each such correlation can be traced back to a published reference.

This database also incorporates more than 10, 000 authentic digital images of plants duly linked to their botanical names. An important feature of this database is a fully-referenced distribution database which provides information on geographical distribution of nearly 6, 000 plant species. Through a system of assigning a unique ID number to each botanical name and linking various aspects of information, for each species, to this unique ID, data relating to several different aspects like propagation, trade, pharmacognosy etc can be quickly accessed for a specific plant entity with search being initiated with the help of a botanical or vernacular name.

This multi-faceted database forms the backbone for undertaking and promoting sustainable use and informed conservation action for native medicinal plant species and also acts as a platform for designing various research projects relating to the management of this valuable natural resource.

This database is also linked to referenced information on the plant materia-medica of traditional systems of medicine as well as to pharmacognosy and pharmacology of the plant entities.

PHARMACOGNOSY DATABASE ON INDIAN MEDICINAL PLANTS

A computerised database called Labguru has been created for storing and retrieving referenced literature on pharmacognosy and pharmacology of medicinal plants. Labguru is a stand-alone database with an easy-to-use interface, linked to the master database.

This database is a valuable literature source for researchers and industry alike. Data compilation is from published sources such as texts and on-line databases. This is an ongoing evolving activity in the laboratory at FRLHT.

Database on metals and minerals used in Indian medicines

Mineral and metal medicine is used by traditional practitioners all over India. These are potent medicinal materials which need accurate identification of materials and careful processing for their proper use.

Therefore it was decided to develop a user-friendly and easily retrievable database on mineral and metal medicine by compilation of relevant references from authentic traditional texts of Ayurveda that are difficult to procure at one place for most users. Correlating the traditional names of metals minerals to modern geological entities helps to understand the identity of the minerals used.

AYUSH Databases

FRLHT in the last 10 years has been documenting and developing traditional knowledge databases on the materia medica of Indian systems of medicine.

Medicinal plant databases have been already initiated on Ayurveda, Siddha, Unani system and Homoeopathy. The current FRLHT databases have screened a limited number of the known medical texts written across the period 1500 BC to 1900 AD and therefore much work yet remains to be done.

In the next 5 years we would also like to initiate new database work on diagnostics and other speciality areas like panchakarma and rasayana, as these fields are critical for effective application of Ayurveda and Siddha. The main goal of the databases is to serve the needs of students and teachers of Indian systems of medicine, medical practitioners, researchers , community enterprises, community health NGOs and pharmaceutical companies.

Database of plants of Susruta Samhita

The database of plants of Susruta Samhita has 9, 650 references. This data has been converted from the previous data environment to the present one to support access to various database tools. A checklist of the plant names was prepared and a report is made available in Sanskrit and English scripts.

Database on plants of Siddha medicine

The bilingual database has an extensive collection of information pertaining to a therapeutic information of plants mentioned in 5 texts of 2, 350 records, simple remedies mentioned in 6 texts of 1, 800 records, formulation data of 3,013 records and 36, 000 records of dictionary file which has Tamil names of plants.

A separate nighantu file in Tamil script and a glossary of the technical terms are also incorporated in this database.

Database on plants of Homoeo medicine

This database could complete compilation of plants and products information of 80 plants mentioned in Homoeo medicine from 15-20 sources as text document.

Database on plants of Unani medicine

A hard copy of the Arabic and Urdu names appearing in the classical texts of Unani medicine was prepared from the FRLHT's nomenclature database. Verification on botanical names and spellings of Arabic names and Unani names were carried out.

DATABASES FOR ASSESSMENT OF LOCAL HEALTH TRADITIONS

The web-based Referral Browser basically aims to provide support for assessment of folk health traditions. This will help to promote best health-related practices in a specific area for human, plant and animal health care. The browser will procure references from Ayurveda, Siddha, Unani and modern pharmacology for a resource used in folk health practice and is subjected to evaluation/assessment.

SPECIALISED REPORTS & CHECKLISTS

FRLHT has come out with state wise checklists and specialised reports on medicinal plants in conservation sites. While specialised reports have been prepared and published on the medicinal plants of Karnataka, Kerala and Tamil Nadu, checklists have been prepared for Andhra Pradesh, Maharashtra, Madhya Pradesh, Arunachal Pradesh, Himachal Pradesh, Meghalaya and Uttranchal. The specialised reports list the species recorded in the state and the species found in the MPCAs, their habit and the system of medicine in which they are used. Specialised reports also has the distribution and the forest type maps of the respective state, the botanical profile of the state and the MPCA and the habit wise analysis of the medicinal plants.

INFORMATION PRODUCTS

CDs on Medicinal plants of southern India

Three CDs on medicinal plants of Karnataka, Kerala and Tamil Nadu have been designed for the use of researchers working in the field of conservation. The CDs incorporate data on checklist of medicinal plants in each of these States. It also provides information on threat status of the species, synonyms, different systems of medicine they are used in and forest type where the plants occur. There are around 900 images. Information is also available on primary health care uses for 128 species and propagation techniques for 200 species. More than 65, 000 regional names have been included, in different languages like Sanskrit, Hindi, Marathi, Telugu, Kannada, Malayalam and Tamil, along with maps to show the occurrence of individual species in various forest types. The search of a species can be done either from botanical or regional name. It can filter the species depending on the forest type, threat status, system of medicine and by the language.

Clinically Important plants of Ayurveda (CIPA)

Clinically Important Plants of Ayurveda is now available as a CD-ROM, which contains detailed information of 3500 pharmaceutical preparations for 200 indications. It has plant pictures, botanical and regional names, Sanskrit synonyms and its complete reference, plant properties and English meaning of all technical Sanskrit terms. This would be useful for pharmaceutical industries, Ayurveda practitioners and researchers.

Plants of Caraka Samhita

This bilingual database incorporates 12, 873 plant references from Caraka Samhita which are grouped into 620 species. This was carried out based on a guideline prepared for grouping plant names as anonyms, synonyms and variant names. In the database, each plant reference is provided with its English translation and all the technical terms are supported with a dictionary of its English meaning. Classification of medicinal plants, 1, 700 formulation information, plant picture, various botanical correlations and its identity status, habit and trade information of selected species, commentator 's opinion of plant identity, etc. are the important features of this database.

A multimedia CD was designed with necessary visual effects highlighting the importance of Caraka Samhita. A brochure on this CD is also available to support dissemination activities.

Database on plants of Ayurveda for BAMS course

All classical information pertaining to detailed and non-detailed list of plants mentioned in the BAMS (Bachelor of Ayurvedic Medicine and Surgery) syllabus were compiled from 20 classical texts. There are 370 plants in the syllabus which are incorporated in the database. Botanical names, regional names, classical references like Sanskrit slokas, interpretation of the slokas into English, and usage of these plants as single drugs are incorporated into this database.

Modern botanical information such as morphology, distribution, propagation methods and pharmacognosy information inclusive of its plant biochemistry and pharmacology are provided. This database is aimed to provide all required information for graduates and postgraduate students of Ayurveda.

Database on Ayurveda formularies

The database of the Ayurveda formularies incorporated in the Ver. 1 of CIPA (Clinically important plants of Ayurveda) CD. The second version of the CIPA will have 4, 000 more Ayurvedic formulation compiled from 7 classical texts covering about 150 plants.

TRIALS FOR ANTI-DIABETIC POTENTIALS OF MEDICINAL PLANTS

Recently the plants and herbs are being used as decoctions or in other extracted forms for their blood sugar lowering potential. There are some useful reviews on Indian medicinal plants having blood sugar lowering potentials. Many useful herbs introduced in pharmacological and clinical trials have confirmed their blood sugar lowering effect, repair of â-cells of islets of Langerhans. Details of some potent Indian herbs, their recently reported pharmacological and clinical hypoglycemic efficacy, active chemical constituents, their mechanism of action and available toxicity status are described chronologically as follows:

AEGLE MARMELOS LINN. COOREA (FAMILY: RUTACEAE)

Hindi name: Bel; Common name: Holy Fruit Tree

The trees grow throughout deciduous forest of India and ripen fruits are commonly use for delicacy. Aegle marmelos is widely used in Indian Ayurvedic medicine for the treatment of diabetes mellitus. Hypoglycemic effect of root bark decoction (1ml/100mg) has been observed in normal fasted rats. Leaf extract produced anti-hyperglycemic activity in alloxan diabetic rats along with decreased cholesterol and blood urea. In diabetic rats leaf extract exhibited insulin like activity. Aqueous leaf extract has been shown to improve the functional state of pancreatic cells in streptozotocin induced diabetic rats. Aqueous leaf extract (250 & 500mg/kg, orally) produced hypoglycemic effect and increased plasma insulin level of STZ-diabetic rats. LD50 (lethal dose) observed greater than 10. 0g/kg at oral administration to rats. Anti-hyperglycemic activity caused by leaf extract (250mg/kg, orally) in glucose fed hyperglycemic rats (Sachdewa et al., 2001). Aqueous fruit extract (250mg/kg, twice daily for one month) produces anti-hyperglycemic effect along with decreasing glycosylated haemoglobin level in STZ induced diabetic albino wistar rats. Hypoglycemic and antioxidant activity of leaves have been observed in diabetic male albino rats. Fruit extract (125 and 250mg/kg, orally twice daily for 30 days) produced anti-diabetic, anti-hyperlipidaemic and antioxidant activity in STZ diabetic rats along with partial repair of damaged pancreatic islets (Kamalakkanan et al., 2005). Treatment of severely (fasting blood glucose level >250 mg/ml) diabetic rats for 14 days with aqueous extract (250mg/kg, orally) of Aegle marmelos seeds reduced the fasting blood glucose by 60. 84% and urine sugar by 75% than their pretreatment levels.

ALLIUM CEPA LINN. (FAMILY: LILIACEAE)

Hindi name: Pyaj; Common name: Onion

The plant is cultivated throughout India. Onion bulb and leaves are the important part of diet. Ether soluble fraction of onion (0. 25mg/kg, orally) has been observed to lower blood sugar level in normal rabbits and exhibited potent antioxidant activity (Auguati, 1973). In a clinical study treatment of diabetic patients by juice of Allium cepa bulb, controlled the blood sugar level. Dipropyl disulphide oxide and onion oil produced significant hypoglycemic effect. Significant blood sugar lowering produced by petroleum ether extract (2g/kg) from onion bulb in glucose, induced hyper-glycemic rabbits. A sulphur containing amino acid, S-methyl cystein sulphoxide (at a dose of 200mg/kg for 45 days) from onion showed potent hypoglycemic activity in alloxan induced diabetic rats. S-allyl cystein sulphoxide from onion significantly reduced blood glucose level of alloxan induced diabetic rats. Prolonged administration of freeze dried onion powder (3%) with a diet produced anti-hyperglycemic, hypolipidemic and antioxidant activity in STZ-diabetic rats. Onion callus cultures showed greater hypoglycemic potential over natural onion bulb. Prolonged administration of a diet containing onion produced hypoglycemic and antioxidant effect in diabetic rats. Allium cepa juice (0. 4g/100g b. w. for 4 weeks) exhibited anti-hyperglycemic and antioxidant effect in alloxan induced diabetic rats, it also repaired hepatic and renal damage caused by alloxan.

ALLIUM SATIVUM LINN. (FAMILY: LILIACEAE)

Hindi name: Lahsun; Common name: Garlic

The plant is cultivated all over India. It is an important part of dietary ingredients. Allicin (0. 25mg/kg, orally) from garlic exhibited pronounce hypoglycemia in mild diabetic rabbits. In alloxan induced diabetic rabbits ethanol, ethyl acetate and petroleum ether extract (0. 25mg/kg, orally) produced antihyperglycemic activity. Treatment of alloxan diabetic rats with the antioxidant s-allyl cysteine sulfoxide isolated from garlic ameliorates the diabetic condition almost to the same extent as did glibenclamide and insulin. It also significantly stimulates in vitro insulin secretion from â-cells isolated from pancreas of normal rats. Extract (500mg/kg/day) of Allium sativum bulb proved to be effective for treatment of l-thyroxine (l-T4) induced hyperglycemia in rats. Alloxan induced diabetic rats fed a diet containing Allium sativum (12.5%) for 15 days were able to reduce blood glucose as compare to control group. Oral administration of a laboratory diet containing 0. 05% of ajoene (derived from garlic) for 8 weeks has been observed to produce anti-diabetic effect in genetically diabetic KK-A(y) mice. The levels of plasma glucose significantly suppressed about 73. 8%. Two garlic compounds garlic oil (100mg/kg body weight) and diallyl trisulfide (40mg/kg body weight) given every other day for 3 weeks to STZ-diabetic rats significantly raised the basal insulin concentration and increased the insulin sensitivity. Herbal extract of garlic (20mg 100 g-1 body weight, orally, daily for 5 weeks) produced hypoglycemia, probably by interfering with food intake of both normal and STZ-diabetic rats.

S-allyl cysteine, a key component of aged garlic, found potent antioxidant and inhibited AGEP (accumulation of advanced glycation end products) formation.

Bis (allixinato) oxovanadium (IV) from garlic found to be the most potent anti-diabetic agent in type 1 diabetic mice on both intraperitoneal injections and oral administrations (Adachi et al., 2006).

ALOE VERA (LINN.) BURM. F. (FAMILY: LILIACEAE)

Hindi and Common name: Aloe

The herbs are cultivated throughout India for its variety of medicinal properties. Dry sap of plant produced prominent anti-hyperglycemic response in type 2 diabetic patients (½ teaspoonful, orally for 4–14 weeks), and in alloxan induced diabetic Swiss albino mice (500mg/kg, twice daily for 5 days). In a clinical study, it was reported that oral administration of aloe might be a useful adjuvant for lowering of blood glucose in diabetic patients. Aloe vera leaf pulp extract showed hypoglycemic activity on type 1 and type 2 diabetic rats, the effect being enhanced in type 2 diabetes as compared with glibenclamide. Plant extract (200 and 300mg/kg, orally) produced hypoglycemic activity along with controlled carbohydrate metabolizing enzymes in normal fasted, oral glucose fed and STZ-diabetic rats. Oral administration of ethanolic extract

(300mg/kg b. w.) to STZ-diabetic rats for 21 days resulted in a prominent reduction of fasting blood glucose along with improved plasma insulin level of diabetic rats. Administration of the five phytosterols from Aloe vera namely, lophenol, 24-methyl-lophenol, 24-ethyl-lophenol, cycloartanol and 24-methylene-cycloartanol to severe type 2 diabetic mice for 28 days decreased the fasting blood glucose levels 64%, 28%, 47%, 51%, and 55% respectively. Oral administration of Aloe vera gel extract (300mg/kg b. w. per day for 21 days) to STZ-diabetic rats resulted in a significant reduction of fasting blood glucose and improved the plasma insulin level.

ANDROGRAPHIS PANICULATA (BURM. F.) NEES (FAMILY: ACANTHACEAE)

Hindi name: Kalmegha; Common name: King of Bitter

This is an annual herb that grows throughout India. Plant extract effectively produced hypoglycemic and anti-hyperglycemic activity in normal rats. Different doses (0. 1, 0. 2, and 0. 4g/kg b. w.) of plant extract effectively reduced the fasting serum glucose level of STZ-diabetic rats. Antihyperglycemic and antioxidant activity of plant extract (400mg/kg b. w, twice a day for 14 days), has also been reported in diabetic rats. The andrographolide from plant increases the glucose utilization and lowers plasma glucose in diabetic rats lacking insulin. Significant reduction in blood glucose level (52. 90%) observed when hyperglycemic rats treated with 50mg/kg body weight aqueous extract of Andrographis paniculata. This effect enhanced when freeze-dried material used at a dose of 6. 25 mg/kg body weight, it reduced 61. 81% blood glucose level. The anti-diabetic potentials of plant restored the impaired estrous cycle in alloxan-induced diabetic rats.

ANNONA SQUAMOSA LINN. (ANNONACEAE)

Hindi name: Sharifa; Common name: Sugar apple tree

The plants grow throughout India and commonly use by tribal communities of Northern India for the treatment of diabetes. Aqueous leaf extract produces hypoglycemic activity in streptozotocin-nicotinamide induced dia betic rats. Ethanolic leaf-extract (350mg/kg b. w., orally 10-day) administration to STZ-diabetic rats has been shown to lower fasting blood glucose level to (73. 3%), and treatment of severely diabetic rabbits with leaf- extract (350mg/kg, for 15 days) reduced fasting blood glucose by 52. 7% and urine sugar by 75%. Annona squamosa fruit pulp extract (2. 5 and 5. 0g/kg b. w.) has been observed to improve the glucose tolerance of alloxan diabetic rats. Further more, fruit pulp (5g/kg b. w.) brought down urine sugar, urine protein and glycol-hemoglobin in diabetic rabbits. Oral administration of aqueous leaf-extract to diabetic rats for 30 days significantly reduced the levels of blood glucose and increased the activity of plasma insulin and antioxidant enzymes.

AZADIRACHTA INDICA A. JUSS. (FAMILY: MELIACEAE)

Hindi name: Neem; Common name: Indian lilac tree

This is an evergreen tree grows throughout India. Aqueous extract is known to produce antihyperglycemic and hypoglycemic activity in diabetic dogs. Fresh leaves decoction induced antihyperglycemic activity and increased the peripheral glucose utilization in normal rats. Leaf extract of Azadirachta indica has been reported to produce the hypoglycemic activity in normal rats without altered serum cortisol level (Chattopadhyay et al., 1999). Crude ethanol extract (250mg/kg, for 2 weeks) potentially lowered the blood sugar level of alloxan diabetic rats.

Leaf extract has been observed to produce anti-hyperglycemic activity in streptozotocin diabetic rats without altered serum cortisol level. Petroleum ether extract of seed kernel (2gm/kg b. w.) & seed husk (0. 9gm/kg b. w.) restricted oxidative stress in heart and erythrocytes caused by streptozotocin in diabetic rats. Dianex, a polyherbal formulation consists of the aqueous extract of Azadirachta indica has been well tolerated in laboratory animals at higher doses (up to 10 g/kg in mice, acute toxicity; up to 2. 5 g/kg in rats, sub- acute toxicity studies for 30 days) without any toxic manifestation. Beta-sitosterol, a steroid obtained from Azadirachta indica, may be responsible for its hypoglycemic property. In a clinical study of type 2 diabetes powdered part, aqueous extract and alcoholic extract of Azadirachta indica at high dose for 14 days exhibited hypoglycemic activity.

CINNAMOMUM TAMALA (HAMM.) NEES. & EBERM. (FAMILY: LAURACEAE)

Hindi name: Tejpat; Common name: Bayberry

The plant is cultivated in different parts of India and use as spice. Aqueous leaf extract induced potential blood sugar lowering effect in 18 hours fasted and glucose induced hyperglycemic rabbits at a dose of 500mg/kg. Oral administration of powdered leaves (20gm for 15 days) exhibited hypoglycemic effect in patients of type 2 diabetes mellitus along with insulin released from pancreatic â-cells. In a clinical study, leave powder produced hypoglycemic response in type 2 diabetic patients. Ethanolic extract (210mg/kg) of leaves induced potential hypoglycemic effect in 18 hours fasted albino rats. Alcoholic extract of leaves produced hypoglycemic activity in alloxan induced diabetic rats when administered orally for two weeks at a dose of 250mg/kg.

COCCINIA GRANDIS (LINN.) VOIGT (FAMILY: CUCURBITACEAE)

Syn. Coccina indica (White & Arn); Hindi name: Kunderi; Common name: Ivy Guard

The plants are wild creepers grow in many parts of India. Blood sugar lowering effect has been observed in patients treated with homogenized freeze dried leaves. Ethanol extract (250mg/kg) of whole plant produced hypoglycemic activity in fasted, glucose fed and diabetic albino rats. Hypoglycemic effect of alcoholic extract (250mg/kg, orally) of Coccinia indica was observed in fasted and glucose fed hyperglycemic male albino rats. Alcoholic leaf extract produced hypoglycemic effect in normal fed and 48 hours fasted rats, response mediated by suppression of gluconeogenic enzyme glucose-6-phosphatase. Pectin (200mg/100gm/day) isolated from fruits, exhibited blood sugar lowering effect and an increase in the glycogen content of liver in normal rats. Ethanol (60%) leaf extract (200mg/kg, orally) lowered the blood sugar level of diabetic rats due to suppressed glucose synthesis, through depression of glucose-6-phosphatase, fructose-1-6-biphosphatase and enhanced glucose oxidation by shunt pathway through activation of glucose-6-phosphate dehydrogenase. Leaf extract was produced hypoglycemic, and insulin secretogouge activity in diabetic patients. Dried extract (500mg/kg, p. o. for 6 weeks), of plant exhibited anti-hyperglycemic activity in diabetic patients. Extract mimic insulin like activity and improved the functional status of enzymes in glycolytic pathway and lypolytic pathway. Potent antioxidant and hypolipidemic activity exhibited by ethanolic leaf extract administered at a dose of 200mg/kg for 45 days to streptozotocin induced diabetic rats.

FICUS BENGALENSIS LINN. (FAMILY: MORACEAE)

Hindi name: Bargad; Common name: Indian Banyan Tree

Plants grow throughout India and in the Indian tradition it is considered as a holy tree. In a chronic toxicity test extract (25 & 250mg/kg), produced reversible hepatic damage while the acute LD50 (lethal dose) found to be 9.47g/kg body weight when given intraperitoneally. Leucocyanidin (3-O-â-D-galactosylcellobioside) a dimethoxy derivative isolated from bark, lowered blood sugar level and increased serum insulin in normal and moderate diabetic rats. It also inhibits the degradation processes of insulin. Alcoholic extract of stem bark at a dose of 25, 50 & 75mg/day/100g, b. w. lowered the blood sugar level 47 to 70%, and also restored the normal levels of serum urea, cholesterol and total protein of alloxan diabetic albino rats.

Glucoside of leucopelargonidin isolated from bark has been reported to induce hypoglycemic, hypolipidemic and serum insulin raising effect in moderately diabetic rats. 3-O-alfa-L-rhamnoside (250mg/kg, single dose study & 100mg/kg/day, long term study), a dimethoxy derivative isolated from bark, lowered blood sugar in fasted and glucose induced hyperglycemic rats, along with enhanced insulin secretion from â-cells.

Leucodelphinidine derivative isolated from bark exhibited hypoglycemic activity in normal and alloxan diabetic rats. 3-O-á-L-rhamnoside isolated from the bark has been showed its median effective dose (ED50) as 100mg/kg with 12% hypoglycemic action in normal rats. Hypoglycemic and hypercholesterolemic effect of aqueous bark extract was observed in alloxan induced mild and severe diabetic rabbits. Lethal dose (LD50) of this was found to be 1gm/kg, when administered orally for 3 months in rats. Leucopelrgonin (100mg/kg/day for one month) isolated from bark lowered the fasting blood sugar (34%) and glycosylated haemoglobin (28%) of alloxan diabetic dogs.

GYMNEMA SYLVESTRE (WILLD) R. BR. (FAMILY: ASCELPIADACEAE)

Hindi name: Gudmar; Common name: Periploca of the wood

Plants are grown in tropical regions of India and used as household remedy for diabetes. Oral administration of a water soluble fraction G-54 isolated from Gymnema sylvestre administered to 27 type 2 diabetic patients reduced their insulin requirement, lowered the fasting blood sugar and glycosylated haemoglobin content. Two water soluble fractions (GS-3 and GS-4) obtained from leaves were found to double the pancreatic islets and â-cell numbers in diabetic rats. Alcoholic leaf extract (500mg/kg, orally) lowered maximum blood sugar in fasted, glucose fed and diabetic rats along with insulin released from pancreatic â-cells. In rats the insulin secretion from islets of Langerhans and several pancreatic â-cell lines induced by alcoholic extract in absence of other stimulus.

Gymnemic acid IV, isolated from leaves produced potent hypoglycemic effect in STZ-diabetic mice. Leaf extract has been observed to produce anti- hyperglycemic and hypoglycemic effects of in corticosteroid-induced diabetes mellitus, without altered serum cortisol concentration. A polyherbal formulation containing aqueous extracts of Gymnema sylvestre produced prominent hypoglycemic activity in normal and diabetic rats at a dose of 100–500mg/kg/day, orally for acute, 6 hours and for long-term, 6 weeks studies.

Gymnemic acid IV isolated from the leaves has been observed to produce hypoglycemic, anti-hyperglycemic, glucose uptake inhibitory and gut glycosidase inhibitory effects.

MOMORDICA CHARANTIA LINN. (FAMILY: CUCURBITACEAE)

Hindi name: Karela; Common name: Bitter gourd

The plant is an annual climber grown mostly in tropical India and commonly use as vegetable. Charantin (50mg/kg, orally) isolated from Momordica charantia has been resembled insulin lower blood sugar level (maximum 42% at 4th hour) of rabbits. In a clinical study of type 1 and type 2 diabetic patients the polypeptide-p isolated from fruit, seeds and tissue exhibited hypoglycemic activity without any side effect.

The subcutaneous injection of (0. 5unit/kg) lowered the blood sugar in gerbils and langurs. Charantin obtained from Momordica charantia induced hypoglycemic effect and also stimulated the insulin release and blocked the formation of glucose in blood stream. Hypoglycemic effect and delayed cataract development was reported in alloxan diabetic rats treated with fruit extract (4g/kg/Day orally for 2 months). Ethanolic extract (200mg/kg) of Momordica charantia was produced hypoglycemic activity in normal and streptozotocin diabetic rats; this was occurred possibly due to inhibiting glucose-6-phosphatase and fructose-1, 6-biphosphatase in liver, and stimulating hepatic glucose-6- phosphate dehydrogenase activities. Oleanolic acid and momordin from plant, produced antihyperglycemic effect by inhibiting glucose transport in intestine of rat. Fruit aqueous extract (200mg/

kg, orally for 6 weeks), and exercise potentially lowered blood sugar of type 2 diabetic and hyperinsulinemic (insulin resistance) rats. Seed aqueous extract produced prominent reduction in blood glucose, glycosylated hemoglobin, lactate dehydrogenase, glucose-6-phosphatase, fructose-1, 6-bisphosphatase and glycogen phosphorylase along with increased hemoglobin, glycogen content and hexokinase, glycogen synthase activity. Anti-diabetic properties of plant such as charantin, vicine and polypeptide-p have the potential to be a part of dietary supplement for patients of diabetes. From Momordica charantia the major compounds, 5b, 19-e poxy -3 b, 25 dihydroxycucurbita-6 , 23 (E)- di ene(4) and 3 b- 7 b , 25dihydroxycucurbita-5, 23(E) -dien-19-al(5) administered at a dose of 400mg/kg produced hypoglycemic effect in ddY mice strain.

OCIMUM SANCTUM LINN. (FAMILY: LAMIACEAE)

Hindi name: Tulasi; Common name: Holy Basil

It is a tropical annual herb grown all over India and use for household remediation. Oral administration of alcoholic extract of leaves of Ocimum sanctum lowered blood sugar level in normal; glucose fed hyperglycemic and STZ-diabetic rats, along with increased insulin release. Ocimum sanctum leaf powder was produced potent hypoglycemic and hypolipidemic effect in normal and diabetic rats. Alcoholic extract of leaves significantly lowered the blood glucose in normal and alloxan diabetic rats. Administration of plant extract 200mg/kg in STZ-diabetic rats for 30 days led to decreased in plasma glucose level by 26. 4%. Plant extract lowered blood glucose level along with inhibited cortisol level. From leaf extract the aqueous butanol and ethylacetate fractions stimulated insulin secretion from perfuse rat pancreas, isolated rat islets and a clonal rat â-cell line in a concentration-dependent manner.

PTEROCARPUS MARSUPIUM ROXB. (FAMILY: FABACEAE)

Hindi name: Vijayasar; Common name: Indian Malabar

Plants grow throughout India and are use as hypoglycemic plant in folklore medicine. Aqueous bark extract lowered blood sugar and improved glucose tolerance of diabetics with no side effects observed. From alcoholic extract of bark the ethyl acetate soluble fraction caused blood sugar lowering and repaired the alloxan induced pancreatic â-cells damage in albino rats. From plant the (-) -epicatechin (30mg/kg, i. p.) produced anti-hyperglycemic effect in alloxan induced diabetic rats. The (-) epicatechin, from bark increased the cAMP content of the pancreatic islets associated with increased insulin release, conversion of proinsulin to insulin and cathepsin B activity in rats. Marsupin and pterostilbene, two phenolic constituents of plant potentially lowered blood glucose at same level as compared to metformin in STZ- diabetic rats. Aqueous extract (1g/kg, orally) of bark has been observed to produce anti-cataract activity in alloxan diabetic rats. Plant extract was prevented the hyper-triglyceridaemia and hyper-insulinaemia (insulin resistance) in type 2 diabetic patients. Aqueous extract (250mg/kg, orally) of dried wood has been reported to produce hypoglycemic effect in acute and sub-acute study.

SWERTIA CHIRAYITA (ROXB. EX FLAM) KARST. (FAMILY: GENTIANACEAE)

Hindi name: Kirayat Chirata; Common name: Bitter Stick

The herbs grow abundantly in Himalayan regions of India and are used for treatment of various ailments by the tribes. 95% ethanol extract (250mg/kg) of plant potentially lowered the blood sugar level in fasted, glucose fed and tolbutamide pretreated animals. Hexane fraction (250mg/kg, b. w. orally for 28 days) of plant, lowered blood sugar of albino rats with increased glycogen content of liver and insulin released from pancreatic â-cells. Swerchirin (50mg/kg, orally) isolated from hexane fraction of plant exerted potent hypoglycemic activity in normal and STZ-diabetic albino rats. A xanthone isolated from the hexane fraction of Swertia chirayita identified as swerchirin (1, 8-dihydroxy-3, 5-dimethoxyxanthone) exhibited blood sugar lowering effect in fasted, fed, glucose fed hyperglycemic and tolbutamide pretreated albino rats. Effective dose (ED50) of Swertia chirayita has been reported to be 23. 1mg/kg/oral, lower maximum 40% blood sugar level of male albino rats of body weight 140–165g. Swerchirin (50mg/kg, b. w. orally) isolated from crude extract lowered maximum 60% blood glucose at 7 hour post-treatment, along with depleted aldehyde-fuchsin stained b-granules and immunostained insulin of islets of Langerhans. Swerchirin isolated from plant was found to be superior blood sugar lowering agent over tolbutamide. Alcoholic extract (250mg/kg, once daily for two weeks) exhibited hypoglycemic effect in alloxan induced diabetic rats.

SYZYGIUM CUMINI LINN. (FAMILY: MYRTACEAE)

Syn. Eugenia jambolana (Linn.); Hindi name: Jamun; Common name: Black

Berry

Plants grow in different parts of India. The ripe fruits are used as part of dietary component. Oral administration of fruit pulp induced hypoglycemic activity in normal and STZ-diabetic rats along with insulin released from â-cells. Seed powder provided good symptomatic relief to 30 patients of diabetes (type 2) and regulated blood sugar level. Increased activity of hexokinase and decreased activity of glucose-6-phosphate in liver produced blood sugar lowering effect at oral administration of aqueous seed extract (2. 5g/kg, b. w. for one month) to alloxan diabetic rats.

Aqueous seed extract (2. 5 & 5g/kg, b. w. for 6 weeks) has been observed to produce hypoglycemic and antioxidant activity, and increase in haemoglobin content in rats. Alcoholic seed extract injection (20mg, intraperitoneally) reduced the blood sugar level to 37. 17% at 3 hour and 46. 68% at 6 hour of administration in alloxan diabetic mice along with enhanced insulin secretion. Decreased plasma glucose concentrations in STZ-induced diabetic mice was observed at oral administration of fruit extract (200mg/kg, for 50 days).

Blood sugar lowering, hypolipidemic activity, increased serum insulin, increased glycogen content of liver and muscles and a fall in glycosylated haemoglobin level produced by ethanolic extract (100mg/kg b. w. orally) of seed.

Ethanolic seed kernels extract (100gm/kg b. w.) has been observed to improve glucose tolerance, and produce hypoglycemic and hypolipidemic effect in STZ-diabetic rats. Syzygium cumini was produced prominent fall of blood sugar in mice. Aqueous and ethanolic extracts of the fruit-pulp has been reported to produce antihyperglycemic effect in alloxan diabetic rats, and 24. 4% raise in plasma insulin level in mild diabetic and 26. 3% in severely diabetic rabbits.

TRIGONELLA FOENUM-GRAECUM LINN. (FAMILY: FABACEAE)

Hindi name: Methi; Common name: Fenugreek

Plants are commonly cultivated throughout India. The leaves are used as vegetable and seeds as spice. Major alkaloid trigonellin from fenugreek seeds produced hypoglycemic activity. Ethanol extract (0. 8g/kg, i. p.) of leaves has been observed to reduce blood glucose concentration in alloxan induced diabetic rats. Lethal doses (LD50) of aqueous leaf extract were 1. 9g/kg at intra-peritoneal and 10g/kg at oral administration. 4-Hydroxyisoleucine, an insulinotropic compound isolated from seeds increased the insulin release in glucose fed hyperglycemic rats and humans.

Seeds powder treatment normalized the enhanced lipid peroxidation and reduced the susceptibility to oxidative stress associated with depletion of antioxidants in liver of rats. Maximum 46. 64% decrease in blood sugar level of diabetic rats was observed at oral administration of seed extract (1g/kg, for one month).

From fenugreek seeds, the soluble dietary fibre (SDF) fraction at (0. 5g/kg, orally administered twice daily, for 28 days) inhibited platelets aggregation in type 2 diabetic rats and produced beneficial effect in dyslipidemia.

Restored activity of glutamate dehydrogenase, NAD linked isocitrate dehydrogenase and D-b-hydroxybutyrate dehydrogenase reported at oral administration of seed powder (5%, for 3 weeks) in alloxan diabetic rats. It also repaired the liver and kidney damage caused by alloxan. 4-hydroxyisoleucine:5, an amino acid, isolated from seeds, produced anti- hyperglycemic effect and decreased the 33% plasma triglyceride, 22% total cholesterol (22%) and 14% free fatty acids.

RECENT RESEARCH ON MEDICINAL PLANTS & REVIVAL OF HERBAL MEDICINE

Being convinced that modern allopathic medicines, though potent, are not safe and also being convinced that these drugs are not sustainable in the context of its incompatibility in the natural system the gamut of modern allopathic drugs is being reviewed differently in recent past. The revival of herbal medicines and its productive blending with modern medical science have been given serious thoughts. The recent findings on the properties of medicinal plants are very amazing. Here we may mention a few of such findings.

A: ON HUMAN

1. SADABAHAR :. The most common Indian plant Sadabahar whose botanical name is Catharanthus rosea syn-Vinca rosea found to contain an important cytotoxic alkaloids vincrystin in smaller quantity and vinblastin in larger quantity. Vincrystin found to be clinically effective against leukemia and vinblastin against Hodkin diseases. The credit goes to USA and Canadian scientist who initiated resJ3arch in 1950s on isolation of alkaloids from common Rosy Periwinckle or Catharanthus rosea or vinca rosea. After the discovery of vincrystin the survival rate of children suffering from leukemia has jumped over to about 80 %. The clinical effectiveness of vincrystin in leukemia among children created a huge demand for Vinca rosea in USA.
2. ASHWAGANDHA: A team of Doctor from Kasturba Medical College, Manipal have reported that an alcoholic root extract of Ashwagandha has shown anti-tumour activity. They have also reported that Ashwagandha Injection can also augment the effect of radiation on tumor regression and delayed its growth.
3. RAKTA CHITRAKA: The same team led by Prof. P. Umadevi also reported that the extract of Rakta Chitraka (Plumbago Indica) a well known herbs in traditional Indian medicine found to have effective anti-tumor property and augmenting the effect of radiation given concurrently in arresting the growth of Tumour. Rakta Chitraka is being prescribed for cancer treatment in Siddha system.
4. MUSTARD : Mustard a popular condiment and oil-seed in India may have potential anti-cancer property according to a preliminary study at the National Institute of Nutrition, Hyderabad. Such anti-cancer property may be attributed to chemical compound phenyl-iso- thiocyanate present in mustard seed.
5. NEEM: Extensive researches in India well as abroad on Neem (Azadiracta Indica) has opened new vistas in Herbal medicines due to its versatile-properties.

Neem extract has shown activity against Rodent-Malaria caused by Plasmodium berghei prevalent in West Africa according to Scientist of University of Nizeria and African Bio-Science Net Work. Researches are being continued to investigate the activities of Neem and other plants against deadly parasite, Plasmodium falcifarum, found in African countries.

Indian researches on versatile applications of Neem are very promising. It is an established fact the chewing of Neem twig fights mouth Bacteria/ protozoa causing tooth decay, Gingivitis and Pyorrhea. India is the first country to manufacture Neem-based tooth paste and soap.

It has been found by the scientist of Defense Institute of Physiology and Science (DIPAS) and National Institute of Immunology (NII), New Delhi that Neem oil acts as an effective spermicidal contraceptive without any hazardous side effects. The contraceptive formulation called Nm-76 prepared from Neem oil extract which is undergoing trials and expected to be a safe and effective vaginal-spermicide. NIL scientist have clinically tried two Neem based products-PRANEEM OIL & PRANEEM POLYHERBAL CREAM which are effective as vaginal contraceptive and vaginal anti-microbial.

A team of Indo-American scientist from NII, New Delhi and Harvard Medical School, USA have shown that a sugar like extract from Neem bark can stop infectivity of AIDS-VIRUS in human blood cells, cultured in laboratories. No doubt, this findings may bring a new hope in the treatment of AIDS.

A group of researchers have shown Neem leaves extract acts as a sedative and anxiolytic in low dose of 10 to 200 mg/kg of body wt. in experimental rate.

Scientists of Malaria Research Institute New Delhi have reported that Neem oil is an excellent and low cost mosquito repellent. 5% Neem oil mixed with kerosene burnt in lamp. repels mosquitoes effectively without causing any harm to human body, unlike mosquito repellent mats and coils. A cream developed from Neem oil when applied to human body nullify the bites of sand fly that spreads Kalazar prevalent in Bihar.

B: ON PLANTS

Recently it has become a serious concern that the chemical pesticide leave high percentage of residual poison in the edible agro-horticultural product leading to serious health hazards. This is one of the bad effects of so called green revolution. Now it is high time that we should seriously think about alternative pesticides and. fungicide which are safe both to human and environment.

It is a matter of pleasure that such alternative pesticides are heading their way by the dedicated efforts of scientist and in near future these will come in a big way and may totally replace the hazardous chemical pesticide. These may be called as bio-pesticide which are of two types: 1) Microbe-based and 2) Plant Extract-based. As we are presently concern about the medicinal plant, we may cite a few examples where plant extracts are processed as pesticides.

1. Extract of marigold leaves (Electra of Ecomax Agrotech) is effective against soil nematodes and it is used as soil spray.
2. Aqueous extract of neem seed powder when sprayed on plants can effectively control a number of plant insects and fungal infections.
3. RÈPLIN-a spray insecticide formulation enriched with neem extract prepared by ITC agro-Industry, Hyderabad successfully tested in the field and found to be effective against steam borer and leaf folders.

C: ON ANIMAL

Even the veterinary surgeon depends upon plant for the treatment of the animal. Scientist from Calcutta have discovered anti-filarial activity in a drug isolated from the plant Acacia auriculoformis. The drug contains two active compounds acaciaside A and acaciaside B. These two saponins at a concentration of 4 mg. per ml. killed 97 percent of micro-filaria-the slender pre-larval forms of the filarial nematode in 100 minutes. The compound could also kill all the adults in 35 minutes. This report is published by the scientists ion the Indian journal of experimental biology.

NATIONAL RESEARCH INSTITUTES ON MEDICINAL PLANTS

Following R & D labs. and institution are engaged specifically on identification, isolation of chemicals and improving agro technique for cultivation of medicinal plants.

1. Central Institute for Medicinal-Lucknow & Aromatic Plants (CIMAP).
2. National Botanical Research Institute. -Lucknow
3. Regional Research Laboratory-Jorhat, Tiruvantpuram, Bhubaneswar, Jammu.
4. Central Drug Research Inst. -Lucknow
5. Council for Scientific and Industrial Research (CSIR) -New Delhi

MEDICINAL PLANTS AS A SOURCE OF RAW MATERIALS FOR ALLOPATHIC MEDICINE

Besides the direct applications of extract, powder, seed powder etc. of medicinal plants on the diseases, as mentioned in traditional system of medicines, many medicinal plants are used in pharmaceutical or drug industries to extract intermediary raw materials in manufacturing of various allopathic medicines.

1. There are sorrye plants which contain 4 to 8 % of diosgenins, the steroidal saponins and examples being Diascorea floribunda, Dioscorea deltoidea the common yam or khamb-alu in Oriya. Diosgenins when subjected to appropriate chemical reactions converted to cortisone a steroidal hormones for therapeutic purposes..
2. Reserpine an alkaloid extracted from Rouwlfia serpentina root (Sarpagandha) is used for manufacturing anti-hypertensive and sedative drugs.

TO CONSERVE AND CULTIVATE MEDICINAL PLANT-A GLOBAL NEED

It is now a need to preserve the medicinal plant which are in this spasm of extinction and to cultivate medicinal plants on commercial basis due to the following reasons.

1. It is being observed that many useful 111edicinal plants have become either endangered or becoming extinct particularly in the

tropical eco- system of developing countries. It is apprehended that the modern allopathic system of medicine will suffer a serious set back if certain medicinal plant species go totally extinct. Therefore, it is high time that our policy makers should seriously think about the preservation of such species in the form of herbarium and Gene Bank.

2. Increased demand for medicinal plants Iike Sadabahar, Rouwlfia, Occimum sanctum, Neem, Ashwagandha, Panax ginseng etc. warrants a development of improved agro-techniques for large scale commercial cultivation in tropical countries. It is interesting to know that there is a substantial demand from Ayurvedic. Allopathic and Homeopathic medicine manufacturers for medicinal plants. The estimated demand of various medicinal plants from leading Ayurvedic medicine manufacturer alone in India like Charak, Zandu. Dabur, Baidyanath etc. amounts to about Rs. 1000 crores per year. The export demand in India for Vinca rosea for preparation of vincrystin in USA is about Rs.5 million.
3. The justification for commercial cultivation for medicinal plants may also be attributed to rampant deforestation.

CULTIVATION OF MEDICINAL PLANTS- A NEW ENTREPRENEURIAL OPPORTUNITY IN RURAL AREAS

Commercial cultivation of most demanded medicinal plant will lead to sustainable employment generation in the rural and tribal areas of India vis-a-vis enormous ur. 1employment problem and secondly it will boost up our forex earning through export ultimately both leading to over all economic development. Therefore, it may be concluded without any doubt and ambiguity that cultivation of medicinal plants offers an opportunity for entrepreneurial venture in a big way, particularly for S & T entrepreneurs.

AN OVERVIEW OF INDIAN NOVEL TRADITIONAL MEDICINAL PLANTS WITH ANTI-DIABETIC POTENTIALS

Diabetes mellitus is the most severe metabolic pandemic of the 21st century, affecting essential biochemical activities in almost every cell in the body and increasing the risk of cardiac problems. It is estimated that in the year 2000, 171 million people had diabetes, and this is expected to double by year 2030. Conventionally, insulin-dependant diabetes mellitus is treated with exogenous insulin and non insulin-dependant diabetes mellitus with synthetic oral hypoglycemic agents like sulphonylureas and biguanides. However the hormone fails as a curative agent for complications of diabetes and synthetic oral drugs produce adverse health effects. Different medicinal systems are using the active plant constituents, which discovered as natural hypoglycemic medicine, came from the virtue of traditional knowledge. Herbal drugs are considered free from side effects than synthetic one. They are less toxic, relatively cheap and popular. In India, medicinal plants have been used as natural medicine since the days of Vedic glory. Many of these medicinal plants and herbs are part of our diet as spices, vegetables and fruits. Historically, in 'Atharva-Veda' (about 200 B.C.) description of medicinal plants was made under a separate chapter 'Ayurveda'. Sushruta (about 400 B. C.) compiled classification of 700 herbal drugs under 37 classes in 'Sushruta Samhita' (A compendium of ancient Indian surgery). Charak (about 600 B. C.) made the scientific classification of herbal drugs based on remedial properties in his renowned treatise 'Charaka Samhita' (A compendium of general medicine). In which he described 50 classes of herbal remedies comprising 500 crude drugs. The medicinal values of plants have been tested by trial and error method for a long time by different workers. Even today great opportunities are still open for scientific investigations of herbal medicines for cure of diabetes and its complications.

❐

Bibliography

Akerele, O.: *Medicinal plants: policies and priorities,* Cambridge, UK; Cambridge University Press, 1991.

Chandrasekar B: *Blood sugar lowering potentiality of selected Cucurbitaceae plants of Indian origin.* Ind J Med Res. 1989.

Chattopadhyay RR: *A comparative evaluation of some blood sugar lowering agents of plant origin.* J Ethnopharmacology. 1999.

De Silva T.: *A Manual on the Essential Oil Industry,* Vienna, Austria; United Nations Industrial Development Organisation, 1996.

Donellan, C.: *Endangered species.* Independence, Cambridge, 1995.

Dutt, Ashwini : *An Introduction to Medicinal Plants,* Adhyayan Pub, Delhi, 2008. Featherly H. I.: Taxonomic Terminology of the Higher Plants, USA, Iowa State College Press, 1954.

Felig G, Bergman M, Felig C.: *The Endocrine Pancreas: Diabetes mellitus,* New York: MacGraw-Hill; 1995.

Fitzsimmons, Judith : *Seasons of Aromatherapy: Hundreds of Restorative Recipes and Sensory Suggestions.* Conari Press, Berkeley, CA; 1998.

Fuller, D.: *Medicine from the Wild.* Washington, DC; Traffic USA, 1991.

Godden G.: *Growing Citrus Trees,* Australia, Lothian Publishing Company Pvt. Ltd., 1988.

Goldsmith, F.B.: *Monitoring for conservation and ecology.* Chapman and Hall, London, 1991.

Harlan, Jack R.: *The Living Fields: Our Agricultural Heritage,* Cambridge: Cambridge University Press, 1998.

Hartley W.: *A Checklist of Economic Plants in Australia,* Melbourne, C.S.I.R.O., 1979.

Hessayon D. G. Dr.: *The Vegetable Expert,* England, PBI, Publications, 1985.

Hill, Clare: *The Ancient and Healing Art of Aromatherapy.* Ulysses Press, Berkeley, CA; 1997.

Janardhanan, K.K. : *Diseases of Major Medicinal Plants,* Daya, Delhi, 2002.

Jeffers P.: *Evaluation of Four Onion Varieties in Montserrat,* Plymouth, CARDI, 1992.

Jerram, M.R.K.: *A Text-Book on Forest Management* : In Agriculture, Horticulture and Forestry, Asiatic Pub, Delhi, 2006.

Kalia Manoranjan : *Post Harvest Technology of Vegetables,* Agrotech Pub, Delhi, 2006.

Kim J.S.: *Sources of Resistance to Viruses of Pepper* (Capsicum spp.): a Catalogue , Taipei, AVRDC, 1994.

Kumar, Supriya : *Amenity Horticulture, Biotechnology and Post-Harvest Technology,* Pointer, Delhi, 2006.

Lawless, Julia: *Essential Oils: An Illustrated Guide.* Harpercollins, London, 2001.

Lewington, A.: *Medicinal Plant and Plant Extracts,* Cambridge, UK; Traffic International, 1993.

Mabberley D.J.: *The Plant-Book : a Portable Dictionary of the Vascular Plants,* Cambridge, Cambridge University Press, 1997.

Madulid Domingo A.: *A Pictorial Cyclopedia of Philippine Ornamental Plants,* Philippines, Makati Metro Manila, 1995.

Matsuoka H.: *Cultivation of Panicum Genetic Resources for Evaluation of Characteristics,* Tokyo, JICA, 1997.

McGilvery, Carole and Reed, Jimi: *The Complete Guide to Aromatherapy. Lorenz Books,* London, 2001.

Mellor, J. W.: *The New Economics of Growth,* Ithaca, Cornell University Press, 1976.

Morton Julia F.: *Fruits of Warm Climates,* Miami, Julia F. Morton Publisher, 1987.

Myers, N.: *The Sinking Ark: A New Look at the Problem of Disappearing Species.* Oxford, UK; Pergamon Press, 1979.

Narayan Das Prajapati: *A Handbook of Medicinal Plants, Agrobios,* Delhi, 2005.

Nayar, M.P.: *Hot Spots of Endemic Plants of India, Nepal and Burma.* The Director, TBGRI, Trivandrum, 1996. 252 pp.

Oka H. I.: *Origin of Cultivated Rice, Elsevier,* Japan Scientific Societies Press, 1988.

Oldham P.: *Cost of Production of Major Tree Crops in Dominica,* Roseau, Ministry of Agriculture, 1991.

Panda S.C. : *Post Harvest Technology and Farm Mechanization, Agrobios,* Delhi, 2008.

Percival John: *The Wheat Plant - A Monograph,* London, Duckworth & Co., 1921.

Peter, K.V. : *Basics of Horticulture,* New India, Delhi, 2009.

Pilgrim R.: *Post Harvest Handling of Minor Exotics,* St. George's, Grenada, 1996.

Raffauf R.F.: *The Healing Forest: Medicinal and Toxic Plantsm, Portland, Oregon,* USA; Dioscorides Press, 1990.

❐

Index

N

O

P

R

S

T

U

V

W

❑❑❑